Cambridge History of Medicine

EDITORS: CHARLES WEBSTER and CHARLES ROSENBERG

Medicine before the plague

This book describes the medical world of the early fourteenth century through a study of the extensive archival material and contemporary writings which exist for eastern Spain in the decades before the Black Death.

It describes the range of medical practice which then existed – a continuum ranging from scattered academic physicians to barbers and empirics – and gives evidence for the levels and numerical growth of these various occupations in early fourteenth-century communities (although it also emphasizes that occupational distinctions were not yet sharply drawn). The newly-translated Greco-Arabic medical learning was beginning to spread through this continuum of practice, and the book argues that public enthusiasm for the new learned medicine led to the "medicalization" of certain social and legal institutions, thus preparing a role for a medical profession in this society before its physicians had shown any consciousness of collective self-interest and identity. The ambitions and expectations of practitioners are examined in archival evidence for individual careers but also in contemporary medical writings, such as those of the famous Arnau de Vilanova, a product of Catalan-Aragonese society. Archives make it possible, too, to study the attitudes of communities and of individual patients to medicine and to health care – from King Jaume II (1291–1327) and his family to his humbler subjects in the countryside. The book thus brings together the world of medical thought and the actual world shared by patients and practitioners.

Cambridge History of Medicine

EDITED BY

CHARLES WEBSTER

Reader in the History of Medicine, University of Oxford,
and Fellow of All Souls College

CHARLES ROSENBERG

Professor of History and Sociology of Science,
University of Pennsylvania

For a list of recent titles in the series, see end of book

Medicine before the plague

Practitioners and their patients in the Crown of Aragon, 1285–1345

MICHAEL R. McVAUGH

Professor of History,
University of North Carolina at Chapel Hill

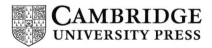

CAMBRIDGE
UNIVERSITY PRESS

Published by the Press Syndicate of the University of Cambridge
The Pitt Building, Trumpington Street, Cambridge CB2 1RP
40 West 20th Street, New York, NY 10011–4211, USA
10 Stamford Road, Oakleigh, Victoria 3166, Australia

First published 1993

Printed in Great Britain at the University Press, Cambridge

A catalogue record for this book is available from the British Library

Library of Congress cataloguing in publication data
McVaugh, M. R. (Michael Rogers), 1938–
Medicine before the plague: practitioners and their patients in
the Crown of Aragon, 1285–1345 / Michael R. McVaugh.
p.   cm. – (Cambridge history of medicine)
Includes bibliographical references.
ISBN 0 521 41235 8 (hardback)
1. Medical care – Spain – Aragon – History. 2. Social medicine –
Spain – Aragon – History. 3. Medicine, Medieval – Spain – Aragon.
I. Title. II. Series.
[DNLM: 1. History of Medicine, Medieval – Spain. 2. Physician-
Patient Relations. WZ 70 M4m]
R557.A7M38 1993
610'.946'.5509023 – dc20
DNLM/DLC
for Library of Congress 92–49626 CIP

ISBN 0 521 41235 8 hardback

For Luis
whose work it is also

Contents

Tables

Preface

Historians of medieval science, even more than their counterparts studying other periods, have been slow to explore the general context of their subject, and have concentrated instead upon understanding and communicating the learned natural-philosophical texts that embody so much of it. When John Murdoch and Edith Sylla published *The Cultural Context of Medieval Learning* in 1975, their exhortations to a broader approach still looked towards a relatively narrow setting, that of the "intellectual community" of the medieval universities whose masters produced and consumed these texts. At that moment I was absorbed in studying and editing the learned medical literature of the Middle Ages, in particular that of the University of Montpellier; the Murdoch-Sylla volume convinced me of the need to set it too into cultural context – but necessarily a much wider one than they had stressed. Natural philosophy may have taken shape in a purely academic setting, but medicine was a learning that justified itself in application to a general public outside the university. It seemed to me obvious that to appreciate the cultural context of medieval *medical* learning it would be necessary to study systematically what today we might call the "health care system" of a medieval society: how did people understand and respond to illness and injury? what kinds of care were available to them, and how effective were they seen to be? what did they want from medicine, and did they feel they could get it? and where did a specifically learned medicine fit into this system?

I originally decided to pursue these questions as they applied to the Montpellier master Arnau de Vilanova (d. 1311), a figure whom I knew well from editing his medical works, and to see whether the society in which he grew up and lived, the Crown of Aragon in northeastern Spain, might have preserved enough documentation to permit a study of the social context of Arnau's practice there. Brief visits to Barcelona in the summers of 1977 and 1979 left me astonished by the wealth of the available records, and through the generosity of the John Simon Guggenheim Memorial Foundation I spent the academic year 1981–2 in Barcelona working my way systematically through royal, ecclesiastical, notarial, and municipal archives. I first concentrated on Arnau's own lifetime, the reigns of Alfons II (1285–91) and Jaume II (1291–1327), but as I proceeded I came to appreciate the extent – perhaps unsurpassed for the medieval West – of the archival materials that survive from the Crown of Aragon, and I began to imagine a study that would go beyond Arnau to examine medicine and society over a somewhat longer period; by the time I returned home I had extended my search to the reign of Alfons III (1327–36) as well, and was planning investigations on a broader scale. I spent the summer of 1983 in the archives of Valencia, and returned in the summer and fall of 1986 to work in the archives of Aragon (Zaragoza and Huesca) as well as in provincial archives in Catalonia (primarily Lerida, Cervera, and Tarragona).

At this point Luis García Ballester (my co-editor of the Arnaldian writings) joined me in the archival investigation, and this led me to think even more ambitiously. Might we not eventually examine medicine and its social relations in the Crown of Aragon for the entire fourteenth century and, in the process, add a new dimension to our understanding of the impact of the plague of 1348? With this as a goal, we spent the summers of 1987 and 1988 in Gerona and Manresa and the fall of 1989 in Barcelona, now carrying our search through the reigns of Pere III (1336–87) and Joan I (1387–95). At the Consell Superior d'Investigacions Científiques in Barcelona the exploration of materials from the later 1300s is still going on, but the principal archival sources from the first half of the century have now been studied fully enough to permit the picture that follows.

For reasons that I hope will be clear, it is a deliberately restricted picture. With one or two exceptions, I do not draw on evidence later than May 1348, when the plague arrived in Barcelona, for fear of distortions; it may well prove that the epidemic had no effect on medico-social relationships, but it seems unsafe to assume it. Likewise I occasionally cite evidence from elsewhere in Europe, but only for comparative purposes: it has seemed more important to try to depict the workings of a particular society than to try prematurely to generalize for all European medicine. Roussillon and the Balearics (though, inconsistently, not Cerdanya) have been excluded from my survey, for while they were reincorporated into the Crown of Aragon in 1343–4, they had previously been ruled by the kings of Mallorca since 1276, under whom a Catalan language and culture but a different law and a different administrative system prevailed. Nevertheless, because of the commonality of culture in southern France and Catalonia, I have regularly quoted the writings of practitioners who trained or taught at the school of Montpellier – Mallorcan territory, nominally, but only 340 kilometers from Barcelona – as witnesses to medical thought in the Crown of Aragon, whether or not they originated in or practiced within the Crown. For medicine, I have depended largely on the works of Arnau de Vilanova, who was Valencian by upbringing and a subject of the Aragonese Crown; for surgery, I have often quoted the *Chirurgia* of Henri de Mondeville, who studied and perhaps taught medicine and surgery at Montpellier before establishing himself at Paris, and who is thus arguably as good a witness as we have for that school and the attitudes and expectations of the surgeons trained there. I have tried to summarize and explain their medical thinking in their own terms as far as possible, without (for example) interpreting their disease concepts or evaluating their drug therapy against a modern framework.

Arnau and Henri are virtually my only literary witnesses to the medical world of the early fourteenth century; primarily this is a study based on archival sources, and this has enforced certain peculiar features of the work. There may seem to be an unconscionable quantity of references to sources, but because almost all my evidence is unpublished I have felt very uneasy about leaving it undocumented. Some features of my practice should be explained. The dates of all documents have been converted into modern terms except where they are necessary to identify the archival location of a document, in which case they have been left in their original Roman form. Where possible, I give manuscript references in a concise form: a number "123–I/45" refers to f. 45 of register 123–I in a given archive. When I transcribe a Catalan source, I do not add the accents that would be required in the modern language.

Proper names have also posed a problem. Both Castilian (strictly, Aragonese) and Catalan were used in the Crown of Aragon, and I have therefore decided to use Catalan forms for people from Catalonia or Valencia, Castilian forms for those from Aragon proper; but having done this it seemed only appropriate that I use Italian forms for Italians, French for French – including Languedoc and Roussillon – and so forth. (I have kept the original Latin form of names whenever a person's place of origin seemed undecidable, and I have left Hebrew names in their medieval transliterations.) If some of the resulting forms seem unfamiliar or incongruous, my practice will at least bring home to the reader the variety of the society I am describing. I have followed the same system with place names *except* for those of regions, rivers, and large cities that are likely to be more familiar to English readers in another form: thus I refer to "Gerona" and "Lerida" rather than "Girona" and "Lleida" or "Lérida," and indeed "Catalonia" and "Aragon" rather than "Catalunya" and "Aragón." Finally, I have used Catalan regnal numbers for the count-kings, so that (for example) Pere el Ceremoniós becomes Pere III rather than Pere IV. I would be the first to agree that this is an imperfect solution to the problem of rendering names in a multi-lingual society, and I am sure that many inconsistencies remain despite my best efforts to eliminate them.

I am very conscious of the extent to which this book has been made possible by the help and advice of others. I have depended upon two people above all others. My friend and colleague Luis García Ballester has been almost another self during the past decade. We have worked side by side in archives and libraries, sharing food, accommodations, a single pair of gloves (in a particularly icy archive in Morella), discoveries, and thoughts. A number of the theses I present here were thrashed out in discussion with him; others with which he may not agree were at least tested in the same way. I am deeply conscious that without his contributions, intellectual and logistic alike, this book would have been utterly impossible. My wife Julie has contributed in ways that include but go far beyond the spousal forbearance that scholars so often thoughtlessly take for granted. Her loving support and active enthusiasm for this project have not kept her from giving my manuscript a dispassionate and chastening scrutiny; both structurally and stylistically it owes a great deal to her professional attention.

Several other friends read all or part of the manuscript for me, and their comments were of great use to me. Vivian Nutton and Nancy Siraisi were kind enough to give it particularly close and thoughtful readings, and their comments have saved me from many blunders while helping me to broaden my treatment. A number of others read all or part of the work in draft, and I have profited from their remarks as well: Monica Green, John Headley, Terence McIntosh, and Seymour Mauskopf. It was Father Robert Burns' early enthusiasm that convinced me that the Catalan archives would be worth pursuing, and he has been an unfailing source of advice and encouragement ever since. Many other people have helped me in a variety of ways, among them Montserrat Arasa, Leila Berner, Asunción Blasco, Carme Batlle i Gallart, Stan Chodorow, George Conklin, Frank Domínguez, Antonio Durán Gudiol, Paul Freedman, Thomas Glick, Christian Guilleré, Alvar Martínez Vidal, Josep Perarnau i Espelt, Josep Maria Pons Guri, Jaume Riera i Sans, Agustín Rubio Vela, Joseph Shatzmiller, John Shideler, and Jill Webster. My map is the careful work of Patricia Neumann. I want, too, to acknowledge a fundamental debt to the several distinguished Catalan historians who in the last hundred years began to uncover and to publish the documentation treating medicine in the medieval Crown of Aragon: Antoni Rubió i Lluch, Josep Maria Roca, Lluís Comenge i Ferrer, Father Martí de Barcelona (whose unpublished papers I was able to examine through the kindness of the director of the Arxiu Provincial dels Caputxins de Catalunya), and Antoni Cardoner. I feel fortunate to have been able to meet and talk with the last of these before his death; the others I have at least met in their writings.

Depending as it does on unpublished documents, this study would have been inconceivable without the whole-hearted cooperation of many Spanish archivists and librarians, who patiently put up with my incessant requests for more and more materials, sometimes rearranging their schedules to do so. I am deeply grateful to them all. It might seem invidious to single any out, yet I cannot let the opportunity go by of thanking in particular the staff of the Archivo de la Corona de Aragón, in Barcelona, for their kindness and generosity manifested in so many ways over the last fifteen years. I owe special thanks, too, to a number of institutions whose financial assistance made the research possible: the American Philosophical Society, the John Simon Guggenheim Memorial Foundation, my own University of North Carolina, and the Spanish Ministerio de Educación, whose grant made possible a six-months' association in the fall of 1989 with the CSIC in Barcelona. And if my parents had not been willing to keep the cat in 1981–2, this project would never have begun.

Finally, let me express a deep debt of gratitude of a different kind to the Orfeó Català. My wife and I have been privileged to sing with this Barcelona-based chorus under four different directors: Lluís Millet i Loras, Simon Johnson, Salvador Mas, and Jordi Casas. From the very beginning we were made to feel unreservedly welcome in this group, which embodies the musical tradition of the Catalan nation, as we delightedly discovered the choral music of Catalan composers like Lluís Maria Millet or Enric Morera. To sing Pau Casals' *Pessebre* on the stage of the Palau de la Música Catalana, looking out into Domènech i Muntaner's marvelous building, is a thrill neither of us will ever forget. Whatever sensitivity to history and place there may be in this study owes a great deal to this opportunity given us by the Orfeó to participate so fully in what remains one of the most important expressions of the Catalan spirit.

Abbreviations

Archives

ACA	Barcelona, Archivo de la Corona de Aragón
ACB	Barcelona, Arxiu de la Catedral
ACFV	Vic, Arxiu de la Curia Fumada
ACSU	Seu d'Urgell, Arxiu de la Catedral
ACV	Valencia, Arxiu de la Catedral
ADB	Barcelona, Arxiu Diocesà
ADG	Gerona, Arxiu Diocesà
AHAG	Gerona, Arxiu Històric de l'Ajuntament
AHAT	Tarragona, Arxiu Històric Arxidiocesà
AHCB	Barcelona, Arxiu Històric de la Ciutat
AHCC	Cervera, Arxiu Històric Comarcal
AHCM	Manresa, Arxiu Històric de la Ciutat
AHCO	Olot, Arxiu Històric Comarcal
AHCP	Puigcerdà, Arxiu Històric Comarcal
AHCV	Vilafranca del Penedès, Arxiu Històric Comarcal
AHMA	Arenys de Mar, Arxiu Històric Municipal
AHPB	Barcelona, Arxiu Històric de Protocols
AHPG	Gerona, Arxiu Històric Provincial
AHPG/CE	Gerona, Arxiu Històric Provincial, fons de Castelló d'Empúries
AHPG/PL	Gerona, Arxiu Històric Provincial, fons de Perelada
AHPT	Tarragona, Arxiu Històric Provincial
AML	Lerida, Arxiu Municipal
AMT	Tortosa, Arxiu Municipal
AMV	Valencia, Arxiu Municipal
ANZ	Zaragoza, Archivo Notarial
ARV	Valencia, Arxiu del Regne
ASZ	Zaragoza, Archivo de la Seo
C	ACA, Cancillería

| CRD | ACA, Cartas Reales Diplomáticas |
| RP | ACA, Real Patrimonio |

Published works

AA	Heinrich Finke, *Acta Aragonensia*
AST	*Analecta Sacra Tarraconensia*
AVOMO	*Arnaldi de Villanova Opera Medica Omnia*
BRABLB	*Boletín de la Real Academia de Buenas Letras de Barcelona*
EUC	*Estudis Universitaris Catalans*
MF	J. Ernesto Martínez Ferrando, *Jaime II de Aragón: Su vida familiar*
RL	Antoni Rubió y Lluch, *Documents per l'historia de la cultura catalana mig-eval*

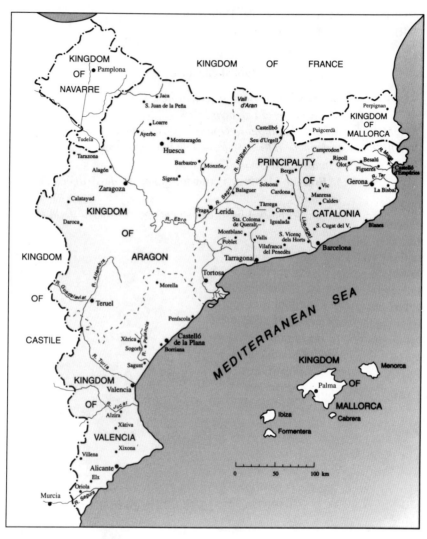

The Crown of Aragon in the early fourteenth century

Introduction

The medieval Crown of Aragon in eastern Spain, the setting for this study, may not be a familiar name to most readers, nor is any of its rulers as famous as Richard the Lion-Heart of England, say, or Saint Louis of France. Until it fused into a larger Spain in 1479, it was often overshadowed and sometimes menaced by two much larger neighbors, the kingdom of Castile to the west and that of France to the north – respectively six and fifteen times as populous. The label, "Crown," suggests its peculiar status as a dynastic union: the count of Barcelona had become betrothed to the heiress to the kingdom of Aragon in 1137, and their descendant reconquered Valencia from Islam two hundred years later and established another kingdom there. As a result, the Crown also brought together significant numbers of three religions: Valencia's population was still predominantly Muslim in the early fourteenth century, and Muslims remained a significant minority in Aragon (its capital, Zaragoza, had only been recaptured from Islam in 1118), while the cities of the Crown permitted communities of Jews to live in relative tolerance. One legacy from Muslim Valencia was the paper mills of Xàtiva, and their output made possible the remarkable series of royal and municipal records whose preservation today means that the Crown of Aragon is one of the most historically accessible late-medieval societies.

In certain respects, the first half of the fourteenth century might be called the most successful period in the Crown's history. Internally, the monarchs were able to maintain stability of rule during the sixty years between the aristocratic reactions to royal authority – the *Uniones* of 1284–7 and 1347–8 – by working through the assemblies (*corts* in Catalan-speaking lands, *cortes* in Castilian-speaking Aragon) to defuse political opposition. Externally, it was a period in which they maintained essentially peaceful relations with their much larger neighbors to the north and west, and instead pushed eastward into the Mediterranean commercially and politically, first trying to succeed the Angevins in Sicily (1282–95), then establishing themselves in Sardinia (1323–4), and finally regaining the Balearic Islands (and mainland Roussillon) from their cousins, the kings of Mallorca (1343–4). This expansion, along with the

1

resettlement of Valencia, helped keep the Crown's population density relatively low. Its inherently limited resources were disguised by the growth of overseas trade, and by the beginnings of banking and of some domestic industries; the Crown maintained strong markets and a strong coinage until the 1340s, when wages and prices began to increase. It may be that the disastrous year of 1333–4, the so-called *mal any primer*, and the social unrest that followed were early signs of the coming decline, but for the most part the first half of the century was, as one historian of the Crown of Aragon has said, an age of "consensus, energy, and optimism, [and] religious *convivencia*."[1]

Among the innumerable aspects of this dynamic, expanding, culturally diverse society that its documentary resources allow us to explore, medicine is of unusual interest. It has long been clear that a learned, rational medicine began to win social acceptance in fourteenth-century Europe, but the process has never been studied in detail. Conventionally, historians have constructed that process about the supposed establishment of university-trained physicians at the top of a diverse hierarchy of practitioners – surgeons, apothecaries, barbers, empirics – whose activities they were thereafter empowered to license or supervise on the strength of their academic qualifications. More recent scholarship on the social history of medicine has altered this picture as it applies to early modern times – by showing, for example, that in England in the sixteenth to eighteenth centuries the learned physicians' control over other practitioners was far from complete, and that a variety of theories and practices were available to patients in a "medical marketplace." For want of narrowly focused research by medievalists, however, our understanding of pre-sixteenth-century developments has remained a relatively diffuse and general one, so that even the most recent account of medicine and society in the Middle Ages, sophisticated and nuanced as it is, has been forced to present the period 1250–1500 as more or less a chronologically undifferentiated unity.[2]

The present book tries to respond to this need for a sharper focus by examining a late-medieval society at a particular moment in time – the Crown of Aragon during the half-century before the arrival there of the Black Death in the spring of 1348 – and it too suggests a modification of the conventional story. It argues that, though the Crown's academic physicians were neither numerous nor self-conscious enough to enforce their standards on medical practice, a learned, text-based medicine did indeed become established there during this period. It diffused rapidly within a community of practitioners who represented a continuum of backgrounds but who were all trying to assimilate what they could of the new medicine. This community was one within which there were still no sharp boundaries dividing one kind of practice from another: surgery and medicine could overlap without fierce rivalry, and traditional remedies could

---

[1] Bisson, *Medieval Crown*, p. 186.   [2] Park, "Medicine and Society."

coexist with Galenic theory in the village empiric as well as the university master.

There is a second argument in this study: that the triumph of a bookish medicine was not led by practitioners, ambitious for their own discipline, but instead owed much to a broad public enthusiasm for the learning that medical education seemed to guarantee. It is possible to speak about a "public" that is more than merely noble patients or municipal councilors because of the remarkable richness of the Crown's documentation, which allows generalization from a much more varied base that stretches out to ordinary people in the villages and countryside. To a certain extent, this public grew to expect more from medicine than practitioners were yet prepared to give: the monopolistic medical profession of a later age was a lay ideal well before its potential for collective advancement occurred to physicians, so that it was the lay community that moved to institute licensing regulations and to "medicalize" certain issues of social concern by setting up medical practitioners as expert judges over them.

A term like "medicalization" may seem like anachronistic jargon, but I have used it and a few other such modern coinages deliberately, to try to bring home the parallels that I see between medico-social relationships in the early fourteenth century and in our own day. We are mistaken if we simply perceive medieval medicine as quaint or foolish or in some sense fundamentally "other." I am convinced that believing in the reality of medical expertise, and agreeing to entrust one's health to someone who claims that expertise, yields similar behavior, similar reactions, and similar consequences in any age, and I suspect that some readers today will recognize something of themselves in the patients – or the practitioners – of the Crown of Aragon.

1

The medical history of a royal family

Jaume II: searching for medical care

In April 1293 the thirty-two-year-old ruler of the Crown of Aragon, Jaume II, wrote insistently from Barcelona to his "faithful *fisicus*" Giovanni Rayner in Messina, urging him to move from Sicily to Spain. Giovanni had served Jaume when the latter ruled Sicily; but in 1291 Jaume had succeeded his brother Alfons II in Aragon, leaving their younger brother Frederic behind as his viceroy in Sicily, and now he wanted his former physician to settle in his new realm. He invited Giovanni to bring his wife and children; promised him a residence in Barcelona or Valencia, whichever he preferred; and offered him a salary of 3,000 *sous* besides – three times what a master-craftsman could hope to earn in a year.[1] A few months later, in September, the king repeated the offer even more insistently, and eventually Giovanni appeared at court. Perhaps the Aragonese-Angevin struggle in Sicily brought about by the Sicilian Vespers (1282) made another country seem temporarily more desirable; at any rate, six months after the peace of Anagni of June 1295 seemed to resolve the conflict, Giovanni asked for and was given permission to return to Sicily.[2]

Giovanni Rayner's decision to return to Messina at the end of 1295 forced Jaume to find another trustworthy physician, and the king wrote immediately to

---

[1] In the early fourteenth century, a master-craftsman in the Crown of Aragon might receive three *sous* per day, a workman half that. A rough idea of the cost of living may be obtained from price levels: 500–1,000 *sous* for a mule (and more for a horse); 60 *sous* for a cow; 20 *sous* for a hectoliter of wheat; and 2 *deners* for a liter of wine. For these and other values, see Dufourcq, "Prix."

[2] Giovanni was in Messina 2 April 1292 when he was rewarded by Jaume for his services (C 260/42r–v); on 13 Oct. 1292 he was given a further grant in support of his daughter's marriage (C 95/139v). On 3 April 1293 the king invited him to move to the Crown of Aragon (C 98/9v–10), and Jaume repeated the invitation 26 Sept. 1293 (C 96/47v). The first evidence of Giovanni's arrival in Catalonia is a document of 25 Sept. 1294 published in Scarlata and Sciascia, *Documenti*, pp. 100–1, 159–62. His plans to return to Sicily are revealed 7 Dec. 1295 (C 102/107v); only a few weeks before he had been made a present of 5,000 *sous* (19 Nov. 1295; C 263/5v).

master Guillaume de Toulouse, at Paris, praising his knowledge and prudence and inviting him to move to the Aragonese court with his family. The king's need for a court physician was all the more pressing since at Christmas he was to marry Blanca, the twelve-year-old daughter of Charles II of Anjou-Naples, as part of the settlement between the monarchs worked out at Anagni six months before. Guillaume had accepted the position but had not yet started for Spain when the queen's pregnancy was recognized in the spring. He arrived at Barcelona over the summer of 1296, was given a grant of 4,000 *sous* yearly as well as the house where Giovanni Rayner had lived, next to the royal palace, and apparently stayed long enough to oversee the delivery of the infante Jaume on 29 September; but he seems to have quit the court and Spain immediately thereafter, leaving the royal family once again without a physician.[3]

In these episodes from the early years of the reign of Jaume II two royal traits already appear that were to grow more pronounced during the course of his life: a desire for continuing medical supervision, and a concern to improve the level of knowledgeable medical care in his kingdoms. Granted that the king may not be fully representative of his subjects, his perceptions of illness and his expectations for medical care do still reflect something of the attitudes of others in the kingdom. Moreover, the king's experience with illness in himself and his family, and its treatment, shaped royal attitudes towards health care and may thereby have affected the form and character of medical practice in his realms. On several counts, therefore, a medical history (in its broadest sense) of Jaume II and his children is a useful introduction to the study of medical culture in early fourteenth-century Aragon, and it is fortunate that archival sources make such a history possible in unusual detail.[4]

The lack of a physician did not leave the monarch without medical personnel in his service. During the 1290s at least three surgeons were simultaneously receiving retainers from the king: Berenguer de Riaria and his cousin Jaume in Gerona, and Bertomeu ça Font in Valencia. But their responsibilities evidently did not include routine supervision of the royal health. They lived away from

---

[3] Guillaume was first invited to the Crown of Aragon on 13 Dec. 1295, as Giovanni Rayner was leaving (C 102/114); we know Guillaume's whereabouts from the letter of instructions given to the royal messenger (C 102/131). Safe-conducts were sent to Guillaume on 10 and 16 May 1296, when he was en route (C 340/100v, 104/25v). After 19 Sept. 1296 he disappears from the record (C 194/257v). Further detail is in McVaugh, "Births," pp. 8–9.

It is conceivable that this is the same man as the Guilelmus de Tolosa who was *medicus* of Puigcerdà 1287–9 (AHCP, Jaume Garriga Liber firmitatis 1286–7, f. 93; AHCP, Bernat Blanch Liber firmitatis 1289–90, f. 14v).

[4] The best biography of the king is that of Martínez Ferrando, *Jaume II o el seny català*. The same author's *Jaime II de Aragón: Su vida familiar* (hereafter MF) focuses on his relationships with his children and wives, and includes in its second volume an important selection of documents pertaining to the royal family. Sablonier, "Aragonese Royal Family," offers a further interpretation of these relationships. J. M. del Estal is preparing a complete *itinerarium* of the reign, but only isolated months have so far been published.

court (although they occasionally accompanied the king in their early years of service) and received much smaller stipends than those promised to physicians: 600 *sous* annually to Berenguer and Jaume, 400 to Bertomeu. Their principal obligation seems rather to have been attendance on the king in his campaigns or military expeditions. Berenguer was present with the unguents necessary to his office on the king's expedition to Murcia in 1300–1; Bertomeu accompanied Jaume to the kingdom of Mallorca in 1293; and both were members of the army in Sicily in 1298–9 and in Almería in 1309–10. Such a relationship was bound to foster royal trust and favor, while leaving the individuals concerned relatively free to further their own interests.[5] It is probably not coincidental that the king came eventually to depend upon both these surgeons primarily as political agents: Berenguer was appointed bailiff (*baiulus*) of Gerona in 1304, while Bertomeu was given charge of the saltworks at Valencia in 1305 and of the castle of Corbera by 1314, and was appointed chamberlain to Jaume's heir in 1318. These men were no doubt useful tools for the king, and used their opportunities to become wealthy and powerful, but they did not provide the daily medical care he felt he needed.[6]

There were other medical practitioners more regularly at court or attending the monarch on his travels around his realms. He always had with him at least two barbers, who not only cut hair but also were responsible for prophylactic bleeding and for cleaning (and extracting) teeth.[7] These medical responsibilities presupposed some basic learning – at what times of the month or year not to bleed, for example – but learning was less important than technical facility. Like his surgeons, the king's barbers – Guillem Martí (active 1298–1303), Pascual López (1302–7), his brother Pedro Martín of Huesca (1307–27), and Juan García of Huesca (1310–27) – came also to be used as royal agents, though at a lower level, and the documents regularly title them *barberius* (or *barbitonsor*) *et portarius*. Again like the surgeons, they proved able to use their position to accumulate considerable property and influence.

5 McVaugh, "Royal Surgeons."

6 For Berenguer de Riaria and his cousin, see below, chapter 2. The career of Bertomeu ça Font, first medical and then political, is well documented and deserves closer study than I can give it here. The first royal grant to him – as "cirurgicus noster" – is dated 12 Jan. 1293 (C 260/173). His expenses for *unguentis emplastris et aliis pulveribus* on the trip to Mallorca are recorded in C 261/73v and 264/21. He accompanied Jaume on a visit to Rome in the spring of 1297 (C 321/37v) as well as to Sicily the next year (C 113/150v). Control of salt production was granted him by Queen Blanca and confirmed by King Jaume 7 Dec. 1305 (C 203/88): the first reference to his position at Corbera is 27 Feb. 1314 (C 241/133). From this time on the curial documentation almost always describes Bertomeu not as "cirurgicus noster" but as "de camera nostra". He was chamberlain to the infante Jaume by 6 June 1318 (C 362/97) but gave up the post 4 Dec. 1319 (C 362/159), two weeks before the infante was allowed by the king to surrender his claim to the throne (see below, p. 26). Bertomeu is last found alive in May 1327 (C 286/148v).

7 An enumeration of tools bought for the barber to the royal heir in the fall of 1319 includes razors, basins, a mirror, and "instrumentis ferreis ad minuendum et ad dentes mundandum": C 362/153v.

Finally, the royal household included an apothecary for much of the time. Queen Blanca appointed Guillem Jordà as her personal apothecary before 1301, and by the next year the king was referring to him as *apothecarius noster* (a title Guillem retained until the king died) and expecting him to follow the court.[8] An apothecary's skills and knowledge were more developed than a barber's, as recognized by his higher rate of pay when accompanying the king in his travels: an apothecary, like a surgeon, received roughly twice a barber's stipend. Guillem could and did prescribe for and treat common ailments independent of a physician – but no more than a barber could he or any other apothecary be expected to treat all the complaints of his customers.

It is surprising that Jaume had begun by seeking a court physician from Paris, for the medical faculty at Montpellier in southern France was at least as renowned and was geographically much closer. The wealthier of Jaume's subjects, if they shared his dissatisfaction with the level of medical care available in his kingdom, might travel to Montpellier for medical consultation and treatment.[9] The city was tied to Aragon culturally and politically. It had come to Pere I, Jaume's great-grandfather, through his marriage with the heiress to the lordship, and had been bequeathed by Pere's son Jaume I to Jaume II of Mallorca, uncle of Jaume II. Montpellier's *studium generale* had come to serve by default as the university for the Aragonese crown, which had no *studium* in its own territories at the end of the thirteenth century.

At that moment, in fact, the outstanding member of Montpellier's medical medical faculty was one of King Jaume's own subjects, Arnau de Vilanova. Arnau had grown up in Valencia and had studied at Montpellier in the 1260s; he had then become physician to Jaume's father, Pere II, until the king's death in 1285, and had returned to Montpellier to teach just before Jaume came to the throne. The extraordinary body of medical commentaries and monographs that

---

[8] Attention has been drawn to Guillem by Sorní Esteva and Suñé Arbussá, "Algunas noticias," pp. 213–16, who trace his career back to October 1302. But he was already in the queen's entourage in April 1301, when he was involved in a fight with two other Barcelonan apothecaries (C 118/101), and he was given a royal privilege for past services in June 1302 (C 199/100v). He is last seen 31 Oct. 1330 (C 496/233v), asking Alfons III for sums due him for medicines he had prescribed for Jaume and the royal family.

It is entirely possible that Guillem originally came to the queen's household from the court of her father, Charles II. Three of Charles' sons, the "princes of Salerno," were made Aragonese hostages in his place by the treaty of Canfranc (1288), but were permitted to be attended by Angevin physicians. In 1286, when their father was still imprisoned, there had been some fear that his physicians might be spies as well, and Alfons II seems to have wanted them replaced by local practitioners: Finke, *Acta Aragonensia* (hereafter *AA*), III: 26–7; and see too C 66/137. By 1291 there was evidently no longer this concern, and master François Andrée regularly went back and forth from Charles' court to the boys, supervising their health, from at least 26 July 1291 (C 85/221); on one of these trips, in 1294, master François brought Guillem Jordà with him as his apothecary (C 97/190v).

[9] Similarly, one of the Angevin hostages left in Barcelona by Charles II was allowed to go to Montpellier when he fell gravely ill (8 Jan. 1296; C 102/153v).

Arnau composed at Montpellier in the 1290s today provides an unmatched picture of medicine as absorbed by university students in the early fourteenth century.[10]

It was to Arnau that Jaume finally turned for medical care after Guillaume de Toulouse left the court. At the beginning of March 1297 the king wrote to Arnau from Rome, asking him to go from Montpellier to Barcelona to look after the queen. Arnau obeyed, staying until November, and pleased both king and queen so much that Jaume began (unsuccessfully) to try to convince Arnau to stay permanently in his realms.[11] In the meantime he asked Arnau to recommend another physician who would be willing to accompany him on a forthcoming campaign to Sicily; his brother Frederic had rejected the peace of Anagni and had been crowned king at Palermo in December 1295, and Jaume had agreed to help his father-in-law Charles II assert his rights to the island. No reply from Arnau to the king survives, however, and we cannot be sure who it was that attended the queen when her second child, Maria, was born in the spring of 1298. The king, queen, and royal household (including the barbers Guillem and Pascual as well as the surgeon Bertomeu ça Font) then left Barcelona, in June, for what would prove to be a little over a year's absence.

Up to this point the king does not seem to have suffered any worrisome acute illness: his most annoying problem was hemorrhoids, and upon learning in December 1297 that Arnau's nephew Armengaud Blaise had "a certain book that treats *de cura infirmitatis emorroydarum*" Jaume wrote to him, asking for the volume and for any advice that Armengaud might have about treatment.[12] The first royal illness of which there is any record attacked him on the Sicilian expedition, early in 1299; three Italian physicians were called to Naples to assist in its treatment.[13] There were by now two physicians in the royal entourage: a master Ugo, who had been appointed physician to the queen upon her arrival in Naples and was to supervise her new pregnancy;[14] and Bernard Marini, the king's physician, who had apparently been picked up in France on the voyage.

---

[10] The extensive literature on Arnau can be approached through the bibliography in Charles C. Gillispie, ed., *Dictionary of Scientific Biography*, I (New York, 1970), pp. 289–91. Paniagua, *Arnau de Vilanova*, is especially good as a general survey of his medical writings, now being given a critical edition in the series *Arnaldi de Villanova Opera Medica Omnia* (hereafter *AVOMO*; 1975–).

[11] Martí de Barcelona, "Regesta," pp. 266–7, docs. 19–26.

[12] Rubió y Lluch, *Documents per l'historia de la cultura catalana mig-eval* (hereafter RL), II:12, doc. 14.

[13] They are named as Johannes de Sist, Rigus de Frisce, and Jacobus de Brandisio: RL, II:xxxii n. 2, who mistakenly gives the date as March 1296 – they were in fact paid 16 April 1299 (C 265/219v). In addition, Giovanni Rayner apparently came over from the island of Sicily and the service of Jaume's brother Frederic to treat his former patient; he returned to Sicily 9 July 1299 (C 113/175v).

[14] I have suggested elsewhere (McVaugh, "Births," p. 10) that Ugo might have attended Maria's birth in Valencia in the spring of 1298, but the documentation does not in fact establish his connection with the royal household before its arrival in the kingdom of Naples.

Both appear to have assisted at the premature birth of the infante Alfons in January 1299 – a "mout beau fil sans grevance de son cors," Blanca's mother wrote Jaume with relief – and both probably joined in attending the king in his illness a few weeks later.[15] We have no details about this illness, but it is tempting to imagine that Jaume had contracted a malarial fever in Naples; in any case, during the next few years he was frequently ill and, not unnaturally, was increasingly preoccupied with the state of his health.

The king returned to Barcelona in the summer of 1299, bringing his physician Bernard Marini back with him. Perhaps the availability of physicians in southern Italy, many trained at the University of Naples, had sharpened his dissatisfaction with the medicine of his own realms; at any rate, within a year Jaume had taken steps to create a university near the center of the Crown of Aragon, at Lerida in Catalonia. Complaining that hitherto his subjects had had to leave the kingdom to study arts, law, or medicine, the king provided for all three disciplines to be taught there, and in 1301 Guillaume Gaubert de Béziers arrived from Montpellier to begin the teaching of medicine at the Leridan *studium*.[16]

In these years the care of the queen in pregnancy continued to be an urgent question. The birth of Blanca's fourth child, Constança, on 1 April 1300, was probably overseen by Arnau de Vilanova, who happened to have arrived at court a few months before, and by Bernard Marini. By the next year there were again two physicians in the king's household: Bernard Marini still served him, while Armengaud Blaise had been brought to court from Gerona as physician to the queen. Armengaud may have tended to Blanca when her daughter Isabel was born in the spring of 1301; he certainly cared for her in the attack of fever she experienced in September of that year. But by January 1302 Armengaud had left the court, and Jaume II had once more to identify a trustworthy physician, since Bernard Marini had left for his French homeland a month before and the queen was again pregnant. The king wrote to Arnau de Vilanova to urge him to come to Valencia, explaining that the birth was expected soon. By late April Arnau had come to court and was preparing to leave again; the delivery (of the queen's sixth child, Blanca) had apparently had no complications.[17]

---

[15] McVaugh, "Births," p. 9, treats Alfons' birth; the letter describing the newborn infante is published by MF, II:1–2, doc. 2. Ugo and "magister Bernardus medicus domini regis" were paid respectively 2,000 and 1,000 *gros tournois* in Syracuse on 8 Jan. 1299 (C 265/128), sums whose magnitude suggests their attendance at the birth. If this is, as I believe, a reference to Bernard Marini, it pushes his association with the court back a year before the date given in "Births," p. 13 n. 22.

[16] McVaugh and García Ballester, "Medical Faculty." For more on the Leridan *studium*, see below, chapter 3.

[17] McVaugh, "Births," p. 10. The most recent account of Arnau's life – Santi, *Arnau de Vilanova* – holds (p. 120) that Arnau refused to come to attend the queen in this pregnancy; however, Santi has overlooked the king's letter of 28 April 1302 (McVaugh, "Further Documents," pp. 368–9, doc. 60a), which permits Arnau to take a horse with him as he returns from the Crown of Aragon to the papal court.

It is impossible not to wonder whether Jaume hoped from the beginning that a medical faculty in Catalonia would guarantee the presence there of physicians who could be called on to serve the royal family as needed. His commitment to a specifically academic medicine was becoming increasingly obvious, for he now began to insist that even his surgeons consult Avicenna's great medical encyclopedia, the *Canon*. And when Armengaud and Arnau had both gone back to Montpellier, the king turned to Lerida as a source of learned medical care, and began to treat Guillaume de Béziers as a household physician. Guillaume cannot have been teaching in Lerida long when in the winter of 1301/2 he was summoned to Valencia to consult with Arnau about the queen's health. Twice more in the next year he was called away from the Leridan *studium* to the court, to Jaca in June 1302 to advise on the king's serious illness, and to Barcelona in September 1302 "on business." Guillaume had evidently proven satisfactory, and the king would not relinquish him; he was subjected to similar demands as long as he remained at Lerida.[18]

The illness that the king contracted in Jaca caught him when Bernard Marini (briefly returned to royal service) was the only physician at court, and it was worrisome, whatever it was. King Jaume told one correspondent that he had been seized by a *discrasia*; *discrasia* meant, strictly, an imbalanced or distempered complexion – a "cold," one might say, except that the medieval term implied a more serious condition than a modern cold, with side-effects ranging from high fever to dysentery.[19] He was troubled enough to call for advice from physicians throughout his realms, and beyond. To Jaca in the hills of northwestern Aragon came not only Guillaume de Béziers but masters Ramon and Francesc from Lerida as well; Juan, Abraffim, and Juceff from Huesca; Guillermo and Rabi Salamo from Zaragoza; and Nicolas and Garsia from Pamplona in the kingdom of Navarre – apparently Jaca itself did not have a competent physician.[20] As the king began to recover, he traveled to Huesca for treatment by master Juan,[21] and then returned to Catalonia (via Teruel, where Guillaume de Béziers was to send a physician to meet the king and treat the infante Alfons' illness) to regain his strength – "pro recreatione corporis nostri" – by resting at Prades in the Sierra de Montsant.[22]

[18] The documentation concerning Guillaume's career will be analyzed more carefully in the study that José María Martínez Gázquez and I are preparing on "Guillaume de Béziers and his *Introductio scolaribus suis.*"

[19] "Discrasia que corpus nostrum arripuat": letter of 25 June 1302 (C 124/220r–v). In ordinary usage, *discrasia* seems to refer to an acute episode and *infirmitas* to a chronic illness, but occasionally they are employed as synonyms. Examples that follow will suggest the range of conditions to which the terms could be applied.

[20] González Hurtebise, *Libros de tesorería*, pp. 56–7, doc. 204, records payment to most of these on 25 June; Guillaume de Béziers and Guillermo of Zaragoza were paid on 6 July, and Juan of Huesca on 7 July (ibid., pp. 61–2, docs. 232–4, 240).

[21] Ibid., p. 65, doc. 258.

[22] Letters of 23 June and 12 July 1302 (C 269/72v, 79).

Perhaps the "business" for which Jaume summoned Guillaume to Barcelona upon his return there in August included advice on whom to appoint next as household physician, now that Bernard Marini had decided to leave the court for good; at any rate, shortly thereafter the king wrote to Jean d'Alès, another master at Montpellier, explaining that his knowledge and skill had been praised by "several members of our court" (presumably Guillaume and Bernard), and asking him to come to Catalonia. The letter was carried by Bernard Marini, returning north for good, who cannot have made the position sound unattractive, for Jean d'Alès made the trip to Spain, finding the king in Figueres; but he stayed only five months before going back to Montpellier – perhaps attending the birth of the infante Joan, which occurred at about this time.[23] All during 1303, therefore, the king and queen were without a personal physician, and made increasingly burdensome demands on Guillaume de Béziers. Jaume tried to get Guillaume to abandon Lerida and move permanently to Valencia, though he did not succeed; but he made Guillaume attend him and prepare electuaries for him on his trip to Castile in June 1303 – and then called him back to the court (at Tortosa) in October to care for both him and the queen.[24]

In the winter of 1303/4 Jaume fell ill in Valencia and, recovering, commanded Guillaume de Béziers, in Lerida, to go to Montpellier and purchase the medicines necessary to improve his health (much to the disgust of the councilors of Lerida, who resented having their medical master so often absent from the school). As the king traveled north in March 1304 his illness flared up again, forcing him to stop in Calatayud. He wrote to Guillaume telling him to finish his business in Montpellier quickly, so that he could return and care for his royal patient, insisting in the meantime that Guillaume send him another competent physician. Before the month was out, Guillaume's candidate, a certain Jaume, had come from Lerida to attend the monarch in Calatayud, as had Guillaume himself from Montpellier (via Lerida) and master Guillermo from Zaragoza. King Jaume was slowly restored to health – in part by taking electuaries and other medicines prescribed by Guillaume, compounded by the apothecary Pere Jutge in Barcelona, and sent to the king in Calatayud.[25]

The onset of the illness had apparently decided the king to renew his search for a permanent household physician, and he had communicated again with Armengaud Blaise, who was back teaching at Montpellier. Armengaud

[23] McVaugh, "Births," pp. 11–14. Jean d'Alès was subsequently physician and chaplain to Pope Clement V and, together with Arnau de Vilanova and Guglielmo da Brescia, advised the pope in his 1309 reorganization of the curriculum at Montpellier. He had returned to Montpellier as chancellor in 1313 and was still alive in 1318; Wickersheimer, *Dictionnaire*, [I] p. 379.

[24] "Ratione infirmitatis . . . regine . . . et discrassie que nostro noviter corpori supervenit": letter of 23 Oct. 1303 (C 130/159v).

[25] C 235/18, 28v, 32v; 258/95v. The letters will be published in McVaugh and Martínez Gázquez, "Guillaume de Béziers."

journeyed to Spain in May 1304, consulting on the way with master Guillermo in Zaragoza about the king's condition, and in the end he agreed to return to court after going back to Montpellier to settle his affairs. He may still have been absent when the king relapsed into illness in July and had to summon a variety of medical assistance once more – Guillaume de Béziers and his protégé Jaume from Lerida, Guillermo from Zaragoza, and, for good measure, Isaac, a Jewish physician from "Barbary." But by September the king was convalescing and Armengaud was at court, styled *fisicus noster* and promised a salary of 8,000 *sous* annually from a variety of sources.[26]

In hiring Armengaud, the king may have been settling for a surrogate for his older and more famous uncle, Arnau, yet he was also acquiring a physician who could boast independent intellectual accomplishments.[27] Armengaud had been master in medicine at Montpellier since 1289 (although the degree was conferred by the bishop of Maguelonne against the wishes of the faculty) and there he had teamed with Jewish collaborators to produce Latin translations of various Arabic medical writings. He continued his scholarly activity in Barcelona, finishing a translation of Maimonides' *De medicinis contra venena* there in 1305 (dedicating it to the new pope Clement V, elected in June), and his own *Tabula antidotarii*, a summary catalogue of compound drugs, may also have been drawn up in Barcelona: in 1306 a Jewish exile to that city, Estori ha-Parhi, encountered the *Tabula* there – "finer than gold and mother-of-pearl," he wrote – and translated it into Hebrew.[28]

Armengaud remained with the king for two years. He seems to have begun his treatment of the monarch by recommending that he take theriac, for in mid-September 1304 Jaume asked three different agents to send him the best and finest specimen of the drug that could be found.[29] Whatever his methods, Armengaud evidently made the king feel secure enough in his medical care to stop summoning Guillaume de Béziers from Lerida; the university there closed for a period in 1305, and Guillaume returned to the faculty at Montpellier (though he attended the king briefly in the summer of 1306).

---

[26] The four physicians are identified in C 294/224r–v, a document of 12 Feb. 1305 recording court expenses of July–September 1304, and in CRD Jaume II, cuenta 61, of July 1304. The Jew Isaac was evidently an immigrant to Aragon from North Africa (already called "Barbaria" in Catalonia by this time); I have found no later trace of him. Jaume speaks of his recovery in a letter to the king of Mallorca 26 Sept. 1304 (C 235/140).

[27] For Armengaud, see Wickersheimer, *Dictionnaire*, [I] pp. 40–1 and Jacquart, *Supplément*, pp. 25–6. I have a fuller study of Armengaud and his medical writings in preparation jointly with Lola Ferre Cano; this will include all the documentary evidence pertaining to his career in the Crown of Aragon.

[28] On the date of Armengaud's translation of Maimonides, see below, chapter 5 n. 100. Estori ha-Parhi's introduction to the *Tabula* (Hebrew text and English translation) is published by García Ballester, Ferre, and Feliu, "Jewish Appreciation," pp. 102–3; his career is sketched in *Encyclopedia Judaica* 6 (Jerusalem, 1971): 918–19.

[29] "Thiriacham de fina et meliori que inveniri poterit": letters of 20 Sept. 1304 (C 258/164).

Eventually Armengaud, like all the royal physicians who had preceded him, gave up his post and left the kingdom; but he was instrumental in arranging for two replacements who stayed with the king as long as he lived and at last gave him continuity of medical supervision. In October 1304, shortly after entering Jaume's service, Armengaud was sent by the king to the *fisicus* Martí de Calça Roja, apparently to persuade him to become a second household physician, and by the end of the year Martí did indeed join the court. These two saw the king through a febrile *discrasia* in March 1305, which they attributed to overwork and to the cold weather of Zaragoza, by advising him to pause and convalesce in that city rather than hasten back to Barcelona; the Catalan *corts* had to be postponed.[30] Then, in June 1306, on the verge of leaving royal service, Armengaud recommended master Joan Amell as his successor, and by mid-October Joan was a member of the household, while Armengaud had disappeared; in January 1307 Joan was granted the income formerly assigned to Armengaud. For the next twenty years Joan Amell and Martí de Calça Roja shared the responsibility for the king's health.[31]

Because the king's attitude towards medical care and his dealings with the world of medicine were bound to change once he had established a permanent relationship with particular physicians, we may pause here and reflect on Jaume as a "health care consumer" at this moment, in his mid-forties. To begin with, he obviously perceived illness as always imminent and always potentially serious, and was convinced moreover that a physician's care *could* make a difference to health. Furthermore, he appears to have believed that learned physicians – academics – were the most effective, since his choice for the royal household fell

---

[30] On the illness and the postponement, letter of 7 March 1305 (C 307/185).

[31] Joan Amell and Martí de Calça Roja will appear frequently throughout this book; here I can only give a brief outline of their careers in royal service. Martí was given a yearly stipend of 1,000 *sous* in 1307, raised to 4,000 *sous* the next year. In 1311 he was given 10,000 *sous* on the occasion of his marriage, and the same year he purchased part of the town (and castle) of Segart west of Sagunt (Valencia); he was allowed to rebuild the castle in 1320, but throughout this period his principal residence remained in the parish of Sant Esteve, Valencia. In 1329 he was promised 4,000 *sous* towards a daughter's marriage (if this is his daughter Johanna, he gave her a dowry of 20,000 *sous*). Another daughter was a nun in Valencia in 1332; a son, Martí, was killed studying in Montpellier in 1335, and another, Jaume, was between fifteen and twenty in 1340. Martí's will was signed 1 Jan. 1338; he died two days later, dividing his property among his three living sons, Jaume, Francesc, and Alfons (ARV, Just. Civil 64/4v–6v). His wife Jacoba Estorna, who had brought him a dowry of 8,000 *sous*, remarried in 1341.

Joan Amell was granted a yearly income of 5,000 *sous* in 1308, and the next year was given another 10,000 *sous* towards his purchase of a *heriditamentum* – Novalles, near Sagunt. In 1313 he was acknowledged as of noble birth. In 1321 Joan bought the village of Xeresa, north of Gandia (Valencia), which he held as a *miles*. His principal residence, however, was in Valencia (parish of Sant Tomàs). His brother Ramon was a monk at Ripoll, and through him Joan purchased the monastery's rents, which kept him involved in a lawsuit throughout the 1320s. He had a natural son, Ramon, by a woman named Valencona, and was able to have Ramon legitimated in 1338; shortly thereafter Joan died. His widow Dulcia and his son Ramon were involved in a lawsuit over Joan's estate in 1344. The documentation on both these men is too extensive to cite here; full biographical studies would be of great interest.

regularly on the members of a medical faculty. But though the advice of one physician might be good, more advice was evidently better, so that in what he felt were serious illnesses Jaume might seek the care of as many as eight or nine physicians from different locales. His diffuse searches also suggest how thinly distributed competent physicians still were in the Crown of Aragon, at least in the king's eyes. This was particularly true of Aragon proper, where the implication is that in 1302 there were no physicians in Jaca, and in 1304 none in Calatayud – none, at least, that the king thought worthy of including in a consultation.

Health problems of a family

The summer of 1306 was a bad one in Barcelona. Jaume mentioned to a correspondent the "grandes enfermedades que son estades en estas partidas," and he himself was attacked by a *discrasia* for a few days in August, one that left him weak just as the queen was coming down with a quartan fever.[32] To his uncle Jaume II of Mallorca, who had invited them for a visit, Jaume apologetically wrote from Barcelona that "according to the advice of our physicians we must go directly to Valencia, due to our illness, which has left our body weak, and to the illness from which our Queen Blanca is suffering at present, a quartan fever."[33] The physicians in question were presumably Martí de Calça Roja and Joan Amell, the latter having just replaced Armengaud Blaise at court. Jaume reiterated the excuse five weeks later, although he and Blanca had proceeded no further south than Tarragona; it is not easy to be sure that this was a medical rather than a social excuse.[34] But for whatever motives Jaume was satisfied with his new physicians' counsel, and he continued thereafter to trust their judgment.

To be sure, Jaume still thought of Arnau de Vilanova as the most desirable physician of all. Arnau had now largely subordinated his medicine to an increasingly heterodox theology, which he was defending stridently at the papal court and elsewhere. He was no longer living in Jaume's realms and could not routinely attend the royal household, but the king found other ways to benefit

---

[32] Letters of 20 and 26 Aug. 1306 (C 236/222, 227). Blanca's fever persisted into the fall, though it was not worrisome: "quartanum patitur de qua aliud non timet periculum ut probatorum . . . tenet assercio fisicorum" (28 Nov. 1306; C 334/170v).

[33] "Propter infirmitatem quam passi fuimus de qua adhuc persona nostra debilis existit, et occurrente etiam infirmitate quo illustris domina Blancha regina consors nostra karissima detinetur, quia patitur quartanam, secundum consilia medicorum opportet nos una cum ipsa domina regina continuo ad partes Valencie accedere": letter of 22 Sept. 1306 (C 236/237). Blanca's father seems to be referring to the same episode in the letter written to Jaume II from Marseille and dated 10 Oct. 1306: ACA pergaminos Jaume II extra-inventario 493.

[34] Letter of 28 Oct. 1306 (C 335/321v).

from his knowledge. When Jaume's *discrasia* of early 1305 had persisted unduly, and Armengaud Blaise had acknowledged his inability to cure it, the king expressed his delight upon learning that Arnau would be visiting Barcelona temporarily and could take over the case.[35] It may have been on this trip that Arnau agreed to prepare for the king the handbook that we now know as the *Regimen sanitatis ad inclitum regem Aragonum*; the deliberately simplified text covered the proper disposition of the various factors responsible for maintaining health in specific application to men with Jaume's temperate, sanguine complexion, and it concluded with a chapter on the treatment of hemorrhoids that responded directly to the king's chronic complaint.[36] Arnau must also have promised the king a more learned work, summing up his scholastic experience of several decades, for in July 1308 Jaume wrote insistently to Arnau asking abut the book he had promised to write to maintain the king in health, the *Speculum medicine*, assuring him that he would show it to no one except (if Arnau agreed) to Martí de Calça Roja.[37] The king repeated his plea six weeks later in a letter entreating Arnau to send him a new supply of an electuary he had used to make up for the king and, if at all possible, to pass on what he had previously been unwilling to reveal, the secret of its composition.[38]

As regards both practical care and the academic learning he valued so highly, therefore, Jaume esteemed Arnau above anyone at court, and his household physicians were selected on his model. Like all their predecessors, Joan and Martí seem to have been trained in a *studium* – the former, indeed, is occasionally styled "doctor in medicina" or the like in royal letters. Perhaps a longer scholastic education explains why the king began to refer to Joan Amell as his "medicus maior" by September 1308, after it had become clear that Arnau would never return permanently, even though Martí had served Jaume two years longer; it was certainly not that Martí lacked Joan's academic orientation, since he was given money by the king to buy his own working copy of Avicenna, five

---

[35] Letter of 6 April 1305 (Martí de Barcelona, "Regesta," p. 278, doc. 85; *AA*, II:872–3).

[36] An edition of the text is being prepared for *AVOMO* by Ana Trías Teixidor. A Catalan translation produced in Arnau's lifetime is printed in Arnau de Vilanova, *Obres Catalanes*, 2:99–200.

[37] Letter of 1 July 1308 (Martí de Barcelona, "Regesta," p. 283, doc. 102; *AA*, II:876–7).

[38] "Meminimus . . . vos dudum ad conservacionem sanitatis persone nostre electuarium seu confeccionem quandam preciosissimam fecisse fieri, que nos usi sumus hucusque et sentimus eam nobis [salubrem] fuisse. Et quia electuarium seu confeccio ipsa expenssa est seu consumata preter modicam quantitatem, que propter vetustatem caret viribus, idcirco dileccionem vestram attente precamur, quatenus de electuario seu confeccione ipsa conficiatis nobis in ea quantitate, qua vobis visum fuerit expedire, et eam nobis mittatis . . . Preterea si discrecioni vestre videretur faciendum, placeret nobis, . . . si nobis in scriptis mitteretis, ex quibus et quo modo dictum electuarium seu confeccio fit et exprimeretis etiam re . . . discreta quam exprimere noluistis, aliis expressis, quando confeccionem ipsam fecistis. Nos enim hec secrete tenemus": *AA*, II:877–8, which I have emended slightly after examining the original (C 149/145v); Martí de Barcelona, "Regesta," p. 283, doc. 103.

years after joining the court.[39] Their success in winning his confidence is apparent from Jaume's household ordinances of August 1308: at meals, his physicians were henceforth to eat at the first table (of eight), along with the sons of barons, knights, and great royal officials.[40]

In the summer of 1309 the king launched a crusade against Muslim Granada, in conjunction with Fernando IV of Castile; Aragonese forces marched south from Alicante to besiege Almería, supported by a fleet of 200 ships. The king and queen arrived with the army before the city on 15 August. Present as well was a considerable body of medical personnel: at least five surgeons, two physicians (Joan and Martí), two apothecaries, and five barbers. Joan and Martí were responsible for the health of the royal couple, of course, but they also contracted to treat the ills of large portions of the army. The siege was unsuccessful, and was breaking up in mid-January 1310 when suddenly Arnau de Vilanova arrived in camp by sea, offering his monarch – just too late – yet one more piece of medical counsel, an impromptu series of thoughts on military hygiene; it had probably been hastily assembled to help distract Jaume from disturbing rumors that Arnau had cast doubt on the king's own orthodoxy in a discourse delivered to the papal court at Avignon a few months before. The king left Almería on 27 January with Arnau still in favor, but within a year he had reacted so sharply to independent reports of the Avignon speech that he would never again have contact with the physician he had so long idealized.[41]

The king seems to have stayed healthy throughout the siege, but he began to feel unwell as the army prepared to leave Almería: he apologized to his brother Frederic III of Sicily that "the illness that we are suffering from does not allow us to write in our own hand," in a letter of 25 January announcing their

---

[39] Martí's Avicenna is mentioned on 12 June 1309 (C 271/39v); the king gave him at least one other (unidentified) book, on 27 July 1326 (C 285/237v–238), which further suggests he shared in a learned culture. To Joan Amell the king gave two books on 13 Dec. 1318 (Martínez Ferrando, "Camera real," p. 137 doc. 100), whose incipits – "Expositio articulorum" and "Celis reddidit" – have not yet been identified; perhaps significantly, the books were given him at the moment when Joan was helping cure Jaume of a grave illness (below, pp. 22–24).

[40] Schwarz, *Aragonische Hofordnungen*, p. 37. Schwarz attributes this honor to the prestige that Arnau de Vilanova had earlier enjoyed at court, but I am inclined to think it is as much a reflection of the trust the king had come to put in Joan and Martí during the preceding years. On the physician's role at court, see also the suggestive remarks of Don Juan Manuel (King Jaume's son-in-law; see below, p. 19) in his *Libro de los estados*, I.96; ed. Tate and Macpherson, pp. 200–2.

[41] This episode is discussed more fully in McVaugh, "Arnau de Vilanova's *Regimen Almarie*." The *Chronicle of San Juan de la Peña* (c. 1370) speaks of "a great sickness . . . breaking out in his host" (p. 97), but I have found no allusion to a general illness in the royal registers. Lluís Cifuentes i Comamala is preparing a thorough study of the medical aspects of the Almería campaign. For the speech at Avignon and its consequences, see Santi, *Arnau de Vilanova*, pp. 134–9.

departure.[42] His slow progress north found him in Teruel in May 1310, where he was struck down with an illness that appeared to be particularly dangerous; he remained there for several weeks trying to recover. He wrote to his brother in early June, when he thought the worst was over, that "when we had returned to our realm and had reached the region of Teruel, we were seized by so painful an illness that for several days we suffered from it in almost every part of our body, but He who sustains kings has brought us back to the health we now enjoy."[43] Actually, the illness was still persisting a week later. Joan Amell had by this time already returned from Almería to Barcelona, and he was hurriedly brought back (together with four pounds of rose syrup and two pounds of *cassia fistula*, a vegetable laxative) to treat the king. Even so, the illness was so disturbing that the king reverted to his earlier practice of collecting as much medical advice as possible in serious illnesses, and did not content himself with his *phisicus maior*. Jaume summoned to his bedside the learned Heinrich of Germany, *medicinalis scientie professor*, from the service of the archbishop of Tarragona; Pedro Cellerer, a disciple of Arnau de Vilanova, from Daroca; Barnabas, a physician, and two surgeons, Bertomeu ça Font and Jaume d'Avinyó, all from Valencia; the Jew Miras, physician to Jaume de Xèrica; and Abraffim and Meyrona, Jewish physicians of Teruel itself. Even with all this advice and support, it was only in July that Jaume felt able to describe himself as recovered.[44]

With the exception of his illness at Teruel in 1310, Jaume seems to have felt in reasonably good health during the decade after 1306. His physicians kept him so by supervising his manner of living. Change of climate played an important role: the chill of the Aragonese hills contrasted with the Mediterranean warmth

---

[42] "In presenti . . . quadam fuimus detenti discrasia que nos propria manu scribere non permisit": Martí de Barcelona, "Regesta," p. 289, doc. 127; quoted in *AA*, II:886. By the treaty of Caltabellotta (1303), Charles II had conceded Frederic the title of king in Sicily for the latter's lifetime.

[43] "Reversi ad regnum nostrum, cum ad partes Turolii venissemus, nos gravi infirmitatis dolor arripuit adeo per plures dies ut quasi omnes nostri partes corporis durissime detineret, set post faciente illo qui regibus dat salutem recepta convalescencia restitui pristine sanitate qua in presenciarum perfruimur gratia saluberris": letter of 3 June 1310 (C 238/156v); or see the letter of 24 July (C 238/185r–v), published in Rubió y Lluch, "Contribució," p. 343, doc. 20.

[44] "Henricus Theutonicus" was summoned at the outset, on 25 May 1310 (C 238/142), and arrived within a week (letter of 30 May 1310; C 297/223). He had been welcomed to Catalonia enthusiastically by Jaume II on 17 Dec. 1309 (C 345/194), and settled in Tarragona. After his treatment of the king, he returned to Tarragona and was rewarded with a grant of 2,000 *sous* yearly (3 Nov. 1310; C 207/162). On 13 June 1311 Jaume II sent him to Fernando IV of Castile, who was recovering from an illness (C 239/92v), and while there he attended the birth of the king's son, who succeeded as Alfonso XI the next year. Heinrich then returned to Tarragona, but in November 1315 Queen María de Molina asked that he be sent back to Castile to care for the three-year-old king, "quia interfuistis sue nativitati et novistis compleccionem eius pro conservanda sanitate ipsius" (letter of 31 Oct. 1315; C 242/262v). Jaume issued a safe-conduct to the physician on 25 Jan. 1316 (C 158/218v–219), and Heinrich seems thereafter not to have returned to the Crown of Aragon.

Evidence for the presence of the other practitioners can be found in C 281/151v; RP 273/56r–v, 67v, 72v; and CRD Jaume II, cuenta 91.

of Valencia, but each had its place in a preventative regimen. For simple ills, medicinal baths could also be prescribed, like the hot springs at Caldes de Montbui north of Barcelona, in use since Roman times. But diet – food and drink – was just as important as the external environment in maintaining a person's health. The king's choice of wines, for example, was implicitly a medical decision, and at least once he was provided with specifically medicinal wines by a medical advisor, his surgeon-counsellor Bertomeu ça Font.[45] A further characteristic feature of Jaume's normal regimen was the astonishing variety of confections prepared by the Barcelona apothecary Pere Jutge and supplied to the royal household once or twice a year. Like wines, confections had a medicinal aspect. Some items in the shipment of December 1312 are more obviously medicinal than others – *cassia fistula*, for example – but even the sweets on the list – *diacitron, rosata novella, sucharo rosato* – were recognized as having medicinal properties, and many could be found in the *Antidotarium Nicolai* that would soon direct every apothecary's practice.[46] When a servant of the infante Jaume became ill away from the court in August 1310, the queen commanded her agent in Zaragoza to provide the patient with 8 *deners* daily – "and whatever else he may need in the way of sugar and other medicines."[47] All these varied items were probably approved or even prescribed by the king's physicians – if not as medicines *per se*, then as part of a balanced and health-directed diet.

The queen's medical situation was particularly delicate. She apparently had no troubling illness after her episode of quartan fever in 1306, but like all women she was at continuing risk during her series of pregnancies. She had borne seven children by 1302, one for every year of her marriage. In the next six years, however, she gave birth to only one child (Pere) of whom there is any record, and it is not impossible that she was beginning to experience difficulties in pregnancy. In August 1308, pregnant for at least the ninth time, the twenty-five-year-old queen drew up her will, dreading "the many dangers that women run before, during, and after childbirth";[48] nevertheless, the infante Ramon Berenguer was born without apparent complications on the last day of the month. In the spring of 1310 Blanca again became pregnant, and this time she lost the gamble her condition entailed. During the summer of that year she was

---

[45] MF, I:259 n. 9.

[46] The full list included *zinziberata, batafalva, dragea deaurata et in pulvere, destemetico deaurato, dactils confits, codonyat, pinyonada, diacitron, marçapa de codonyat, sucaro rosato, rosada novella, camamilla, cacia fistola, cimiama* (C 298/179v–181v); on such confections, see below, chapter 5.

[47] "Et quicquid etiam in succaro et aliis medicinalibus ipsum vobis constiterit ydonee" (21 Aug. 1310; C 289/163). The normal *per diem* expenses provided to an incapacitated servant were 8 *deners* per day (cf. letter of 14 Oct. 1309, C 344/108).

[48] "Partus nostri periculum obstupentes ob multa pericula que emergent femineo sexui ante partum et in partu similiter et post partum": MF, II:34, doc. 57.

traveling constantly – to Teruel in June, Zaragoza in July, Lerida in August, Tarragona in September – before returning to Barcelona for the expected birth. The infanta Violant was delivered there on 11 October; Blanca ("racked by terrible pains brought on by childbirth," wrote her sorrowing husband) died two days later.[49]

Women were in special danger during childbirth, but children were susceptible to illness at any time, and Jaume was continually supervising his children's health from delivery to maturity and even beyond.[50] Typically the infantes spent their first two years or so with a wet-nurse.[51] As they grew older, they would often leave the court and be placed in the charge of a tutor (alumnus).[52] From 1304 to 1311, and perhaps beyond, the Valencian physician Berenguer des Far appears to have been charged with the medical care of the young children who remained in the royal household,[53] while the king kept himself informed of the condition of the others through communications from their alumni, sending back advice and physicians from the court as necessary.[54] Some of the children caused more concern than others; of the girls, Isabel seems to have been sick much of the time, while Joan and Ramon Berenguer were the weakest of the boys. The latter developed a facial condition (infirmitas) that needed surgical intervention in 1315: Guillem de Valls boasted that he could cure it without cutting or burning, but evidently vainly, for a month after Guillem saw the boy another surgeon, Bernat de Pertegaç, was paid to treat him.[55]

The delicate health of the infanta Constança gave the king particular reason for concern. At the age of six, in 1306, she was betrothed to Juan Manuel, uncle to the young Fernando IV of Castile, as part of her father's plans to intervene in

---

[49] McVaugh, "Births," pp. 14–16.

[50] Sablonier, "Aragonese Royal Family," pp. 221–2, interprets the king's preoccupation with his children's health as an expression of political (dynastic) concern as well as of parental affection, but the preoccupation as nonetheless real.

[51] Miret y Sans, Sempre han tingut, II:13–29, assembles some material on the wet-nurses to the royal family. His indictment of "la voracitat eterna de les dides," which he bases on the gifts made them by the monarchs, seems to me overstated.

[52] MF, I:36–54.

[53] Berenguer des Far fizich was a witness in Valencia on 19 April 1300 to the Arnaldian document in Martí de Barcelona, "Regesta," p. 268, doc. 36. Perhaps his association with Arnau brought him to the attention of the queen; on 15 Feb. 1304 she granted him 1,000 sous annually while in her service or that of her children (confirmed shortly after her death, 22 Feb. 1311, by the king; C 207/202). He was attending the infanta Maria on 2 July 1311 (quoted 26 July 1320, C 282/53, by which time he was dead); his will was drawn up 30 Dec. 1318 (ARV, Just. Civil 36, f. 121). In 1317, when his responsibilities had nearly disappeared, the king cut the amount of his grant in half (C 214/23v, 278/134).

[54] MF, I:54–63. Cf. the king's fussy letter (MF, II:245) to his fifteen-year-old daughter Blanca, in the monastery of Sigena: "feyt todo al que la priora e los fisigos vos consellaran."

[55] The king permitted Guillem to treat Ramon ("absque ferreo cissura et igne") on 16 April 1315 (C 242/128v); despite his failure in this case, Guillem was still practicing surgery in and around Manresa thirteen years later (AHCM 118, 4 kls. Dec. 1328), when he was a surgeon of second resort. Bernat de Pertegaç's bill was presented 13 June 1315 (C 300/1).

the Castilian succession, and she was sent from her native Valencia to Juan Manuel's castle of Villena in the care of her governess, Saurina de Béziers. At Saurina's insistence the following June, Jaume II requested a Valencian physician, Guillem de Barberà, to travel the 110 kilometers to Villena to restore Constança's health.[56] Guillem did so, made the same trip a year later, and then visited the infanta more or less regularly as her personal physician. When her marriage to Juan Manuel was celebrated in 1312, Constança was taken to live in the Castilian province of Cuenca, still only 150 kilometers distant from Valencia but in its dry emptiness a region worlds away from the luxuriant Mediterranean surroundings in which she had grown up. Here Guillem de Barberà continued to care for her, taking medicines to her in 1314, and in early 1315 he became gravely concerned about her health. He sent word of his concern to Jaume II, advising him that she was in serious condition from her many illnesses, especially a hectic fever, and urging that she be sent back to Valencia and the coastal lands in which she had been born and brought up. Jaume proposed the plan to Juan Manuel immediately, saying that in Valencia Constança "would have plenty of physicians and all sorts of medicines, which are easier to find here than there." Nothing came of the proposal, however, and by April Constança wrote that she was well.[57] From this time on neither Guillem de Barberà nor any other physician sent by Jaume II seems to have attended Constança in Cuenca.[58]

In one significant instance Jaume personally oversaw the health of a child – his first-born, the infante Jaume – even after he was nominally adult, or at least independent, and could have been expected to control his own health care. Of course, the king would naturally have been concerned to maintain the health of his eldest son and heir. In 1313, when the infante Jaume was not quite seventeen, he contracted a fever that called for medical attention, and his father sent Joan Amell to him in Valencia to treat it. Joan reported his diagnosis – "the infante has a simple tertian [fever], suffering four bouts, but now, by God's grace, he has been restored to health" – to his patient but also to the king, who was in Lerida. Jaume returned strict instructions to Joan to keep the infante from hurrying back to work in the heat of a Valencian August, so as not to provoke a

---

[56] Letters of 16 June 1307; MF, II:30, docs. 50–1; the first of these exists in draft in CRD Jaume II extra-series 1002.

[57] "In gravi condicione sue persone propter plures infirmitates quas paciebatur, signanter propter eticam"; King Jaume's response to Guillem's concern quoted here, repeating the diagnosis, is dated 9 Jan. 1315 (C 242/74v–75); his letter to Juan Manuel, written the same day, was extracted by Giménez Soler, Don Juan Manuel, pp. 463–4, doc. 320, and published in full in MF, II:115–16, doc. 170. Constança had recovered by 2 April (C 242/122v).

[58] I have found no sign of Guillem's further involvement with the court, though he continued to practice medicine in Valencia. He was still there on 17 Jan. 1332, when he and his wife Àgata de Castellar acknowledged a debt of 100 sous; ACV, perg. 1496. (The summary of this document given in Olmos y Canalda, Pergaminos, p. 217, doc. 1831, transcribes both his name and his wife's incorrectly.)

relapse.[59] But as time went on the king felt particular concern at the infante's disturbingly erratic behavior as procurator-general of the realm.[60] In 1315 Jaume II agreed to the request of Bertomeu de Bonells (who had previously been physician to the infanta Maria, succeeding Berenguer des Far, at the time of her marriage in 1312) and appointed him physician to the infante Jaume,[61] warning him to use the greatest possible care in supervising the boy's health; Bertomeu was expected to report back regularly to the king.[62] Moreover, the king's one-time surgeon, Bertomeu ça Font, was made the infante's chamberlain. But medical supervision or no, he continued to act unpredictably. In the spring of 1318 he announced to his father that he wished to withdraw from his betrothal to Leonor of Castile, renounce his succession to the crown, and enter a religious order. His father was understandably infuriated, and tried unsuccessfully to talk his heir out of the decision. Then in August the infante developed an abscess (*apostema*), for which Bertomeu de Bonells treated him aggressively with *cassia fistula* and other laxatives into the winter.[63] Young Jaume chose to use his condition as an excuse for not visiting his father in the severe illness that attacked the latter that fall, and his apparent lack of concern for his parent seriously aggravated the relations between the two.

For Jaume II had begun to be concerned again about his own health in his mid-fifties. At Montblanc, in July 1316, he experienced a *discrasia* that momentarily convinced him of the need for additional medical help. Martí de Calça Roja was with the court at the time, but Joan Amell had been given permission to travel to Valencia to manage his affairs conditional upon his promise to return if needed, and the king now recalled him. Two days later, afraid that Joan might not arrive in time, the king summoned Barcelona's leading physician, Pere Gavet, to Montblanc for consultation with Martí.[64] Even more disturbing was the illness the king suffered in January 1318, when in Xàtiva he was attacked by "a serious febrile *discrasia* which, together with other complaints, has kept us down for several days." He wrote these words in February, convalescent but still feeling

---

[59] "Dictum infantem egrotasse simplici terciana et aflictum fuisse ex eadem quatuor paroxismis, sed tandem per dei graciam fere sanitati pristino restitutum": letter of 17 Aug. 1313 (C 241/28); MF, II:98, doc. 142.

[60] On these strange events, see MF, I:83–8; and Miret i Sans, *Forassenyat primogènit*.

[61] Payment to him for service to Maria in January 1312 is recorded 3 Feb. 1312 (C 298/55–56v). Bertomeu was practicing in Lerida in 1306 (C 236/112) but was in Huesca in 1312 when he was called to Maria's service. He planned to move to Vilafranca del Penedès while serving the infante Jaume (18 Oct. 1317; C 215/171), though he was still spoken of as "of Huesca" in 1320, after returning to private practice. He was dead by 1329, when his son Bertomeu, also a physician and living in Vilafranca, tried to get an accounting of the estate (18 July 1330; C 437/211v–212).

[62] The king thanked Bertomeu for keeping him informed on the infante's health 18 July 1316 (C 243/133v).

[63] Letter of 5 Dec. 1318 (C 362/118v).

[64] Letters of 25 and 27 July 1316 (C 243/138v–139).

too unwell to travel, and he had to defer the planned meeting of the Catalan *corts*.[65]

In June 1318 the king called Martí to his side once again.[66] If he was imagining another attack, it proved a false alarm, but the summons ensured that Martí was with the king in the fall, when he was struck by the most terrible illness of his life.[67] He was on his way to Perpignan in September to visit his sister-in-law, the queen of Mallorca, when he was attacked in Figueres by a series of fevers that utterly incapacitated him. There was no question of continuing his trip: he had to be transported in a litter from Blanes in the last stage of his return to Barcelona, where he was prostrated for weeks.[68] By mid-October he had temporarily recovered enough strength to describe the episode to the infanta Constança: "we have just suffered a *discrasia*, an erratic fever that turned into a quartan from which we have not yet recovered; but we trust in God, and besides we have excellent physicians around us, so we should get well, by God's grace."[69] For good measure, Jaume brought in other physicians to supplement his household staff: Geraldo de Sapiach, the infirmarian to the cathedral chapter at Zaragoza; a Jewish physician from Fraga, Juceff Alfogoyl; and probably others as well.[70] All agreed that it would be terribly dangerous for the king to think of venturing into a colder region, and the scheduled meeting of the Aragonese *cortes* was therefore put off until fifteen days after the coming Easter.[71] Then the king's recovery began to reverse itself. He continued to suffer bouts of fever two days in three, and with such intensity that he began to accept the likelihood of his death. In *ordinationes* issued in mid-November,

---

[65] "Febrilis discrasia nimis gravis que cum aliis gravis accidentibus nos per dies aliquod tenuit graviter impeditos": letter of 8 Feb. 1318 (C 308/216). See also the letters of Feb. 1318 published in *Cortes*, I:238–40; or Jaume's explanation that "fueramus corporea invalitudine graviter impediti . . . set prout fisicorum nostrorum tenebatur opinio nullum ex infirmitate ipsa nobis suberat periculum" (letter of 13 Feb. 1318; C 244/232).

[66] Letter of 21 June 1318 (C 244/308).

[67] The illness was first studied carefully in MF, I:255–60.

[68] The litter from Blanes is recorded in C 259/157–8, listing court expenses of Dec. 1318.

[69] "Vos fazemos saber que destos dios en yendo a Perpinyan a visitar la reyna de Mallorcas vuestra tia en el camino oviemos discrasia de fiebre [e]ratiga de la qual somos caidos en quartana e no somos aun librados della, mas fiamos de dios e otrosi que avemos a nuestro regimiento buenos fisicos que guarescremos bien con la gracia de dios": letter of 16 Oct. 1318 (C 245/44v). Elsewhere he was already speaking of it as a double quartan (letter of 13 Oct. 1318; C 245/40v–41). "Febris erratica" was for Montpellier's Bernard Gordon *c.* 1303 a class of compound fever, as were *causonides* or *emitriteus*: *Lilium medicine* I.8; f. 6va.

[70] Accounts make explicit that these two physicians were helping to treat the king: C 259/157–8, 162v; RP 282/74, 83, 85; RP 283/31v, 32, 68v. Geraldo de Sapiach had been the Zaragozan *infirmarius* since 1316: Beltrán, Lacarra, and Canellas, *Historia de Zaragoza*, p. 297.
It seems likely that others, too, were involved in the case: Bernat de Pertegaç, at court from mid-October to December (RP 283/45v); Bafiel Costantí of Zaragoza (RP 283/66v); and Jaffuda Bonsenyor of Barcelona (RP 282/74; RP 283/31v). Bafiel had long served the royal house (*AA*, III:524–5), while Jaffuda had translated medical works for Jaume II (below, chapter 2). On Bernat de Pertegaç, see below, chapter 7 n. 34.

[71] Letter of 3 Oct. 1318 (C 308/239).

Jaume provided for compensation to anyone whom he might have injured by establishing a commission to hear complaints against him and depositing treasure with the bishop of Barcelona to dispense to the victims of royal injustice – doing this, he explained, so as to obtain the health of his soul and to enter more easily into the kingdom of God.[72]

Expecting death, the king nevertheless extended his desperate search for medical help. In mid-November he wrote to Pablo de Gualdo (physician in Valencia to his son Jaume's betrothed, the infanta Leonor of Castile), commanding his presence by virtue of his "knowledge and experience."[73] In December he looked outside his kingdom to summon another physician to his staff, Jordan de Turre, a Montpellier master with a reputation for successful practice. And by the middle of that month his physicians were at last able to hope that he might be improving and out of danger; the electuaries prescribed by Jordan, Martí, and Joan and prepared by Guillem Jordà (notably one made from powdered pearls and gold) had had their effect.[74] In January 1319 the king spoke with more assurance of his recovery, writing to his brother-in-law the king of Portugal that "the double quartan that we had has reverted to a simple one," and to the queen of Portugal in February that "we now have only a little of the quartan fever that we used to have, and we trust to God that we will be cured of it within a few days more."[75] He did not relinquish his grasp on his physicians, however, and in that same month wrote to the justices at Morvedre (present-day Sagunt) that Martí de Calça Roja could not be allowed to attend a court case there, since he was unable to do without Martí for the moment.[76] And the fevers lingered on into late April – "we still have the simple quartan, though not with such strong bouts as before," he wrote his son Pere[77] – so

---

[72] MF, 2:189–91, docs. 268–9.

[73] "Nos iam sunt dies febre quartana duplici fuisse et esse vexatos, adeo quod in corpore nostro plurimum nos extenuavit atque oppressit. Et licet nos phisicos habeamus nobiscum, considerantes tamen plurimum de sciencia et experiencia vestris, volumus atque vobis dicimus et mandamus quatenus . . . ad nos continuo veniatis": letter of 13 Nov. 1318 (C 245/50r–v). Pablo de Gualdo had apparently come to the Crown of Aragon from Castile with the infanta Leonor, for when he first turns up in the documentary record it is already as her physician; this is 16 April 1312 (ACA pergaminos Jaume II 2930), three months after her arrival – aged three – in her future father-in-law's realms (MF, I:87). His responsibilities were always to Leonor, though in 1319 the king did ask him, exceptionally, to visit the infanta Maria, sick at Almansa (C 245/212). He was still physician to Leonor in 1330, by which time she had married Jaume's brother Alfons and had become queen (C 438/239v–240). Pablo died shortly before 5 March 1335 (C 471/78v–79).

[74] McVaugh, "Two Faces," p. 312. The electuary is referred to in RL, II:30, doc. 37. Jaume wrote cautiously of his returning health on 18 Dec. 1318 (C 245/66v) and somewhat more positively on 30 Dec. (C 245/67v).

[75] "La quartana que soliamos haber dobla es tornada a simple": letter of 16 Jan. 1319 (C 245/85). "Avemos ya muy poqº de la febra quartana que soliamos aver, ed a questa esperamos en dios que seremos dentro pocos dias guaridos": letter of 22 Feb. 1319 (C 245/97v–98).

[76] Letter of 12 Feb. 1319 (C 167/25v).

[77] "Aun avemos la simple quartana, pero no avemos tan fuertes accessiones como soliamos": letter of 23 April 1319 (C 245/117).

that it was not until June 1319 that he dared say joyfully that he was fully recovered.[78]

The experience marked Jaume psychologically and medically. Three years later he still remembered the "grave et diuturna infirmitate quam passi fuimus" as a milestone in his life,[79] and his sensitivity to possible ailments became increasingly obsessive. He had been adjudged cured only two months when he detected the onset of a rheum, and he immediately wrote Pablo de Gualdo to return to care for him. Feeling better the next day, he wrote another letter to Pablo, telling him his presence was not needed after all – and then after another twinge called back the messenger and tore up the second letter.[80] Tormented by doubts about his health, increasingly on the lookout for the first signs of an illness, the king had become a valetudinarian as he entered his sixties.

Aging and death

For the last eight years of his life Jaume II accepted an invalid's status. The "gravis infirmitas" of 1318/19 left its mark in his belief in his own frailty, his fear that a fatal illness could strike at any time. His health had now to be protected by the unbroken attention of the best physicians, even at his own family's expense. In the summer of 1323 the court was at Tortosa and included the eighteen-year-old infante Pere, Count of Ribagorça. When Pere left his father to return home through Aragon, he was unwell, and King Jaume sent Martí de Calça Roja along with his son to look after him; at the same time, he wrote to his *phisicus maior*, Joan Amell, to come back to court, "since we cannot be without you both." Joan must have replied that he was unable to return, for two weeks later the king wrote urgently to Martí ordering him back immediately – "our dear son the infante Pere," the king said a little callously, "can probably find some competent physician in Zaragoza or Huesca."[81]

The counsel of Jaume's doctors confirmed his tendency to self-protectiveness, exemplified particularly in his absolute unwillingness to risk climatic changes. In March 1320 he suffered a few bouts of fever, and because of the inclement weather he stayed in Montblanc rather than travel.[82] Thenceforth, however, it

---

[78] He so described himself to his son Joan on 2 June 1319 (C 245/134). Two days later he spoke of himself as "sanitati pristine restituti" to his daughter Isabel (C 318/19v).

[79] MF, I:256.

[80] "Jacobus etc. dilecto phisico nostro magistro Paulo etc. Licet pridie vobis scripsimus ut pro reuma quam patimur ad nos veniretis, quia vidimus quod adventum vestrum excusare possumus significamus vobis quod non opportet vos ad presenciam nostram venire ad presens. Dat. Barch. 9 kls. Sept. anno domini 1319." Below this letter, copied in C 245/179, the scribe has written: "Predicta litera licet fuisset expedita et tradita cursori fuit recuperata et laniata quia fuit ordinatum quod non mitteretur."

[81] Letters of 29 June and 17 July 1323 (C 247/302 and 308). Jaume's action is the more striking because less than a year before Pere had seemed in danger of death (MF, I:161 and 57).

[82] Letters of 23 March and 5 April 1320 (C 246/4, 8).

was chronic infirmity, not acute illness, of which he usually complained, and which he consistently made a not wholly unwelcome excuse for delaying meetings of the Catalan *corts* or Aragonese *cortes*. In February 1321 he told the Catalans that "the advice of many skilled physicians" was that he stay in Valencia to avoid the intemperance of a wintry climate.[83] In October 1322 he wrote the Aragonese that "our condition at present is not such as can bear a strain of this sort or can tolerate so cold a region";[84] he wrote them again to the same effect in November 1323, again attributing the decision to his physicians' recommendation.[85] In July 1324 he delayed the Aragonese *cortes* until Michaelmas, claiming a *gravis discrasia* and explaining that the summer heat was bad for him; in late August he spoke of another *discrasia corporalis* and put them off until All Saints'; and at the end of September wrote again that his physicians had advised him not to travel to Aragon, because of its cold winters, but to seek out a warm climate, and that therefore it was necessary to defer them until Ascension 1325.[86] Naturally, by the next June it was again too hot to stay in Aragon, and the *cortes* were put off once more.[87]

And Jaume may have been suffering from more than recurrent fevers and *discrasie*. Writing in December 1326 to delay a meeting of the Catalan *corts*, he explained that "we are prevented by the sickness from which we have long suffered in the leg [*tibia*], and by general bodily disorders."[88] A problem with the leg suggests a surgical, not a medical, problem, and for this reason it may be significant that during these last years Jaume was making repeated demands on surgeons – especially on one Bernat Serra, who joined the king's service in November 1317 and remained in it until the king died. Jaume's concern for his new surgeon's skills was made apparent during the first months of his grave illness, when he arranged for Bernat to be given the extensive library and tools (*ferramenta*) of another surgeon who had just died.[89] During 1320–3 and again in 1326 Bernat was regularly at the king's side, and in the fall of the latter year two additional surgeons, first Bertomeu Valentí of Mallorca and then Salamon

---

[83] He was, he explained on 13 Feb. 1321, "nondum tunc a longa et periculosa infirmitate qua lacessiti diu fuimus sinceriter liberati" (C 308/221).

[84] "Status persone nostre non patitur ad presens huiusmodi subire labores, nec existere etiam in frigida regione": letter of 1 Oct. 1322 (C 308/243).

[85] Letter of 5 Nov. 1323 (C 308/246).

[86] Letters of 7 July, 30 Aug., and 24 Sept. 1324 (C 308/247v, 249, 250v).

[87] On Jaume's reluctance to meet his Aragonese *cortes*, see Sarasa Sánchez, *Cortes*, pp. 37–40, and González Antón, "Cortes," p. 601; the latter believes that "sus razones no pasaron de ser meras excusas dilatorias."

[88] "Infirmitas quam in tibia (non absque tocius corporis nostri affliccione) diu passi sumus et patimur ut potuistis audisse nos impedit": letter of 10 Dec. 1326 (C 308/269). A letter from the infante Joan to his father asks about "infirmitatem vestram quam in tibiis passi estis," dated simply "19 October" (CRD Jaume II 12991); the infante subscribes himself "Archbishop of Toledo," so that the letter could have been written at any time from 1320 on (the pope approved his election in November 1319; Vincke, "Trasllat," p. 127).

[89] See below, chapter 3.

Avenforna of Alagón (northwest of Zaragoza), were summoned to help care for him.[90]

The king's preoccupation with his own health did not prevent him from continuing to supervise the health of his children.[91] Some gave him particular cause to worry. He had eventually allowed his heir Jaume to renounce the succession in favor of his second son, Alfons, but even in orders the infante Jaume continued to trouble the king with his instability and licentiousness.[92] The health of the king's daughters Isabel and Constança – in 1325, twenty-three and twenty-five years old, respectively – presented more specific problems. After Isabel married Friedrich the Handsome of Austria in 1312 and left for Germany, her father had tried to ensure that her health would still be looked after, and had encouraged her to put herself in the care of her husband's physician, Giovanni de Verona: "Since it is the part of wisdom to follow the advice of prudent physicians for the sake of health, we urge you to follow the regimen and advice of your doctor sensibly so as to avoid illnesses and stay well."[93] His advice encapsulates the respectful attitude towards medicine that Jaume himself never lost. But if Isabel followed it, her faith must have been sorely tested. She began to suffer severe headaches shortly after her husband's army was defeated at Mühldorf in 1322, and then problems with her eyes that brought her closer and closer to blindness: when her husband was released from captivity in 1325, she could barely make out his face. In June 1326 she finally let her father know of her condition: "It is an illness of the eyes that the doctors call 'cataract,'" she wrote, and on the chance that it was of a curable type she asked him to send her an expert from Aragon, someone more skilled than the German masters. The king replied immediately, asking for a fuller account of her symptoms so that he could pass them on to his surgeons. Simultaneously he summoned a Zaragozan eye-doctor (*metge de mal de uyls*), Jaime de Rocha, presumably with the idea of sending him to Isabel when further information had arrived; but in October 1327 the king was still asking pathetically for a fuller account of his daughter's condition.[94]

---

[90] Documents of 4 Nov. and 1 Dec. 1326 (C 303/132v–133v, 137r–v).

[91] The king's concern to keep informed of their condition is reflected in the five letters sent him during four weeks in the summer of 1326 by his son Pere, dutifully reporting on the course of a febrile *discrasia*, from onset to recovery: CRD Jaume II 8977, 8999, 9000, 9026, 9047.

[92] Miret i Sans, *Forassenyat primogènit*, pp. 36–46; MF, I: 88–101.

[93] "Sane cum sapientis sit, ob bonum sanitatis adquiescere prudencium consilio fisicorum, ortamur et suademus vobis ut regimini atque consilio dicti fisici prout frugi et salubria fuerit pro evitandis infirmitatibus et adipiscenda salute efficaciter intendatis": letter of 5 Aug. 1315 (C 318/10). (I have examined the original document and slightly modified the text published by Zeissberg, "Register," p. 34 doc. 26.)

[94] Isabel's letter to her father announcing her illness (4 June 1326; CRD Jaume II 8791) is published in *AA*, I:379–80, and by Zeissberg, "Register," pp. 89–90. On the course of the blindness, see the references cited by Zeissberg, p. 88. Jaume instructed Joan Amell to compose a letter for Jaime de Rocha with an account of Isabel's condition, and summoned Jaime to court 19 Oct. 1326 (C 286/30v–31); he had arrived by 1 Jan. 1327 (C 303/140; RP 294/96v).

Constança's situation was even more unfortunate. Still living – perhaps one should say immured – in her husband's castle of García-Muñoz, she had seen two of her four children die soon after birth, and her young daughter Constança was taken from her to the Castilian fortress of Toro in 1325, to be betrothed to Alfonso XI of Castile. Subsequently her brother Joan, then archbishop of Toledo, visited her for five weeks and wrote in distress to their father about her condition:

> She often weeps, and, what is worse, she will take almost no food or medicine, asking instead for me and that we send her to Valencia. I fear either her death or damage to her mind . . . If you were to see her, you would be horrified at her appearance. Let it please you then to think on these things and to reply what seems best to you and your physicians to do.[95]

King Jaume felt too insecure of his own health to make the journey, but he was kept informed of Constança's condition by a physician in her brother's entourage, Pedro Cellerer, and at one point during the second half of 1326 the king even made plans to send Joan Amell to look after his daughter.[96]

At the beginning of 1327 Constança's husband, Juan Manuel, wrote to Jaume II from García-Muñoz, saying that physicians had diagnosed "a certain melancholy [*alguna tristeza*] that she has taken"; though she was better at present, so that he hoped that "soon she will be free of all those fancies she has had," he urged that the king send Joan Amell and other physicians from the Crown of Aragon, "the best there are," to Constança.[97] But the king now felt too ill to risk sending his doctors to Castile, though he promised he would do so

---

[95] "Flet frequenter, et quod peius est, nichil medicinale vult recipere nec etiam cibum, nisi in valde modica quantitate, petens pro me et quod mandamus Valentiam. Multum dubito de ea vel de morte vel de diutina intellectus lesione . . . Si videritis eam, distraeretis solum ex aspectu. Placeat itaque vestre dominationi circa hec cogitare et rescribere, quid vobis et medicis vestris videretur agendum." The letter is published in *AA*, II:867, dated only "die lune post festum Corporis Christi"; Giménez Soler, *Don Juan Manuel*, pp. 675–6, republishes it from this source. MF, I:137–8, dates it 24 Sept. (!) 1325, and assumes that the visit occurred that summer. However, it is perhaps more likely that the letter should be dated [26 May] 1326, since Joan refers there to current Castilian distress at the plans for the marriage of Juan de Viscaya, which was in the air in that year; Joan gave more details to his father about Castilian unhappiness on this matter in July (*AA*, III:518).

[96] Jaume asked Amell to make the trip early in the summer, and his physician consented to go, though he complained of the rigors of summer travel in Castile and of the expense it would entail (5 July [1326]; CRD Jaume II extra-series 521). Jaume thanked Pedro Cellerer for his news of Constança's improvement in a letter of 31 July 1326 (C 249/197v), and the same day wrote to Amell, telling him to ask for a safe-conduct for the trip (C 249/198; MF, II:328, doc. 452, mistakenly dates it as 1327 and places it in C 294). On 25 Sept. 1326, however, the king told Amell that he himself had need of his physician and that he should present himself at court if an envoy from Castile had not yet arrived (MF, II:318–19, doc. 438; and cf. doc. 437).

[97] Giménez Soler, *Don Juan Manuel*, pp. 533–4, doc. 422 (2 Jan. 1327), who does not identify the source; the document is now CRD Alfons III 31.

when he had recovered further.[98] During that spring Constança added her pleas to her husband's, imploring her father to send her medical help or at least visit her, and wondering whether his neglect meant that "you have forgotten me, or don't want me to get well,"[99] and finally Jaume instructed master Junta de Nucerio to travel south from Zaragoza to attend the infanta and care for her.[100] It was too late, however, for Constança had only a few months more to live; the king sorrowfully reported her death to her brothers in mid-August 1327.[101]

The king's habitual reluctance to be separated from his medical staff had been reinforced by the appearance of a new febrile *discrasia* at the beginning of 1327. By March he felt better, although, as he told Juan Manuel, "still weakened by the illnesses we have had,"[102] but even so he decided to bring Martí de Calça Roja back from Valencia to join in overseeing his case.[103] The improvement did not last. At the beginning of October, pleading a "gravis et longua infirmitas," he postponed once more the Aragonese *cortes*, scheduled to meet at All Saints'.[104] And by All Saints', indeed, Jaume was aware that he was about to die. On the last day of October 1327 his son Ramon Berenguer wrote to his elder brother Alfons, the king's heir, holding out a little hope: "Last Friday night at midnight he took so great a rheum that the doctors gave him up; then Saturday morning following he was a very little bit better, but since the moon is turning the doctors say he is still not out of danger."[105] The king himself, without illusions, wrote the next day to tell Alfons that he was dying, and his death came one day later, on 2 November.[106] As the chronicler Zurita wrote, it had ended "una larga indisposición y enfermedad."[107]

Like father, like son: Alfons III

Perhaps because Alfons' expectation of succession to the throne came so late, or perhaps because he seemed a stabler personality, his father Jaume did not

[98] Jaume describes this illness to Jaume of Mallorca as a "febrili discrasia," 8 Feb. 1327 (C 249/288; MF, II:321–2, doc. 442).

[99] "Si es por que me avedes olvidado o porque no es vuestra voluntat que yo guaresca deste mal": Giménez Soler, *Don Juan Manuel*, p. 541, doc. 433 (4 May 1327); MF, II:323, doc. 445.

[100] MF, II:325, doc. 448.

[101] Letter of 23 Aug. 1327 (C 250/51v). MF, I:137–41, gives an account of Constança's last illness that differs slightly in detail.

[102] "Ahun flaco por las enfermedades que havemos havidas": letter of 23 Mar. 1327 (C 250/5v).

[103] In two letters of 18 and 23 March 1327 (C 250/5v–6).

[104] Letter of 1 Oct. 1327 (C 308/254).

[105] "Senyor sapia la vra. altea quel molt alt senyor Rey pare nre. comu havent alguns dies precedents cadarn, divendres anit prop passada al punt de la miya nit li vench tan gran reuma que vench al punt axi quels metges ho tamien per fet; puys al dissapte mati saguent pres fort poch de mallorament, mas per tal con es la luna en lo contorn dien los dits metges que encara no es fora de sospita": CRD Jaume II 12994 (31 Oct. 1327).

[106] Letter of 1 Nov. 1327 (C 250/74v).

[107] Zurita, *Anales* 6.75, ed. Canellas López, II:282. Cf. Muntaner, *Crònica*, cap. 292: "a ell venc malaltia tal e tan gran, que en soferí molt de treball" (in Soldevila, *Cròniques*, p. 933).

supervise his health as closely or as long as he did that of his first-born. Alfons' marriage in November 1314 (at the age of fifteen) to Teresa de Entença, the heiress to the county of Urgell, made him independent of his father and master of his own health. He does not appear to have had a household physician at first, but was content rather to summon medical help when it was needed – as he summoned a physician from Cervera and a surgeon from Tàrrega to treat "patients in our household" at Agramunt in October 1318,[108] or as he summoned Guillaume de Carcassonne and Ramon de Vilalta from Lerida and the Jew Mosse Avinardut from Huesca to treat him personally in Alcoletge in the fall of 1319.[109] Shortly thereafter Mosse – and then Mosse's son Alazar – became physician to Teresa, who was less fortunate in her pregnancies than Blanca, losing a son Alfons in 1319, the same year that her second child, Pere (the future Pere III), was born. Alfons finally selected Bertomeu de Gauders as his personal physician in 1322, at Joan Amell's recommendation, advising him to consult Joan and Jaume II before taking up attendance. But he made no very heavy demands on Bertomeu or the remainder of his medical staff in the three years Bertomeu remained with him.[110] When Alfons broke his leg boar-hunting in Valencia early in 1323, he hired two local surgeons – Pere Correger and Jaume d'Avinyó – to set it.[111] In his early twenties Alfons seems to have outgrown his sickly childhood and to have become a normally and unconcernedly healthy individual.

Heinrich Finke suggested that the ill health of Alfons' later years was touched off by his year of campaigning in Sardinia to establish his father's rule over the island (1323–4).[112] Certainly epidemic disease was widespread among his troops

---

[108] The physician Pere d'Odena and the surgeon Bertomeu de Pau (accounts of 5 Dec. 1318; C 418/68). Pere had come to Cervera from Huesca in 1301, attracted by the offer made him by municipal authorities, and was still there 6 Aug. 1341 (C 616/115v). Bertomeu had treated the infante once before, in 1315 (C 416/17), and would be called back to his side again in 1333 (C 534/143v).

[109] On Ramon and Mosse see below, pp. 73 and 56. Ramon's attendance here is established in accounts of October 1319 (RP 556/82v), while Mosse's can be inferred from the grant made him 6 Sept. 1319 (C 425/121). Guillaume's service to the king is rewarded in accounts dated 9 Nov. 1319 (C 425/117ff.; and see RP 556/84v). He had been in practice in Lerida since 1309 (C 475/104r–v), had treated the infante in 1317 (C 418/28), and continued to obey summonses to attend Alfons throughout his reign; Guillaume was at the king's deathbed in December 1335 (RP 307/80v). Subsequently he treated his widow Queen Leonor (RP 312/59, for July–Dec. 1338), and was still in Lerida, a member of the municipal council, in 1344–5 (AML, Llibres de Actes, 397/2).

[110] The letter of appointment is 22 Sept. 1322 (C 386/124v). Bertomeu was not in continual attendance on the infante; twice in the spring of 1323 he traveled from Valencia to Barcelona to see Alfons (C 388/115v; RP 560/70v), perhaps helping prepare for the expedition to Sardinia, in which he seems to have taken part: he was sold an income of 2,000 *sous* from Sardinian property 4 May 1325 (C 398/127).

[111] Accounts of 15 Jan. 1323 (C 387/198).

[112] Finke, "Nachträge," AA, III:632. Jaume II had been promised the kingdom of Sardinia by the pope in the treaty of Anagni (1295), and he had been invested with the title in 1297.

there – not unnaturally, given their wretched living conditions; during the sieges of Iglesias and Cagliari the rotting bodies of the dead were stacked up about the camp. Alfons had repeatedly to grant permission to the sick to leave the army and return home to recover. The few physicians with the army could do little, apparently, and were not themselves immune: at least one, Mosse Avinardut (who had come in the king's immediate entourage), died during the campaign.[113] Whether Alfons himself was seriously affected is uncertain. His son Pere later wrote that his father had not passed a day in Sardinia free of fever, but Alfons' accounts and correspondence from the expedition do not bear this out.[114] The first clear indication of the serious sicknesses that would become recurrent during his brief reign came in the summer of 1327, as his royal father lay dying in Barcelona. About St. John's day, he was attacked on his way to Zaragoza by a dysentery that weakened him terribly. He was cared for in the first, most frightening stages of the disease by Gracia Orlandi, physician to a powerful Sardinian dynast, who had been on a mission to the court from his lord when Alfons fell ill; Orlandi remained with the infante day and night.[115] Alfons finished his journey in daily stages of a league or two that were all his body could support, and once at Zaragoza his physicians insisted he rest for at least two months, "for they believe that due to certain side-effects of our illness it could be very dangerous for us to travel."[116] At the beginning of September he was still abed in Zaragoza; seven months later he was to be crowned king in the same city.

For the first few years after his accession, Alfons' health seems to have remained stable.[117] He continued to maintain Mosse Avinardut's son Alazar as his personal physician. His wife Teresa had died in childbirth only a week before his father,[118] and his second marriage – in 1329, to Leonor of Castile – added a

---

[113] A full analysis of the medical evidence from the Sardinian campaign is included in Cifuentes i Comamala, "Medicina." The resettlement of Sardinia by the Catalans and Aragonese was made more difficult by its reputation for unhealthiness: "per pahor de les grans enfermedats de Cerdenya les gens dupten de venir" (CRD Alfons III 3673; 13 Nov. [1327]).

[114] "E lo dit senyor infant emmalatí tan fortment que null temps, aitant com en Sardenya estec, no fo sens febre" (Pere el Ceremoniós, *Crònica*, I.22; in Soldevila, *Cròniques*, p. 1011); while Muntaner wrote that Alfons was so ill that only the care of his wife kept him from dying (*Crònica*, cap. 274; in Soldevila, *Cròniques*, p. 915). However, Alfons' letters from Sardinia show only that he had a few bouts of tertian fever in September 1323, from which he had recovered by the beginning of the next month, and a second brief siege in December; see Arribas Palau, *Conquista*, pp. 214–15.

[115] The infante praised him for "non parcendo persone vestre, varios die noctuque pro corporis nostre quiete sustinendo labores": letter of 10 July 1327 (C 403/104v–105v).

[116] "Car entenen que per alcuns accidens qui's son mesclats in nostra malaltia poria esser a nos molt perillos lo moviment": letter of 31 Aug. 1327 (MF, II:330, doc. 456).

[117] Although Zurita says (*Anales* 7.27; ed. Canellas López, III:397) that "después que sucedió en el reino y se casó segunda vez [in 1329], vivió muy enfermo."

[118] After the birth of Pere (the future Pere III) in 1319, Teresa had given birth to Jaume d'Urgell and Constança, the future queen of Mallorca, and a son Frederic who died. Twins, Isabel and

further doctor to the household, for she brought with her a Jewish physician, Salomon Abenpater (who converted to Christianity and changed his name to Pere Ferrandi within a year after his arrival in the Crown of Aragon).[119] With one or both of these two at hand to advise and prescribe, Alfons rarely felt ill enough to need outside medical assistance, although he did call on Junta de Nucerio for help in November 1328 and June 1330.[120]

As his father Jaume had done, Alfons kept himself informed of his heir's health, expecting notice of even apparently trivial ills: "last Monday," wrote the dutiful fourteen-year-old Pere to his father in April 1334, "I began to feel a certain feverish heat in my body, though not a very severe one, from which I have not yet been entirely freed."[121] Alfons also took on his father's task of supervising the health of his brothers and sisters. When his brother Ramon Berenguer was sick with fever, his brother's wife Blanca anxiously notified the king of the disease's course; when in turn Blanca became seriously ill after childbirth, Ramon Berenguer wrote Alfons asking for the loan of Joan Amell, since his wife had "great faith in his skill."[122] To his sister Isabel, in Germany, Alfons tried to send the surgeon she had asked their father for. Jaime de Rocha was supposed to visit Isabel in the summer of 1329, but apparently did not; he set out at last in September 1330, only to find on his arrival in Graz that his patient-to-be had died on 12 July.[123] His brother Joan's perennially poor health was also a concern to the king, and he arranged for reports from his brother's

Sanç, were born to her on 23 Oct. 1327, but both soon died – Sanç on the 24th – and Teresa followed them on the 28th (CRD Jaume II 9744; Zurita, *Anales* 6.75; ed. Canellas López, III:281).

[119] He first appears in accounts of July/Aug. 1329, six months after the marriage, and he converted at some point between 22 Feb. (C 522/254v–255) and 17 Sept. 1330 (C 482/35). He is last in evidence at the moment of the king's death, 2 Jan. 1336 (C 530/259).

[120] Junta de Nucerio, who practiced in Zaragoza from at least 1315 (C 352/141r–v) until 1340 (C 869/95), was in constant demand by the royal family, as much as any other medical practitioner in the Crown of Aragon. He had attended Jaume II in 1321 (C 246/322v), the infante Alfons in 1324 (C 427/1v), and Alfons' wife Teresa in 1326 (C 426/56), and was sent to the infanta Constança in 1327 (above, n. 100); Junta would subsequently treat not only Alfons III but his brother Joan, his wife Leonor, and his sons Pere and Jaume d'Urgell.

[121] "Sensimus primo in corpore nostro aliquem febris calorem, non tamen nimium excedentem, de quo nondum perfecte existimus liberati": letter of 25 April 1334 (C 578/223). Pere was assigned his own barber in 1330, when he was ten (C 532/67v).

[122] Letters of 15 Sept. (no year) and Monday 5 Nov. [1330] (respectively CRD Alfons III 3446 and 3488).

[123] Alfons' first attempts to make the arrangements came on 28 July and 15 Aug. 1329 (C 521/127v–128 [published in *AA*, III:551–2]; C 560/82), but it does not seem that Jaime made this trip. Alfons tried again the next year, 16 Aug. and 2 Sept. 1330 (C 523/100v, 115v–116 [the latter published in *AA*, III:555–6]), and this time Jaime made it to Germany, for he was paid 1,000 *sous* expenses on his return in November 1330 (RP 298/95). He was still alive in late 1333, imprisoned in Vic for forgery (C 468/28r–v, 501/126r–v; ACFV 223, kls. Dec. 1333; ACFV 286, 6 kls. Feb. 1334).

physicians.[124] During Joan's final illness in August 1334 the archbishop wrote his royal brother that "we suffer from a continued fever, as well as an intermittent one that sometimes strikes us twice a day," but expressed confidence that the attacks were growing weaker; the archbishop's physicians reported more pessimistically in a private letter that "since his lordship is of a weak complexion, his illness is not without danger," and indeed the infante Joan died only fifteen days later.[125] Joan's death meant that besides the king only five of the children of Jaume II were left alive, for the unhappy eldest son, Jaume, had died just a month before.[126]

Meanwhile, in Montblanc in the early summer of 1333, Alfons had had an illness that seems decisively to have altered his condition, in a manner reminiscent of his father's illness fifteen years before. It was not so psychologically traumatic, perhaps, for speaking of it in late July he said merely "we suffered from a fever and a certain *discrasia*, but now we are better"; his son Pere spoke more circumstantially of "the fever and violent dysentery that you suffered."[127] But it clearly seemed severe and extraordinary when it attacked, for Alfons summoned to Montblanc Pere Gavet from Barcelona; Guillaume de Carcassonne and the aging Joan Amell from Valencia; Berenguer ça Coma from the infante Joan's archiepiscopal household at Tarragona; and a surgeon, master Bertomeu of Tàrrega – despite the fact that Alazar, Pere Ferrandi, and Gracia Orlandi (on yet another mission from Sardinia) were already with him. The apothecary Mateu Sola was brought from Solsona with various electuaries, plasters, and comfits for Alfons, while two more apothecaries in Barcelona, Felip Jutge and Lorens des Soler, sent down additional drugs. Montblanc's physician, Borraç Alanya, was allowed to help during the convalescence.[128]

Alfons now had thirty months to live, and they were marked by a preoccupation with his health that recalls his father's last years. In March 1334, with Alazar and Pere still held tightly at court, Alfons felt a need for a healthful purge; but rather than have it administered by the physicians of the household,

---

[124] Jaume II had earlier supervised Joan's health in the same way: for his response to an illness of Joan's in the spring and summer of 1321, see Avezou, "Prince Aragonais," p. 362 (to the documents quoted there as bearing on the illness can be added C 246/276, 291v).

[125] "Febrem patimur continuam et eciam interpolatum que quandoque nos affligit bis in die" (CRD Alfons III 3765). "Cum . . . dictus dominus sit debilis complexionis, egritudo eius non est sine periculo" (CRD Alfons III 3764). Both letters are dated 4 Aug. 1334. CRD Jaume II 12220, of the same date, is a lay observer's detailed report to Alfons III on his brother's condition.

[126] MF, I:101.

[127] "Passi fuimus febrem et aliqualem eciam discrasiam set iam convaluimus"; "febre et valido fluxu ventris quibus fuistis afflicti": letters of 27 and 29 July 1333 (C 578/148 and 528/156).

[128] Junta de Nucerio was summoned 23 June 1333 (C 577/141v), though it is not clear that he was able to come. The others are rewarded in accounts dated July 1333 (RP 303/32–35v), except for Gracia Orlandi, whose service is recorded in a letter of 20 Sept. 1333 (C 535/1). The king wrote to the queen of his recovery 3 July 1333 (C 577/145v). For Berenguer ça Coma (or de Cumba) see below, chapter 7.

he wrote peremptorily to Joan Amell in Valencia, bidding him come immediately with the appropriate wherewithal. When Joan did not instantly respond, the king wrote again even more insistently, hedging his bets with a similar letter to Domenico de Crix in Falset, a Neapolitan physician whom Alfons had salaried in 1332.[129]

Joan Amell did eventually attend the king, diagnosing an overheated liver and obstructed spleen, and stayed until Michaelmas 1334.[130] Within a month after his departure, however, a new crisis occurred that again forced the king to consult widely: physicians Abraham des Castlar from Besalú, Junta from Zaragoza, and Berenguer ça Coma from Tarragona all came to Alfons at Tortosa in October; so did surgeons Arnau ça Riera from Gerona and Domènech Gargila from Tortosa itself.[131] After the crisis had passed, in March of 1335, the king let Domenico de Crix know that he had been dismissed for failing to come immediately to his patron when summoned;[132] he was replaced in royal service by Arnau ça Riera, who remained with Alfons to the end.[133]

The nature of Alfons' last illness, like that of previous stages, cannot be determined, partly because he referred to his physical condition very little in his personal correspondence, much less than had his father. His son Pere, writing much later, attributed Alfons' death to dropsy.[134] A summons of April 1335 to Junta says that the king "suffers seriously in his ear";[135] the previous August he had complained that "we suffer in one of our feet."[136] Whether these ailments – literally from head to foot – were largely imaginary, or whether they were symptomatic of underlying problems, we cannot say. It was in the hopes of improving his health that in June 1335 the king paid two visits to the hot springs

---

[129] Alfons first wrote to Joan Amell 19 March 1334 and then four days later commanded that he come "sub pena nostre gracie," writing the same day to Domenico de Crix (of Cres? C 529/8v, 10). Domenico, described as "peritum in medicinali sciencia," had on 28 June 1332 been given a salary of 2,500 *sous* annually for as long as he remained in Alfons' service (C 485/210v).

[130] Joan treated "excedenti calore jecoris et opilacione splenis . . . per quoddam medicinale poculum": letter of 8 May 1334 (C 578/235r–v). Two documents (C 536/19, 19v) of 30 July and 1 Aug. 1334 suggest that the medicines prescribed were rose sugar and *conserva rosarum*.

[131] From accounts for Oct.–Nov. in RP 305/70, 73v, 79, 91, 94, 101. The volume is labeled "1333" in error for 1334.

[132] "Scire vos volumus quod nos, propter necessitatem infirmitatis persone quam passi fuimus et moram quam reveniendi ad nos traxistis, alium recepimus medicum et domesticum loco vestri": letter of 10 March 1335 (C 530/152; quoted in part in *AA*, III:632).

[133] For Arnau and Alfons, see McVaugh and García Ballester, "Medical Faculty," p. 6; and McVaugh, "Royal Surgeons."

[134] "Lo dit senyor rei, pare nostre, no visqué sinó huit anys aprés que fon rei, car partida del temps que visqué fon malalt, e finalment fon hidròpic, del qual mal morí . . . Mas, per accident de la malaltia, com fos hitròpic, agreujà-li la malaltia e finà sos dies en Barcelona": Pere el Ceremoniós, *Crònica*, prol., 6, and I.54; in Soldevila, *Cròniques*, pp. 1006, 1022.

[135] "Patitur in aure graviter": letter of 11 April 1335 to the infante Pere (C 536/51r–v), forwarded to Junta 20 April 1335 (C 579/121).

[136] "Altero pedum nostrorum patimur": letter of 12 Aug. 1334 (C 536/21v).

at Caldes d'Estrach, north of the capital,[137] but the first signs of the final crisis appeared in September, when the king brought Jordan de Turre back to Barcelona to attend him – perhaps remembering that Jordan had been present when his father Jaume II had begun to recover from his *gravis infirmitas*. Alfons made Jordan the gift of 100 gold florins (equivalent to perhaps 1,500 *sous*) on top of his expenses.[138] After Jordan left, in November, Alfons called in four more physicians to assist Alazar (Pere Ferrandi had been allowed to go to Huesca on royal business): Berenguer ça Coma from Tarragona, Guillaume de Carcassonne from Lerida, Guerau de Sant Dionis from Gerona, and Jaume de Vallerio from Mallorca.[139] And in mid-December Alfons spoke hopefully of his illness as "passing off."[140] He was mistaken. A new order of "plasters, syrups, unguents, and other medicinal items" supplied early in the new year by the Barcelonan apothecary Pere Janer did no good, and on 24 January 1336 the young king died, within a few days of his thirty-seventh birthday.[141] His son Pere's reign would last more than half a century.

As I have already said, it would be reckless to claim that the medical history of these two generations of the royal family is fully representative of the experience of their subjects. Both biologically and socially they enjoyed advantages that set them clearly apart from most of their society: they had all they wanted to eat, for one thing, and they could expect continuing access to the best medical care, for another. Yet having acknowledged this, we may not find it so obvious that they were very different – from the urban middle and upper classes, at least – in their attitudes towards health and illness, physicians, and medical care: in what they feared, and in what they expected. The fact remains that for lack of comparable personal documentation it is impossible to construct even this much of a medical biography for any other inhabitants of the Crown of Aragon in the first decades of the fourteenth century. Hence it will be useful to keep in mind the experiences of Jaume II, Alfons III, and their families, as we consider the mass of more purely social data that our sources give us. We will find that the royal family's personal involvement with the medical culture of its time can often make more meaningful what would otherwise be mere abstract generalizations.

---

[137] His physicians had decided by February 1335 that his illness of the foot, which they attributed to the stress of a journey, required him to visit a medicinal bath (CRD Alfons III 3154, of 20 Feb. [1335], and by April they had settled on Estrach (C 558/19). Miret y Sans, "Itinerario," p. 123, dates the visits themselves.

[138] McVaugh, "Two Faces," p. 319 n. 8.

[139] Letters of 30 Nov. 1335 (C 530/246r–v). For Guerau de Sant Dionis see below, chapter 6.

[140] Letter of 2 Dec. 1335 (C 530/247).

[141] RP 308/52v; on the date of Alfons' death, see Mutgé Vives, *Ciudad de Barcelona*, p. 325 n. 2.

2

Medieval health manpower

Defining the questions

One obvious feature of the medical history of the Aragonese kings is the number and variety of health providers they were increasingly able to call upon as time went on. Does this variety imply a differentiation of medical services within the realm? Does the apparent increase in the availability of medical assistance over time mean that the number of physicians in the kingdom was actually growing during the first third of the fourteenth century? A number of attempts have recently been made to measure the presence of practitioners in other fourteenth-century societies, in England, France, and Italy: was the Crown of Aragon better or worse supplied than these?

At the outset we must recognize that no single answer is likely to be given to any of these questions, inasmuch as the Aragonese count-kings ruled over three distinct societies. The kingdom of Valencia, mountainous to the west and north, had long enjoyed extensive agricultural development in its rich coastal plain: a variety of crops in its market garden, the *horta*, and rice in the *albufera*, the lagoon south of Valencia city. Aragon, on the other hand, is high country, relatively arid throughout – except for the valley of the Ebro, which cuts across it from west to east and along which most of its population lived, cultivating the cereals that were the region's principal exports. Catalonia too has its mountain ranges, but they isolate it less sharply (it maintained close cultural ties with southern France), and the ports of Barcelona and Tarragona – and the outlet of the Ebro at Tortosa – gave it a commercial outlook that Aragon never attained. By the early fourteenth century, Catalonia had assumed political and cultural leadership in the confederation.[1]

Opinions vary widely on the population of these lands in the early fourteenth century; the first data of any reliability come after the demographic calamity of

---

[1] A convenient brief survey is Bisson, *Medieval Crown*; placing it in a wider context, Hillgarth, *Spanish Kingdoms*.

mid-century, the epidemics of plague. But, lacking any census, most historians would still probably agree that figures of 100,000 for Aragon, 200,000 for Valencia, and perhaps as many as 550,000 for Catalonia cannot be badly off the mark.[2] Settlement in Valencia was primarily along the coast, where Valencia city may have had as many as 30,000 inhabitants. The smaller population in Aragon was established along the river valleys – in Zaragoza and Calatayud – and further north in Huesca.

Catalonia's much larger population was spread through a greater number of population centers, and it is therefore of some interest to try to get some sense of its distribution. Historical demographers of medieval Catalonia have at their disposal a series of *fogatges* drawn up in the second half of the fourteenth century: enumerations of hearths (*focs*) to be assessed a tax to aid in the war with Castile.[3] The most valuable of these surveys was prepared in 1365, but it shares the limitations common to all as an index to population: most crucially, it counts households rather than individuals, so that one must guess at a multiplier (4.5 or 5 is often chosen) to convert it into a census; and it excludes Jews and the clergy, who were not subject to the tax, as well as certain enfranchised Christians.[4] According to this *fogatge*, the principal towns of Catalonia in 1365 fell by size into three reasonably distinct groups: Barcelona alone at the top with 6,668 hearths; four others (Gerona, Lerida, Cervera, Tortosa) with between 1,000 and 1,600; and another nine with 400–1,000.[5]

To assess the size of these towns in the first half of the century, we would hope somehow to be able to measure the demographic impact of two intervening catastrophes, the plagues of 1361–2 and especially 1348–50. Not surprisingly, municipal records were rarely kept up during the epidemics, and lacking data from most communities we still have no good estimates of their population losses. However, the town of Vic (592 hearths, perhaps 3,500 inhabitants, in 1365) is unique in preserving records that seem to show that perhaps a sixth of its inhabitants died during 1348–50, so that we might guess that in the 1340s Vic had a population of a little over 4,000.[6] On this basis, we probably will not be too

---

[2] Dufourcq and Gautier-Dalché, *Historia*, p. 179; Hillgarth, I:29–30, with somewhat lower estimates for Valencia and Aragon; Russell, *Medieval Regions*, p. 175, with twice my estimate for Aragon; Bisson, *Medieval Crown*, p. 163, who suggests as many as 250,000 inhabitants in Aragon at this time.

[3] Pons i Guri, "Fogatjament," surveys all the known *fogatges*, dating them and establishing their interrelation. It should be used to correct Smith, "Population Records," which nevertheless still contains conclusions of interest.

[4] Iglesies Fort, "Fogaje." Iglesies Fort calls attention to a *fogatge* of 1553 that did survey the clergy and listed 74 monasteries, 6 hospitals, and the households of 4,260 priests, and infers (p. 275) that the church probably represented between 5 and 10 percent of the Catalan *focs* in the fourteenth century.

[5] Iglesies Fort, "Fogaje," pp. 317 et seq.; for a partial list, see below, table 2.5.

[6] The data are provided by Bautier, "Nouvel ensemble." I base my calculations on his report of the excess of recorded burials in the town during August 1348–December 1350 and January–

far off if we suppose Barcelona to have had 30,000 inhabitants in the 1340s, and Lerida and Tortosa, Gerona and Cervera 8,000 or so; and that the next group of nine smaller towns had populations of 2,500–6,000. In any case, for certain purposes it will be enough to keep in mind the hearth totals from the 1365 *fogatge*, for if we assume that the order of Catalan towns as ranked by number of hearths stayed roughly constant before and after the plague, that number will serve as an index to their relative importance in the first half of the century.

Still harder to judge is the size of the non-Christian populations present in the three divisions of the realm.[7] Valencia, so recently reconquered from Islam, may have been as much as two-thirds Muslim (virtually all a rural peasant class), with 5,000–10,000 (primarily urban) Jews; Aragon had a sizable Muslim element – perhaps one-third the total – and a Jewish population of less than 10,000. Only in Catalonia were Christians overwhelmingly predominant: the population there has been estimated as no more than 5 percent Jewish and 3 percent Muslim, the latter almost entirely in the lower Ebro valley. Even though these numbers are only informed guesses, they provide an approximation against which to assess the availability and distribution of medical care.

The three constituents of the Crown of Aragon were linked together through their count-king, and consequently the royal archives – still preserved in Barcelona, in the Archivo de la Corona de Aragón (ACA) – furnish information about them all. The 338 chancellery registers surviving from the reign of Jaume II (1291–1327) contain an estimated 300,000 documents;[8] the 157 from the reign of Alfons III (1327–36) an additional 120,000. The royal chancellery organized its records under a variety of headings, the most important of which are *commune* (administrative documents of all sorts, including appeals from lower courts), *gratiarum* (royal grants and privileges), *pecuniae* (commanding curial payments and recording expenses), *sigilli secreti* (documents under the secret seal), and *curiae* (the political and personal correspondence of the king). Still other volumes incorporate similar material generated by the secretaries of the

December 1362 over a normal death rate of perhaps 3 percent (here I am following the model for early modern Europe sketched out by Flinn, *European Demographic System*, ch. 2). Freedman (*Origins*, p. 162) interprets Bautier's data as yielding a higher death rate for Vic but accepts a figure of 20 percent for Catalonia as a whole. Russell, *Medieval Regions*, pp. 168–9, argues on quite different grounds that "the cities [in the Crown of Aragon] lost a sixth of their population by 1352 in the initial epidemic." Pladevall, "Disminució," argues for an enormous drop in population (by two-thirds) in the region of which Vic was the center. However, his study compares population over a much longer period (from the years before the plague to the early fifteenth century), and examines, not Vic, but the villages around it, which would have lost population not only to disease but to emigration to the urban center. Our understanding of the effects of the plague on the Spanish kingdoms remains very limited. For a recent survey, see Sobrequés Callicó, "Peste negra."

[7] On this, see Hillgarth, *Spanish Kingdoms*, I:31–2; Dufourcq and Gautier-Dalché, *Historia*, p. 179.

[8] "De Jaime II se decía en la curia romana que solo él escribía mas que todos los restantes soberanos juntos de Europa": Martínez Ferrando, *Archivo*, p. 34.

queens and of the infantes. A further forty volumes of financial accounts in the section of the Real Patrimonio record actual payments by the two kings' treasurers.[9]

This combination of private and public-administrative material mirrors the monarchs' involvement with each of the three regions constituting their realms. An exhaustive search of this documentation has generated a list of medical practitioners throughout the whole of the Crown – the series *commune* revealing those who came into contact with the royal administration for a variety of (ordinarily non-medical) reasons, the other series generally identifying those summoned by or rewarded by the monarch. In what follows, this list will be treated as amounting to a random sample of the medical practitioners in the Crown of Aragon. No doubt it is only crudely and roughly random, biased by royal priorities and problems of reportage, but its use in this way will allow us to generate and test some hypotheses about the distribution of the health occupations in the realm.

That medical practitioners can be singled out as such in the documents is owing to the common scribal practice of labeling individuals by their occupations as well as by their names. Four such labels denote occupations that could supply health care to the public, and we can summarize their activities here, though they will be examined more carefully at a later stage.

Both (1) the physician (*phisicus, fisicus*) and (2) the surgeon (*cirurgicus*) normally had no other occupation, but they routinely engaged in commercial activities on the side. Broadly speaking, the surgeon treated fractures, wounds, abscesses, skin ailments, and external complaints generally, while the physician attended to internal or systemic illness, though there was some overlap and confusion between their spheres of competence.[10]

(3) The apothecary (*apothecarius, speciarius, herbolarius*) prepared medicines for physicians but also made independent recommendations or gave drugs directly to the sick, and might normally be called to attend them day or night; it was not unusual for an apothecary to be pressed into service by municipal authorities when no *phisicus* was available.[11] But, unlike the

---

[9] The collection is described analytically by Udina Martorell, *Guia histórica*, whose terminology I follow in referring to its subdivisions. Finke, *AA*, I:xxv–clxxxx, explains in detail the character of the various classes of material available from the reign of Jaume II; see also Sevillano Colom, "Apuntes," and Conde y Delgado de Molina, "Análisis." Burns, *Society and Documentation*, is an indispensable guide to the development of the archive, though its focus is on the thirteenth century.

[10] See below, chapter 4.

[11] For examples of visits to the sick, see below, chapter 4 n. 94. For medical activity, see examples below: an apothecary of Castelló hired by the town to read urines (below, chapter 7 at n. 11); an apothecary of Nules (Valencia) permitted to treat patients in the absence of a town physician (below, n. 39). A further case is that of a Geronan apothecary who had crossed the line into medical practice while still maintaining his old trade (ADG, Sèrie G [Libri Notularum], 19/109v, 2 Aug. 1347).

physician and surgeon, the apothecary had an occupation that normally involved more than medical activity; filling prescriptions brought in only small sums, and most therefore chose to deal in many things besides drugs.[12] In Barcelona, apothecaries belonged to the confraternity of *candelers e tenders e especiayres* (chandlers and grocers and druggists) – not mutually exclusive occupations but one and the same, for apothecaries did much of their trade in the wax or candles needed for funeral ceremonies as well as more broadly in general merchandise.[13] Because their business required a certain capital, some developed into merchants on a fairly large scale, investing their own money and that of others in cargoes or tax revenues, and selling drugs wholesale throughout the region (or Crown);[14] rarely they even exchange the title *apothecarius* for that of *mercator*. But even the most prosperous apothecaries seem to have maintained a retail outlet for medicines.[15]

(4) The barber (*barberius*, *barbitonsor*) provided routine medical care of a prophylactic character; the phlebotomy that he offered kept the body healthy by removing excessive or diseased humors.[16] While in principle his activity might be subject to a physician's advice, in practice many people followed a barber's recommendation or their own judgment in having blood drawn.[17] Barbers of course also shaved and cut hair, and might pull teeth as well, as lists of their belongings show,[18] but such services were rarely if ever able to support them completely. Barbers typically supplemented their income with a wide range of

---

[12] For a survey of their activities, see Batlle i Gallart, "Apotecaris." Other aspects of the apothecaries' role are treated below, chapter 4.

[13] Consider Pere Ahinardi of Castelló d'Empúries, active 1321–36, who described himself variously as "tenderius" and "apothecarius" and dealt not only in medicinal preparations but in barley, figs, paper, rice, pepper, cheese, honey, almonds, and ginger.

[14] See below, chapter 4.

[15] A case in point is Joan de la Geltrú, nephew of a prominent Barcelonan apothecary, Pere Jutge. Joan first appears in business in the year that Pere died, 1316, associated with his uncle's son and heir, Felip Jutge. Soon Joan had launched out on his own, selling drugs and comfits to the royal court. By 1319 he had taken an assistant, a year later he was trading in naval stores, and in 1324 he was able to loan the infante Alfons 4,500 *sous* for the conquest of Sardinia. In 1325 Joan begins to be called "mercator" as well as "apothecarius"; over the next few years he had important dealings in grain and took in big sums in deposit, but he continued to supply medicines and comfits to the royal family until at least 1339, and he was still alive in 1343. (In contrast, his uncle's heir, Felip, was far less successful.)

[16] The rationale is summarized by Voigts and McVaugh, *Phlebotomy*, pp. 5–6.

[17] See the document (of 14 July 1332) cited in García Ballester and McVaugh, "Nota," p. 88.

[18] See above, chapter 1 n. 7, for a barber's possession of dental tools. A barber's equipment varied very little: typical are the contents of a shop rented by a Barcelona barber from an absent barber's wife, which included "quatuor bassinos de lautono idoneos et sufficientes ad exercendum officium supradictum et tres cuces et unum speculum de banussio et duo paria forficum et .vii. rasoria et duas cathedras de fuste et unum scannum et duas curtinas et unum calffedor de cupro et unum cogomar et tres ventoses et tria manilia ac duas peccines de borio": document of 24 March 1337, in AHPB, manual de Jaume de Comarmena, Oct. 1336–Aug. 1337, f. 70v. The *curtina*, when hung at the door, proclaimed that a barber was open for business: Bofarull y Sans, "Gremios," pp. 274, 279 (from the year 1408).

other minor dealings – mule-trading or iron-selling or cloth-dyeing[19] – and their precarious economic situation no doubt helps explain why they eventually began to offer surgical treatments for which nominally they were unqualified. They were the lowest, socio-economically speaking, of the health professions, with least to gain from the *status quo*; it was a barber who captained the Valencian mob that taunted King Pere III in the revolt of the Unió and forced him to dance before them (1348) – and who eventually suffered horribly for his insolence.[20]

In addition to these four labels, a fifth, *medicus* (Catalan, *metge*), is sometimes used. Historians are still trying to understand the changing implications of this term in the Middle Ages.[21] Some scholars have concluded that as an occupational label *medicus* means simply "physician,"[22] but in the early fourteenth-century Crown of Aragon, at least, the two terms were not synonymous, for there "medicus" can be found being used to describe either a physician or a surgeon; perhaps the best way to think of it is as equivalent to "healer" or "doctor." Sometimes it appears with a qualifier – "medicus phisice" or "medicus cirurgie" – suggesting an attempt at precision in labeling; and indeed, as the fourteenth century goes on the bare title "medicus" becomes noticeably less frequent. At the same time, the title "phisicus et cirurgicus" comes into occasional use, another indication that distinctions were coming to be insisted upon. As we shall see, attempts at enforcing occupational definition were eventually introduced (to a limited degree) in the 1330s.

One other health provider in the Crown of Aragon needs to be acknowledged: the *infirmarius*, who was normally to be found in every monastery or cathedral chapter. A particularly full account of his responsibilities as already defined in the mid-thirteenth century is set out in the cartulary of Zaragoza cathedral: his duties were by no means merely custodial, but actively interventionist. He was charged with the regular bleeding and purging of his fellows in health, and the provision to them of diet and medicines when ill, though under medical supervision. He was to make up a syrup (*exarop*) for any sick canon "following the advice of a physician [*medicus*], based on violets or roses or vinegar, as the physician may think best," and must likewise follow a physician's advice in

---

[19] For example, Berenguer de Santa Cruce, *barbitonsor* of Igualada, who contracted to dye cloth for Manresan manufacturers in his *tintoreria* in the former town (AHCM 105, 4 id. Oct. 1326); or Monachus Petri, barber of Daroca, who as a "mercator publicus" is found selling iron in 1347 (C 650/97).

[20] In his *Crònica*, IV.42 (in Soldevila, *Cròniques*, pp. 59–60), King Pere speaks only of "un barber apellat Gonçalva," but this man can now be probably identified as Gonçalvo de Roda, active in Valencia since at least 1326 (ARV, Just. Val. 19/64v), and elected to represent the barbers on the municipal *consell* in 1329 and several times thereafter (AMV, Manuals de Consells, A-3).

[21] See Bylebyl, "Medical Meaning," for the earlier emergence of *physica* from *medicina*, and their relationship.

[22] This is the approach of Jacquart, *Milieu médical*, pp. 31–4. See also her discussion of the perplexing French term, *mire*, which presents some parallels to *medicus/metge* in the Crown of Aragon.

giving food and drink to the patient.[23] Secular practitioners were already being contracted to give continuing as well as occasional medical assistance to cathedral chapters before 1300 – in 1289 the Zaragoza chapter decided that "the best *barbitonsor* in the city" should be hired to take over the task of prophylactic bleeding[24] – but this still left *infirmarii* with considerable responsibility, and many took that responsibility seriously: the infirmarian at Poblet had a pharmaceutical dispensary and library, which he did his best to keep off-limits to the king's retinue on royal visits to the monastery.[25] Hence someone like Arnaldo de Zaidín, who was *infirmarius* at Zaragoza for over fifty years (1258–1314), was bound to acquire some medical expertise in the course of time – and perhaps, as well, a certain reputation in the outside world, judging from Jaume's appeal to Arnaldo's successor, Geraldo de Sapiach. But ordinarily the *infirmarius* tended to the not-inconsiderable fraction of society that lived in the cloister; lay practitioners treated the secular world.[26]

Drawing up a census of medical practitioners from materials of this kind means, of course, that we are liable to overlook anyone who provided some sort of health care without claiming an occupational label. To be sure, such people do occasionally surface in the archives – like Gueraula de Codines of Subirats, who diagnosed her neighbors' complaints by reading their urines, or Pere Nicolau of Lerida, who made up medicines for his sick friends – but it is impossible to know how widespread such domestic healing was.[27] Whatever its frequency, however, it was a healing socially distinct from what self-proclaimed *medici* promised; the generally anonymous, unlabeled healers were always at the professional margin and were ordinarily not treated as economic or occupational competition by *phisici* and *cirurgici*. Gueraula de Codines, for example, swore always to send her clients to "real physicians" (*medicos maiores*) for treatment, and a leading Barcelonan *phisicus* agreed that in that case she might be allowed to continue counseling her neighbors, as long as she didn't prescribe for them.[28] In effect, a distinction was tacitly recognized between domestic healing and the practice of *medici*; those who presumed to call themselves "medicus," who

---

23 "Secundum consilium medici, sive violatum vel rosatum vel acetosum, prout medico videbitur quod expediat infirmo": ASZ, Cartulario mayor, fol. 236r (2 id. June era 1268 = 1230). See Requejo Díaz Espada, "Vida conventual."

24 ASZ, Cartulario mayor, f. 236v.

25 Letter of 1 Aug. 1346 (C 887/36v).

26 For more on clerical involvement in secular medical practice, see below, chapter 3.

27 For Gueraula, see further below, chapter 5. Pere was accused in 1344 of "having given medicines to people who didn't know how to use them," perhaps including abortifacients, and was convicted and banished despite testimony that some of his cures had worked (AML 774/15–20).

28 On this physician, Bernat ça Llimona (active 1294–1316), see Perarnau, L' "Alia informatio," pp. 118–19; and McVaugh, "Royal Surgeons," n. 8. Further documentation of his medical activities and his association with other practitioners can be found in C 254/194v; ACB, manual de Bernat de Vilarrúbia, April–Sept. 1295, f. 64, and Aug.–Nov. 1315, ff. 116v–117v; and Rius Serra, *San Raimundo de Penyafort*, pp. 224–5, 242–6.

Table 2.1.* *Practitioners identified in Barcelona, 1300–40*

	Phys.	Surg.	Apoth.	Barb.	Total
From ACA	21	17	32	13	83
Added from other sources	14	16	54	34	118
Total	35	33	86	47	201

*Here and in subsequent tables people labeled as "medicus" are included with physicians, those as "phisicus et cirurgicus" with surgeons.

adopted the occupational label, were making certain claims for their knowledge or skill that justified their demand for a fee.[29] In the main, these are the practitioners revealed by our census, and they embody what their own society was coming to recognize as the best care available; at the same time, we must acknowledge that there was always another level of care available, though one of unmeasurable extent.

Counting medical practitioners

If we carry our search for secular practitioners from the archives of the Crown to those of the largest cities of the kingdom, we can get a particularly good reading of the availability of medical care, for two of these cities preserve early fourteenth-century materials that furnish an important supplement to the documentation of the ACA. Barcelona possesses not only scattered municipal and ecclesiastical records from this period, but also a remarkable series of notarial manuals that furnish information about the lives of many more citizens than ever came to the attention of the royal bureaucracy.[30] All told, these materials more than double the number of Barcelonan health practitioners known from the royal archives alone (see table 2.1). They are particularly useful in expanding our acquaintance with the minor health occupations, with apothecaries and barbers. The availability of judicial and municipal records from this same period in Valencia has the same effect for that city (see table 2.2). Apparently the ACA records by themselves would lead us to underestimate the number of physicians practicing in the cities by at least one-third, of the surgeons by one-half, and of the apothecaries and barbers by two-thirds or more.

Combining these sources of information makes it possible for us to follow careers over an extended time, and to obtain a minimum figure for the number of health providers in individual cities on a year-by-year basis. The results (given in table 2.3 for Barcelona and Valencia as well as for Zaragoza, the third capital

[29] For an instance when this tacit distinction was made explicit, see below, chapter 3 n. 130.
[30] The papers in Brezzi and Lee, *Sources*, suggest something of the rewards and problems inherent in such materials.

Table 2.2. *Practitioners identified in Valencia, 1300–40*

	Phys.	Surg.	Apoth.	Barb.	Total
From ACA	22	12	21	13	68
Added from other sources	10	22	35	62	129
Total	32	34	56	75	197

of the realm, though the Zaragozan material is much less comprehensive) have a number of curious features. Barbers, for example, seem to have been far more common in Valencia than in Barcelona, while to a lesser extent the reverse was true for apothecaries. In the quarter-century after 1310, the number of practitioners in each city grew by 50 percent, a growth due almost entirely to an increase in the number of apothecaries and surgeons. The swelling number of apothecaries is probably to be explained by the expansion of Catalan trade in the first part of the century, since they were so deeply engaged in commercial activities; why surgery should suddenly have prospered so, however, is not yet clear. If we assume that both Barcelona and Valencia had populations of 30,000 in 1330, they each had about seven major health providers (physicians and surgeons) and twenty practitioners of all sorts per 10,000 inhabitants.

The most obvious feature of table 2.3 is the contraction of the practitioner population in the capitals that begins gradually in the early 1330s and then continues more sharply in the 1340s. The latter collapse is perhaps only apparent, an artifact of data collection,[31] but the earlier decline and general downward trend may be real. The year 1333 was the Valencian *mal any primer* that began the economic decline of the Crown of Aragon, and service occupations like medicine would have become less profitable in the later 1330s and 1340s; the fields that shrank most were barbering, the most marginal of the health occupations, and surgery, which had to retrench after its burst of growth in the 1320s. Furthermore, the mid-1330s were also the moment when licensing requirements were first introduced, and this too could have helped to restrict medical practice in the biggest cities, where competition had earlier caused complaints about the proliferation of physicians and had made self-interest most intense.[32] It seems not unreasonable to imagine that the practitioner levels I have computed for the late 1330s represent the actual conditions in Barcelona and Valencia during the decade immediately before the arrival of plague.

Significantly, no such shrinkage is to be seen in the smaller cities and towns

---

[31] See remarks in the appendix.

[32] I might add that at the very moment when my computed number of Barcelona surgeons begins to decline, in 1334, the city was actually complaining of a lack of surgeons ("cirurgicorum inopiam"); the occasion was the request that an ex-slave be allowed to stay in the city after the death of his surgeon master (C 571/69r–v).

Table 2.3.* *Urban practitioners identified, 1310–45, in Barcelona, Valencia, and Zaragoza (all sources)*

	Barcelona					Valencia					Zaragoza				
Date	P	S	A	B	Total	P	S	A	B	Total	P	S	A	B	Total
1310	10	2	12	9	33	10	3	4	19	36	4		1		5
1311	9	2	12	9	32	9	4	3	21	37	4	1	1		6
1312	10	2	12	8	32	10	4	6	15	35	4	2	1		7
1313	10	3	11	10	34	9	5	5	15	34	3	2	1		6
1314	9	4	14	12	39	9	5	6	19	39	3	3	2		8
1315	8	3	16	8	35	10	6	5	23	44	4	3	2		9
1316	9	3	18	8	38	8	8	6	22	44	3	3	2		8
1317	8	5	17	8	38	8	7	8	19	42	4	3	2		9
1318	8	5	20	9	42	10	7	13	24	54	4	3	2	2	11
1319	6	6	23	8	43	10	8	13	24	55	5	4	2		11
1320	6	6	22	8	42	9	10	17	27	63	5	4	2		11
1321	6	8	23	8	45	11	13	17	26	67	4	4	2		10
1322	6	8	24	9	47	13	14	16	23	66	6	4	2		12
1323	6	7	28	8	49	13	13	16	18	60	6	4	2		12
1324	6	10	30	9	55	13	12	16	17	58	7	4	2		13
1325	5	14	30	7	56	13	12	16	20	61	8	6	2	5	21
1326	8	11	29	7	55	12	13	17	19	61	11	6	2	4	23
1327	6	12	27	10	55	12	12	17	19	60	10	6	2	4	22
1328	8	12	26	9	55	11	11	18	21	61	10	5	2	4	21
1329	7	11	25	10	53	11	11	21	20	63	10	5	2	4	21
1330	8	12	26	11	57	11	9	17	17	54	15	5	5	6	31
1331	8	11	24	11	54	11	10	18	18	57	11	6	5	8	30
1332	7	10	24	11	52	11	12	18	20	61	8	6	7	6	27
1333	10	11	25	12	58	10	12	24	20	66	8	6	7	6	27
1334	10	8	25	12	55	10	9	20	18	57	6	6	5	6	23
1335	7	6	23	13	49	11	10	18	18	57	5	5	6	7	23
1336	8	4	23	11	46	10	9	16	16	51	3	4	5	6	18
1337	7	3	26	12	48	10	10	14	13	47	3	4	6	9	22
1338	8	4	26	9	47	10	10	14	10	44	2	3	5	5	15
1339	7	3	26	9	45	9	10	17	10	46	1	4	4	3	12
1340	6	4	27	8	45	9	9	13	7	38	1	3	5	4	13
1341	6	4	27	8	45	9	9	14	6	38		3	2		5
1342	10	3	26	10	49	11	8	13	6	38		3	2		5
1343	7	4	21	8	40	10	7	11	6	34	1	3	2		6
1344	6	5	21	9	41	8	7	9	6	30		3	1		4
1345	7	5	15	5	32	8	7	7	6	28		2	1		3

*The figures given here and below supersede those already presented in García Ballester and McVaugh, "Nota," and in García-Ballester, McVaugh, and Rubio-Vela, *Medical Licensing*.

of the kingdom, where there appears to have been a slow increase in the (much smaller) number of practitioners until a stabilization, rather than a decline, in the early 1330s (see table 2.4). Particularly full series of notarial manuals survive from three Catalan towns of quite different size: Gerona (1,590 hearths in 1365), Manresa (691 hearths), and Santa Coloma de Queralt (188 hearths). In each case the supply of practitioners grew steadily until 1335 or so, and then remained

Table 2.4. *Practitioners identified in selected Catalan communities, 1310–45 (all sources)*

	Gerona					Manresa					Sta. Coloma de Queralt				
Date	P	S	A	B	Total	P	S	A	B	Total	P	S	A	B	Total
1310		3	4		7	1	1		5	7	1			1	2
1311		1	4		5	1	1		4	6	1			1	2
1312		1	4		5	1	1	1	4	7	1			1	2
1313		1	4		5	1	1	1	4	7	1			1	2
1314			4		4	1	1	1	5	8	1			1	2
1315			4		4	1	1	2	5	9	1			1	2
1316			5		5	2	1	2	5	10	1			1	2
1317			5		5	1	1	2	5	9	2			1	3
1318	1		5		6	1	1	2	5	9	2			1	3
1319	1		5		6	1	1	2	5	9	2			1	3
1320	1		5	1	7	1	2	2	5	10	3			1	4
1321	1	4	9	1	15	1	2	2	5	10	2			1	3
1322	1	4	7	1	13	2	2	2	6	12	2			1	3
1323	1	5	6	1	13	1	2	2	5	10	3			1	4
1324	1	4	9	1	15	1	3	2	5	11	3				3
1325	1	4	8	2	15	1	3	2	5	11	3			1	4
1326	1	5	10	1	17	1	3	2	5	11	2			1	3
1327	2	4	10	3	19	1	2	2	5	10	2			1	3
1328	2	4	10	3	19	1	2	2	5	10	2			1	3
1329	3	5	12	4	24	2	2	2	7	13	2	2		1	5
1330	3	8	12	7	30	1	4	2	5	12	2	2		1	5
1331	4	6	10	8	28	1	5	2	4	12	2	2		1	5
1332	5	4	10	6	25	2	4	2	5	13	2	2	1	1	6
1333	4	4	11	6	25	2	5	2	5	14	2	2	2	1	7
1334	4	4	15	7	30	2	5	2	4	13	2	2	1	1	6
1335	3	5	16	6	30	2	5	2	4	13	2	2	3	1	8
1336	3	5	13	8	29	2	5	2	4	13	2	2	3	1	8
1337	3	6	14	8	31	2	5	2	5	14	2	2	3	1	8
1338	3	5	16	9	33	2	5	2	4	13	2	2	4	1	9
1339	4	5	13	8	30	2	4	2	4	12	2	2	4	1	9
1340	4	4	14	8	30	2	4	3	4	13	1	2	4	1	8
1341	4	4	14	8	30	3	4	4	4	15	1	2	4	1	8
1342	3	3	15	7	28	4	4	4	4	16	1	2	4	1	8
1343	3	3	13	6	25	3	5	3	4	15	1	2	5	1	9
1344	3	3	13	6	25	3	4	4	7	18	1	2	5	1	9
1345	3	4	12	6	25	3	2	3	2	10	1	2	5	1	9

at that level for another decade. In 1335 Gerona had perhaps nine major practitioners and thirty-five of all types per 10,000 inhabitants, and was thus slightly better off, proportionally, than Barcelona had been five years before.

At first glance the figures for small towns like Manresa and Santa Coloma de Queralt seem even more favorable – twenty and forty major practitioners per 10,000 inhabitants, respectively, and twice those ratios for practitioners of all kinds. But these figures are deceptive. If we look closely at the ACA sample of practitioners in Catalonia, 1300–40 (table 2.5), it suggests not only that, as one would expect, practitioners generally were rarer in the smaller communities, but also that people calling themselves "physicians" were virtually non-existent in towns of fewer than a hundred or so families; on the other hand, the middle-sized towns show a tendency to attract surgeons and especially physicians disproportionately, who would use their town as a base from which they would serve the area for twenty or twenty-five kilometers around. Investigations in municipal archives confirm this tendency. Pere de Fontanet, for example, a surgeon active in Manresa 1325–45, can be found treating patients from nearly a dozen villages as much as thirty kilometers distant from his nominal place of practice.[33] Joan de Rivis, serving the town of Vic in 1319, must have had just as dispersed a practice, for he had to ask the town fathers for fifteen days' grace to get back to town from his treatment of patients in the district (Osona) of which Vic is still the center.[34]

In contrast, outlying villages could usually support no more than a resident barber, and even here they were often dependent on a nearby town to supply or train their personnel. In 1308 a resident of Fortià – a hamlet two kilometers south of Castelló d'Empúries, the latter a town of several hundred hearths northeast of Gerona – apprenticed his son Bernat Leto to a barber of Castelló to learn the craft during a two-year period. The contract provided that every Friday young Bernat could go back to his village to cut hair, though he was required to give his master all his profits. By 1319 Bernat had returned to Fortià and was in business for himself as a barber.[35] The Castelló archives record the activity of barbers not just from Fortià but from several other small villages within a radius of ten kilometers (Sant Pere Pescador, Palau-saverdera, and Torroella de Fluvià), and of one surgeon from a similar community (Garrigas), but not of village physicians or apothecaries. If a villager wanted specifically medical care, therefore, he had to look to the nearest town, and this means that the high practitioner:patient ratios for middle-sized communities like Manresa conceal the extent to which the countryside too was served by the town physician (see below, chapter 6). Santa Coloma's physicians presumably cared for the whole of the mountainous region – a triangle formed by Tàrrega/Cervera, Montblanc/Valls, and Igualada, forty kilometers on a side – of which this small town was the hub.

How then might one assess the level of health-care availability *outside* the cities and larger towns? It is possible to make a rough approximation by

---

[33] They came from Santpedor and Pont de Cabrianes, both within ten kilometers of Manresa; Castellfollit del Boix, Rajadell, Sant Pere Sallavinera, and Castellar, all within twenty; Igualada and Calaf, twenty-five kilometers distant; and Gavadons, thirty kilometers away – and much closer to Vic than to Manresa. See below, chapter 6.

[34] ACFV 72, document of 8 id. Feb. 1319.

[35] AHPG/CE 2035 bis/50v (21 Aug. 1308); APHG/CE 98/67 (18 Dec. 1319).

Table 2.5. *Practitioners identified (by town) from ACA, 1300–40 (number of hearths in 1365/1378 in parentheses)*†

	P	S	A	B	Total
Barcelona (6,668)	21	17	32	13	83
Gerona (1,590)	2	8	5	1	16
Lerida (1,213)**	10	4	6	6	26
Cervera (1,057)	3	2	4	1	10
Tortosa (991)**	1		2	2	5
Tarragona (860)**	1	1			2
Puigcerdà (833)		3			3
Vilafranca del Penedès (820)	2		1		3
Manresa (691)	1	2		2	5
Vic (592)	1	2			3
Valls (569)					
Berga (556)	1	1			2
Montblanc (457)**	2	1	1		4
Tàrrega (426)	2	2		1	5
Balaguer (344)*	1				1
Besalú (238)	1	2			3
Solsona (212)*			1		1
Sant Cugat del Valles (207)	1				1
Sanahuia (200)		1			1
sa Reial (194)*	1				1
Santa Coloma de Queralt (188)		2			2
Sant Celoni (177)		1			1
la Geltrú (135)			1		1
Tamarit (80)		1			1
Agramunt (67)*				1	1
Copons (57)	1				1
Ullà (43)*		1			1
Martorell (26)			1		1
Pallerols (25)					1
Socarrats (9)		1			1

† Values marked with either one or two asterisks (see Appendix) are from the *fogatge* of 1378, while the remainder come from that of 1365. I do not include the towns of Roussillon in this list – the most important being Perpignan, credited with 2,675 hearths in 1365 and 1,640 in 1378 – because this territory did not make up a part of the Crown of Aragon until its conquest from the king of Mallorca in the 1340s, though I do include Puigcerdà in Mallorcan Cerdanya.

searching the random collection provided by the ACA and comparing the level of city practitioners identified there with the level in the rest of the kingdom. In Catalonia, for example, we find roughly the same number of physicians and surgeons in its five largest cities combined as in the rest of the country, three times as many apothecaries, and six times as many barbers; and they are serving a population one-seventh the size (table 2.6). The comparable figures for Valencia, where the city made up perhaps one-sixth of the population of the kingdom as a whole, are even more striking, for they suggest that the density of medical care in the countryside was only one-twentieth that in the capital (table 2.7). On the other hand, in Aragon, where the largest city (Zaragoza) probably had a population of no more than 15,000 in the mid-fourteenth century,[36] the difference, though still significant, is less impressive: Zaragoza and Huesca seem to have enjoyed perhaps three times the physician density of rural Aragon, but no more than that, and the higher density of practitioners in Aragon outside the cities than in rural sections of Valencia and Catalonia suggests that the Aragonese population was less widely diffused than in the other two realms – not improbably, given a landscape that was almost all either mountainous or terribly arid.

To find medical practitioners thus concentrated in the cities, especially the larger cities, is not particularly surprising. In pre-modern as in modern times, once the effectiveness of medical expertise has been admitted, urban wealth and population density create a market for health care that in prosperous times draws practitioners to the city – and, more generally, encourages the ambitious to turn to medicine as a career. The European "urban revolution" that began in the twelfth century had shaped "a new social environment" in which medical occupations could flourish after they had proven themselves; but with unhappy consequences for the countryside.[37] In the early fourteenth century, while Barcelona and Valencia were enjoying high levels of medical care, a variety of documents reveal the need of one small town after another for medical help, throughout the Aragonese Crown. In 1324 Jaume II allowed Bernat de Ulmis to practice surgery in Besalú (Catalonia: 238 hearths in 1365) at the request of the town fathers, who reported that otherwise there would be no surgeon in town.[38] Eight years later Jaume's son Alfons III permitted an apothecary of Borriana (Valencia) to practice medicine in nearby Nules, "where there is no physician or surgeon and it would be . . . tiresome, a danger and a burden . . . to have to go to the city of Valencia [forty kilometers down the coast] . . . for advice and assistance."[39] But there are reasons why some rural areas were probably more poorly served than others, and in particular why the Valencian countryside appears to have had the lowest level of practitioners. To understand these reasons, we must begin by examining the role of the two religious and cultural minorities in shaping the health-care system of the Christian Crown of Aragon.

---

[36] This is an inference from the hearth figures for the later part of the century given by Ledesma Rubio and Falcón Pérez, *Zaragoza*, pp. 121–2. My estimate of the population of Huesca as 7,000–8,000 is based on Utrilla Utrilla, "Monedaje."

[37] Park, "Medicine and Society," p. 75; and, for a case study of urban attractiveness to the late-medieval physician, see Park, *Doctors*, pp. 142–50.

[38] "Cum nos intellexerimus pro parte procuratorum seu sindicorum dicte ville quod in villa Bisuldini non est cirurgicus aliquis": letter of 7 Feb. 1324 (C 181/162).

[39] "Ubi non est aliquis phisicus sive cirurgicus et sit . . . tediosum periculum et onus . . . recurrere ad civitatem Valencie . . . pro consilio et remedio": García-Ballester, McVaugh, and Rubio-Vela, *Medical Licensing*, pp. 19–20.

Table 2.6. *Catalan practitioners identified in ACA, 1300–40*

	P	S	A	B	Pop.	PS/10K	All/10K
In five largest towns combined	37	31	49	23	70,000	9.7	20
Elsewhere	29	31	16	4	480,000	1.3	1.7

Table 2.7. *Valencian practitioners identified in ACA, 1300–40*

	P	S	A	B	Pop.	PS/10K	All/10K
In Valencia city	22	12	21	13	30,000	11.3	22.7
Elsewhere	3	7	0	7	170,000	0.6	1

Table 2.8. *Aragonese practitioners identified in ACA, 1300–40*

	P	S	A	B	Pop.	PS/10K	All/10K
In Zaragoza	14	5	6	4	15,000	12.7	19.3
In Huesca	9	3	5	4	8,000	15	26.3
Elsewhere	25	18	7	8	80,000	5.4	7.3

Muslim practitioners

At the beginning of the fourteenth century, Islamic medical thought was greatly admired in the Crown of Aragon – by the king himself, among others.[40] The value that Jaume placed on Avicenna's *Canon* has already been noted (above, p. 10) and illustrates his interest in having the best of Islamic medicine readily accessible in his kingdom; so does his support of medical translations from the Arabic. In November 1313, for example, he commanded his treasurer to pay 1,000 *sous* to Jahuda Bonsenyor for translating into Catalan "a certain book of medicine called 'halçahahuy'" – if, as has been suggested, the word is a transliteration of the *nisbah of* Abū 'l-Qāsim al-Zahrāwī, known to the west as Abulcasis, it may refer to his great medical encyclopedia, *al-Taṣrīf*.[41] What portion Jahuda was expected to translate for the king we cannot tell; Antoni

---

[40] Much of what follows is based on McVaugh, "Islamic Medicine."

[41] RL, II:22, doc. 29. Jahuda Bonsenyor, son of Astruch, had been responsible since 1294 for preparing all Arabic-language documents and contracts drawn up in Barcelona; he was also a physician (*metge*), and a friend of the king's own physician, Joan Amell. On his career, see Cardoner Planas, "Nuevos datos." Only a few sections of the *Taṣrīf* had been translated in Jaume's day, even into Latin: the surgery by Gerard of Cremona in the twelfth century, the pharmacology by Simon of Genoa and Abraham Judeus (as the *Liber servitoris*) at the very end of the thirteenth.

Cardoner has proposed that he translated only a small part of the text, perhaps the section dealing with bloodletting, but the considerable sum with which the translator was to be rewarded – twice as much as the entire *Canon* might have sold for – suggests that he may have translated a larger portion of the work.[42]

The physician whom King Jaume most esteemed, Arnau de Vilanova, was himself a notable Arabist. His earliest appearance in the historical record is in Barcelona, in 1282, as the translator of Ḥunain ibn Isḥaq's Arabic version of Galen's short work *On tremor*; Arnau's translation is in general a faithful and quite competent one.[43] Two other translations from Arabic to Latin can also be securely attributed to Arnau: a translation of Abu 'l-Ṣalt's *Kitāb al-adwiya al mufrada* and another of Avicenna's *Kitāb al-adwiya al-qalbīya* (under the title *De viribus cordis*) – the Avicenna, like the Galen, prepared in Barcelona.[44] When Arnau died in 1311, the inventory of his belongings included works by Arabic-language authors in Latin translation as well as eight codices written in Arabic script – one of them a work on anatomy, with figures, another a *Synonima*, perhaps the work of Yūḥannā ibn Sarafyūn.[45]

Arnau was not unique in Jaume's realms as a translator of Arabic medicine for a Latin-reading audience: Armengaud Blaise – Arnau's nephew, and also (as we have seen) for a time a royal physician – was responsible for translating Avicenna's *Cantica* with Averroes' commentary in 1284. A generation or so later, Berenguer Eymerich of Valencia prepared a Latin version of the dietary sections of al-Zahrāwī's *Taṣrīf*.[46] Nor was Arnau unique as an educated

---

[42] Jahuda's translation seems not to have survived. Another example of Jaume's support for such translations is his agreement in 1295 to pay 2 *sous* per day to Benvenist Abenvenist, a Zaragoza Jew, to translate from Arabic to the vernacular "varis llibres de medicina . . . molt necessaris" (Rubió y Lluch, "Notes," p. 395); fifteen years later the king further rewarded this translator, by which time Benvenist had moved to Vilafranca del Penedès (4 Feb. 1310; C 351/135r–v). Cardoner i Planas, *Història*, pp. 38–41, discusses translations made in this period from Latin and Arabic into Catalan. On the monetary value of the *Canon*, see below, chapter 3, nn. 93–4.

[43] The translation has been edited (with an introduction) in Galen, *De rigore*.

[44] Paniagua, "Traducciones." Arnau's translation of *De viribus cordis* is being edited by Kristin Peterson for *AVOMO*.

[45] Chabás, "Inventario," esp. nos. 48, 65, 76, 93, 115, 150, 173, 183; Carreras Artau, "Llibreria," pp. 68–9. The identification of the *Synonima* with the work of ibn Sarafyūn is suggested by García Ballester, *Historia social*, p. 18.

[46] The copy of this work in MS Vienna, Nationalbibliothek 5434, explains (f. 283) that it was "translata de arabico in vulgare cathalanarum et a vulgari in latinum a Berengario Eymerici de Valencia ad instanciam magistri Bernardi de Gordonio." Eymerich was evidently a medical student at Montpellier (where Bernard Gordon is known to have taught as late as 1308; Demaitre, *Bernard de Gordon*, p. 31). He was practicing in Valencia from at least 1318 (ARV, Just. Val. 24/437) until 1356, and was selected five times between 1337 and 1353 as a municipal examiner of physicians and surgeons. See García-Ballester, McVaugh, and Rubio-Vela, *Medical Licensing*, pp. 56–7; and García Ballester, *Historia social*, p. 25 n. 31. Wickersheimer, *Dictionnaire*, [I] p. 69, records the same translation in MS Torino H.IV.29, which however does not make mention of Bernard's role; here Wickersheimer mistakenly identifies Berenguer Eymerich with Berenguer de Thumba (also ça Coma or de Cumbis), a Catalan physician active 1334–48 (on whom see below, chapter 7).

Christian physician able to read such works in their original language: when master Joan, physician of Barcelona, died in 1302, his estate included "decem libros Sarracenicos de fisica," which his executors then turned over to another physician, Matheu de Suria.[47] We may conclude that in the early fourteenth century the value of Islamic medicine was widely acknowledged by Christian physicians in the Crown of Aragon, and by knowledgeable patients (like the king) as well.[48]

This high estimation placed by Latin physicians upon Islamic medical thought, combined with the long history of Islamic civilization in the Iberian peninsula, might lead us to expect to find a number of learned Muslim physicians active in the Aragonese kingdom, celebrated for their knowledge and rewarded for their skill. Yet, surprisingly, only about 1 percent (twelve) of the more than one thousand medical practitioners identifiable in the kingdom from the ACA records for the years 1300–40 are Muslims – a much lower percentage than that of Muslims in the population as a whole – and they are far from being a distinguished group. Six of the twelve were barbers, with only a limited medical role and no sign of special skills; one was an empiric; and the remaining five were surgeons, none of whom seems to have had a significant practice.

Indeed, the kings themselves, eager though they were to attract the best of medical care, were unable to locate trustworthy and capable Muslim physicians. There is no record that Jaume II was ever treated by a Muslim, though he regularly consulted learned Jewish practitioners. His son Alfons III drew no distinction between Jewish and Christian physicians, either – his most trusted physician was a Jew, Alazar Avinardut – yet he only once consulted a Muslim practitioner, a female surgeon who treated him during one episode of illness in 1332/3 and never returned. That this lone practitioner was a woman again suggests that learned Islamic medicine (far more likely to be embodied in men) was hard to find.[49]

Because there is so little evidence of the presence of Islamic practitioners in the Crown of Aragon, there is understandably little concrete that can be said about the nature of their practice. In only a few cases do we find any evidence of

---

[47] ACB, manual de Bernat de Vilarrúbia, April–July 1302, f. 110r–v. Matheu de Suria is known in practice as late as 1319 (ACB, manual de Bernat de Vilarrúbia 1319–33, f. 34v).

[48] On the spread of learned Arabic medical literature in Latin translation, see further below, chapter 3.

[49] In December 1332 Alfons made a grant to "Olmocat Sarracenam domesticam nostram in presenti infirmitate nostra ex officio suo cirurgie . . . pro labore in infirmitate ipsa" (C 500/146); in February 1333 there is reference to "Cahat Sarracena Valencie cirurgica nostra" (C 486/12), who is surely the same person; I have altered the opinion expressed in McVaugh, "Islamic Medicine," p. 18. On 12 June 1346 (C 881/11v–12) the children of "Macahat Sarracenam quondam in arte medicine expertam" were granted an extension to them of the enfranchisement given their mother by Alfons III for her care of him.

the sort of medical care offered by a Muslim in the kingdom. In December 1311 the king commanded that an investigation be launched against Ali de Lucera, a "Saracen" of Daroca in Aragon, on the grounds that

> when the late Menga Menguez of Daroca was suffering with pains in the head, you promised to cure her of this illness so that you could extort money from the said Menga and her son Bartolome; and that acting diabolically you made the said Menga wear talismans [*caractes*] and did other wicked things, because of which she is said to have died.[50]

The king had pursued the investigation in order to keep his subjects free from diabolic beliefs, not to punish medical malpractice, and he agreed in April 1313 that Ali (who had hastily left Daroca when the investigation began) would not be harassed further by the charge.[51] Nevertheless, the royal reprieve is implicitly critical of Ali for treating illness with talismans or seals, and it might be noted that this quasi-magical remedy is far removed from the wholly materialistic intervention recommended for headache by Islamic medical authorities like Rhazes or Avicenna; the latter, for example, variously prescribes ointments and embrocations, remedies to be taken internally, and bleeding from veins in the head as treatments for headache.[52]

Here let us turn back to reflect again on the level of health manpower revealed in the Crown of Aragon (table 2.9). One would expect Christians to be subjects of the surviving documentation more often than Jews or Muslims, but the enormous predominance of Jews over Muslims is less easy to explain as due to a bias of the sources. It is particularly curious that in Aragon, where Jews may have been outnumbered three to one by Muslims, we find ten times as many Jewish as Muslim practitioners; and that in Valencia, where the Muslims were perhaps ten times as numerous as Jews, there are a few more Jewish

---

[50] "Promisisti eidem quod tu eam curares de infirmitate predicta, et . . . tu operando eciam diabolica opera faciebas portare dicte Mengue caractes et alia opera maligna qua de causa mortua fuisse dicebatur." I interpret the word "caractes" as cognate with Catalan "caracter" and referring to graven symbols which, as the text shows, were to be worn ("portare") by Maria; hence, I suggest, "talismans" or "seals." Evans, *Magical Jewels*, p. 109, makes clear this meaning of "caracter." The full text is printed by Perarnau i Espelt, "Activitats," p. 54 n. 26, who does not comment on "caractes."

[51] An inquiry was commanded 2 Dec. 1311 (C 239/181v); by 20 Dec. Ali had left Daroca, though the inquiry was not yet concluded (C 240/124); and on 7 April 1313 Ali was given a quittance, since nothing had been proven (C 210/34v).

[52] Avicenna, *Liber canonis*, III.1.2; ff. 173–80. It may be, however, that some learned Islamic physicians would have taken a less restrictive approach to the treatment of headache. Dols, *Black Death*, pp. 121–42, shows how widely talismans, symbols, and incantations were used in Islam to ward off or to treat the plague, though he seems also to suggest that in this case magical practices were to some extent accepted even by a learned tradition in response to the unprecedented character of the epidemic. It should also be acknowledged that for some Jewish and Christian physicians (including Arnau de Vilanova) the use of seals and talismans was thought to be of medicinal value, though this was a matter of some controversy in the fourteenth century; see below, chapter 5, pp. 162–4.

Table 2.9. *Practitioners identified in the Crown of Aragon, 1300–40*
(male:female; all sources)

	Christian	Jewish	Muslim	Total
Catalonia	684:4	54	0	738:4
Aragon	85:1	53	5	143:1
Valencia	222:1	9	5:2	236:3
Total	991:6	116	10:2	

practitioners recorded than Muslims.[53] We must conclude, I think, that there were disproportionately few Muslim physicians at work in the Crown of Aragon, and that those who could be found lacked the familiarity with their medical heritage that their Jewish and even Christian counterparts possessed – it was a Barcelona Jew, after all, to whom King Jaume had had to turn for a translation of the work of al-Zahrāwī.

On the face of it, the intellectual poverty of the Islamic practitioners in the Crown of Aragon is cause for surprise, but we can understand the reason for it if we consider the career of one learned Muslim surgeon who chose not to live in King Jaume's lands: Muḥammad al-Shafra. Al-Shafra's birthplace was Crevillent, a Muslim enclave surrounded by Christian Spain – Valencia to the north and Murcia to the south – which maintained an independent existence until 1318. Born about 1280, al-Shafra studied surgery, not with a Muslim master, but with a Christian, a certain master Bernat;[54] he criticized the Muslim surgery of his day as being the province of mere empirics. At about the time that Crevillent was absorbed into the Valencia of Jaume II, in 1318, al-Shafra moved south to the Muslim kingdom of Granada; later he shifted to Algeciras, and when it too was reconquered by Christians, in 1344, he moved across the straits of Gibraltar to Fez. In his repeated moves from Christian territory he was doing what most other members of the learned professions in Islamic Spain seem to have done: so long as there were Muslim lands with wealthy patrons to the south, it was more to a Muslim physician's advantage to sell his services there.[55]

---

[53] The "escassedat de metges sarraïns" and the much more extensive practice of medicine by Jews was recognized impressionistically long ago by Rubió i Lluch, "Cultura catalana," pp. 238, 239.

[54] García Ballester, *Historia social*, pp. 21–2 n. 22, suggests that this master may have been the Montpellier physician Bernard Gordon; however, that Bernard is not known to have practiced outside southern France. Of the Valencian physicians I have so far identified as active in the appropriate time period, the most likely possibility is Bernat Frayre or de la Grassa (active at least 1321–33). On the other hand, it would seem more probable that al-Shafra learned his art from a surgeon than from a physician: in that case, his master might have been Bernat Borraç or Bernat de Molla, both practicing surgery in Valencia by at least 1321. I have found no trace of a Valencian surgeon named Bernat at an earlier date.

[55] Renaud, "Chirurgien musulman"; Franco Sánchez and Cabello García, *Muḥammad aš-Šafra*; Burns, "Spanish Islam," p. 102.

This emigration of the learned is more an indication of the wider opportunities open to them in an Islamic society than it is of the repressiveness of Christian rule. It seems clear that, at least in the longer-established territories (Aragon and Catalonia), Muslims were not particularly disaffected: they enjoyed many rights, had a certain independence within their enclaves (*morerias*) safeguarded by the king, and were in large measure acculturated.[56] Occasionally a Muslim physician might even migrate *into* these realms, as did Faraig, a surgeon who was granted permission to move from Agreda (in Castile) to Daroca (in Aragon) with his family and household in the 1320s.[57] However, Granada and North Africa were far more attractive to the able, the learned, and the ambitious, with the result that Muslim medicine in Christian Aragon was soon represented by poorly educated or empirically trained practitioners. There are many signs of this decline in medical knowledge among Muslim physicians in Aragon. There is the case, for example, of Mahomet Peix, a carpenter of Zaragoza, who claimed a knowledge of medicine and surgery but was brought to trial in 1340 for having caused many deaths in his practice.[58] Equally suggestive is the case of Hamet Acequia of Xàtiva in Valencia, accused in 1342 of practicing medicine without undergoing a required examination; "he has no knowledge of the medical art," the king wrote, "yea rather depends on necromancy and divination."[59]

On the basis of isolated references to Muslim healers in documents of later date, John Boswell concluded that "Muslims and Jews seem to have played an important – perhaps disproportionate – role in the practice of medicine under the

[56] Burns, "Spanish Islam," examines the process of acculturation in Valencia during the first generation after the reconquest. For a discussion of the situation of the Muslim communities in the Crown of Aragon in the mid-fourteenth century, see Boswell, *Royal Treasure*, which concentrates on the period 1355–66 and looks at the Crown as a whole. Burns, "Muslims," carries its story well beyond 1300 and emphasizes the contrasts among the Crown's three constituent realms.

[57] C 569/38v. Faraig d'Agreda was still in Daroca enjoying royal protection in early 1335 (further documentation in C 441/17r–v and 31, 569/38v, 464/54r–v, 488/87v).

　　Ali de Lucera (above, p. 52) was probably also an immigrant; presumably he had come to Spain as a refugee after the destruction of the Muslim colony at Lucera (in Apulia) by Charles II of Naples in 1300. This event was brought to my attention by Abulafia, "Monarchs and Minorities," The fate of Lucera is alluded to more briefly in Abulafia, "End of Muslim Sicily," pp. 130–1 (with references).

[58] The text describes Mahomet as "fingens se scire in arte cirurgica et medicina, curas aliquas in se sumere non formidat, propter cuius magnam imperitiam aliquos interfecit," and goes on to state that he has been accused of being a poisoner, a diviner (*sorcerius*), and an adulterer (C 1057/28r–v; partly quoted in Rius Serra, "Aportaciones," pp. 340–1). It seems probable that this is the same man as the *barbitonsor* Hahametum Peix who had earlier been made free of certain financial dues in return for his professional services to the Franciscans of Zaragoza (11 Oct. 1330; C 482/14v–15).

[59] Hamet had asked to be allowed to practice in March 1338 (García-Ballester, McVaugh, and Rubio-Vela, *Medical Licensing*, p. 19), but apparently had never taken the required examination. The accusation of 1342 is published by RL, II:67–8, doc. 67.

Crown of Aragon in the fourteenth century."[60] As we have now seen, this is untenable as far as Muslims are concerned. It is not true even of the later fourteenth century: a systematic survey of the royal archives from the reign of Joan I (1387–97) has identified only two practitioners (out of some 220 mentioned) as Muslims.[61] A previous study of the Muslim medical tradition in Christian Spain has suggested that its original vigor was weakened when public authority began to impose licensing requirements on physicians and surgeons, in the 1330s;[62] but the figures presented and discussed here seem to show that a learned Islamic medicine had disappeared from the Muslim communities in the Crown of Aragon long before that date, so that the licensing laws would have had little effect on the healers who were left.

Healers of some sort there must still have been. In the (largely Muslim) population of rural Valencia, and in Aragon as well, there were obviously empirics still to be found, men and women for whom medicine was not a principal occupation and whom we do not find identified by the professional label. Only accidentally do we learn of the medical activities of individuals like Mahomet Peix, the carpenter of Zaragoza; or the anonymous Muslim slave (*servus*) owned in 1342 by the town of Vilafranca del Penedès, who was reputed to be expert in the treatment of eye diseases.[63] Such people rarely came to the attention of Christian society, which was looking for the learning for which Islam had been so famous.

Jewish practitioners

With the Jewish minority the situation was altogether different. To begin with, they were primarily an urban rather than a rural society, though their numbers were everywhere small. Estimates of the population of the various Jewish communities (*aljamas*) have varied wildly, but the five largest were probably those of Valencia city (1,500–1,700), Barcelona and Zaragoza (each 1,200–1,500), Calatayud (750–1,000), and Huesca (500–700).[64] Yet these tiny societies apparently supported an astonishing number of physicians.[65] In the four decades after 1300 there are traces in the ACA of eleven Jewish physicians in the Barcelona *aljama*; the Christians of Barcelona, nearly twenty times as

---

[60] Boswell, *Royal Treasure*, p. 58. In contrast, Burns' brief discussion of medicine acknowledges the fourteenth-century disappearance of learned Arabic-language medicine and treats it as an aspect of Mudejar ruralization ("Muslims," pp. 90–2).

[61] I am grateful to Jaume Riera i Sans for his kindness in making available the results of his systematic examination of this material.

[62] García Ballester, *Historia social*, pp. 46–50.

[63] Rius, "Més documents," pp. 162–4, docs. 57–9.

[64] Baer, *History*, I:194–5, and notes thereto.

[65] A first survey was made by R[ubio] y B[alaguer], "Metjes"; Pita i Merce, "Metges Jueus," is much fuller but still based entirely on printed sources.

numerous, give evidence of only twice as many. Three of the ten or so physicians we can find practicing in Valencia city during the 1320s were Jews. And there are signs that these impressive levels were viewed as inadequate outside and perhaps even inside the biggest cities. The *aljama* of Morvedre tried to lure the physician Abraham Tauell away from Valencia in 1329 by promising him lifetime exemption from all taxes imposed on the community, but it lost out when the *aljama* at Valencia promised him the same privileges.[66]

If we look more closely at a small but relatively well-documented town, Huesca in Aragon, it becomes clear that the strength of medicine in the Jewish community was guaranteed by occupational tradition within families.[67] Important contributions to medicine by the Jews of Huesca can be followed back at least to the beginning of the twelfth century and the Christian recapture of the city: Pedro Alfonsi, the translator of astronomical works who was physician to King Henry I of England, was a *conversus* baptized in Huesca in 1106, at the age of forty-four.[68] Here, while the Jews constituted 150 households and perhaps 10–15 percent of the population, they contributed over half of the physicians and surgeons discoverable in the archives: the four physicians known to have been practicing in the city in 1310–11, indeed, were *all* Jews.

Of the Jewish families in Huesca in which medicine was a customary occupation,[69] the best documented is the Avinardut line. Mosse Avinardut, the earliest-known of these physicians, already had a wide reputation within the Christian world by 1310, when he was in receipt of a yearly grant of wheat from the abbot of Montearagón for medical services, and was sent to Luesia by Queen Blanca of Aragon to treat the daughter of the lord of Ayerbe. By 1319 Mosse was in the service of the young infante Alfons, and by 1322 he had been named physician to Alfons' consort Teresa. In 1321 he expressed his conviction that he could cure the intractable illness of Ruggiero II di Loria (see below, p. 110). In the summer of 1323 Mosse accompanied his patron Alfons on the conquest of Sardinia, and died there.

Mosse's son Alazar Avinardut soon surpassed his father's achievements. In June 1323, with Mosse about to leave for Sardinia, Alazar, then physician to the infante Blanca, prioress of Sigena (50 kilometers southeast of Huesca), was sent

---

[66] Letter of 23 May 1329 (C 434/120v). Abraham Tauell, son of Omar Tauell (also *fisicus* of Valencia; active 1297–1330), is found practicing 1318–32.

[67] Emery, "Jewish Physicians," p. 116, similarly emphasizes the persistence of medicine as a family occupation among the Jews of fourteenth-century Perpignan, and Jacquart, *Milieu médical*, p. 171, makes the same generalization for France as a whole.

[68] Kealey, *Medieval Medicus*, pp. 75–80 and references there.

[69] These included the Abnarravi, Abulbaca, and Avinardut families; see Durán Gudiol, *Judería de Huesca*, pp. 34–6. Durán's reference to "David" Abulbaca *médico* (p. 34) should be to "Vidal"; however, in further speaking of this individual as (p. 35) "el médico Vidal Abulbaca hijo de Jucef" he has misinterpreted his source (Régné, *History*, doc. 2918): Jucef Abulbaca, not Vidal, is the physician named there. Martínez Loscos, "Orígenes," has much to say about the Jewish physicians of Aragon, and of Huesca in particular, but all based upon printed sources.

to give *his* opinion on the condition of the young Ruggiero II. Shortly thereafter Jaume II began to give him occasional administrative responsibilities, as well as the corresponding rewards: freedom from having to contribute to the *aljama*'s assessments; possession of the scrivenership of Huesca; 1,000 *sous* yearly; and the promise that no *elongamentum* (permission to defer repayment of debts) should excuse debts owed to him. In his role as physician, Alazar followed his father into the service of the infante Alfons, becoming physician to Teresa and then, when she died in 1327 (a week before Jaume II), physician to Alfons himself, now king. He soon became, in effect, the crown's principal minister for matters having to do with the Jews of the Crown of Aragon, first for Alfons and then (after 1335) for Pere III, but his medical role was not abandoned. When the new king's sister Blanca was afflicted simultaneously by scabies (*sarna*), stomach-ache, and fever, she appealed to Alfons to send Alazar to her: no one else would do, and besides, she added, he understood her health better than anyone.[70] Other scattered documents show him providing medicines to the court in 1337, accompanying the king on the recovery of Mallorca and Roussillon in 1343 and 1344, and supplying drugs to the royal household at the siege of Argelers in 1345. And in his turn Alazar trained two sons as physicians: Jucef, who was practicing in Huesca already in 1333 and was still doing so in 1360 (though by 1351 he too had received the post of royal physician), and Vidal, who served the king during at least 1348–52.[71]

Family traditions like this one suggest that it was unremarkable for two generations to be practicing at once in the community, and it is thus not surprising to find, as we have, that there could be at least four Jewish physicians at work simultaneously in Huesca in 1311. The resulting density deserves comment, however; it gives the Jewish *aljama* a physician/population ratio of fifty-seven per 10,000, fifteen times as great as the ratio for Barcelona in the same year and as high as those we find today in practice-intensive cities in Europe or the United States. What makes this understandable is the realization that Jewish physicians did not practice medicine only within their own quarter; as the careers of the Avinarduts make plain, they routinely practiced within Christian society as well.

For despite discriminatory laws and policies that marked Spain as well as the rest of Western Europe, Jews found the Crown of Aragon a relatively tolerant world during the thirteenth and fourteenth centuries.[72] The period before 1283

---

[70] CRD Jaume II sin fecha 1200.

[71] The ACA documentation on the family is not exhausted by two fundamental collections: Cardoner Planas and Vendrell Gallostra, "Aportaciones," and Rius Serra, "Aportaciones." Durán Gudiol, *Judería de Huesca*, pp. 76–7, shows that the family could boast physicians as late as 1415.

[72] The indispensable accounts are Baer, *History*, and Neuman, *Jews in Spain*. See too the recent overview by Romano, "Juifs."

may have been something of a golden age, but later monarchs from Jaume II to Pere III continued a generally enlightened policy towards them. The expulsions of Jews from Gascony (1288), Anjou (1289), and England (1290) produced an influx into France, whence some passed on into Aragon in the 1290s under royal protection.[73] The great expulsion of Jews from the lands of the French king, however, in 1306, affected the Crown of Aragon much more deeply. The Jews of Languedoc and Catalonia had long had close intellectual and social ties, which made it natural for families of Carcassonne, Béziers, Narbonne, and even Montpellier to move south across the Pyrenees when King Philippe IV the Fair ordered them to leave their homes. This massive exodus made a forcible impression on the consciousness of Catalan Jewry; only a few Jews returned to France when Louis X permitted them to do so in 1315, and the number affected by the next expulsion (1321) was correspondingly small.[74]

King Jaume II made no difficulty about permitting – for a price – the resettlement of Jewish families from Languedoc into the communities already established in the Crown of Aragon. Reports suggest that the 1306 arrivals increased by about 10 percent the Jewish population of the largest Catalan cities – sixty families settled in Barcelona, for example, and ten each in Lerida and Gerona – and certainly included some physicians.[75] But the influx would not have affected the nature of the medicine being practiced: the history of intellectual exchange between Languedoc and Catalonia, exemplified in immigrations of Jewish physicians from the north even before the expulsions,[76] had ensured a common medical culture. And as far as can be determined, the number of Jewish medical practitioners who settled in the Crown of Aragon after 1306 was not large; no more than half-a-dozen can be identified with any confidence.[77] The most prominent of these was undoubtedly Abraham ben David des Castlar, whose history shows how a few refugees at least were able to establish themselves quickly in a new land. Abraham and his father David were expelled from Narbonne in 1306 and came to the Catalan province of Gerona; they eventually settled in Besalú, where David des Castlar died in 1315 or 1316.[78] Abraham

---

[73] Assis, "Juifs de France," pp. 290–1; Jordan, *French Monarchy*, chapter 11.

[74] Assis, "Juifs de France," pp. 309–12.

[75] Ibid., pp. 294–5; and see Romano, "Juifs," pp. 180–1.

[76] The physician Bendit was encouraged by Alfons II to move from France to the Crown of Aragon 5 March 1288 (C 72/16, where it was scratched out as inappropriate to the volume, to be reregistered in C 74/91v).

[77] In addition to Abraham des Castlar and Estori ha-Parhi (though the latter eventually moved on to Egypt and then Palestine), both of whom are discussed elsewhere, the clearest case is perhaps that of Bonenfant, on whom see Miret y Sans, "Massacre," pp. 255–6, and Régné, *History*, doc. 2870.

[78] Emery, *Jews of Perpignan*, p. 24, finds David ("Davinus") at Perpignan 1273–7; he had come to Narbonne by the 1280s. He seems to have translated at least one medical work into Hebrew, Galen's *De malitia complexionis diverse*; Steinschneider, *Hebraeischen Übersetzungen*, p. 653.

had by this time become well known for his medical skills, and had contracted to serve the count of Empúries and his town of Castelló, though he continued to live in Besalú; he married into another prominent Jewish medical family of the region.[79] In the 1320s and 1330s he was called to attend at least three of the children of Jaume II.[80] Abraham's visibility should not mislead us, however; there is no evidence to support the idea that the refugees included so disproportionately many and brilliant physicians as to threaten the livelihood of those already established in the Catalan *aljamas*.[81]

David Romano has emphasized that for the "ordinary" Catalan Jew (as distinguished from eminent personages like Alazar Avinardut), urban living still involved normal and uncomplicated relations with Christians: "the Jew would leave his quarter, which was not a ghetto, to draw water at the public fountain, buy bread, chat . . . "[82] Yet it might seem that for the "ordinary" Jewish physician, medical relations with Christian patients could not be entirely normal. During the thirteenth century secular and ecclesiastical legislation in both France and Spain had begun to reveal a mistrust of Jewish medical practice, not simply on abstract theological grounds but for the practical reason that it might allow the Jew to realize his presumed desire to poison his Christian patient.[83] The *Siete partidas* of Alfonso X of Castile, for example, command that Christians may not take medicines compounded by a Jew, though a Christian practitioner may prepare a drug that a Jew has prescribed.[84] A similar suspicion apparently lay behind contemporary ecclesiastical provisions. Provincial councils began to prohibit taking drink or medicine from Jews (Trier, 1227), or provided more broadly for the excommunication of "Christians who when sick commit themselves to the care of Jews for treatment" (Béziers, 1246; Albi, 1254).[85] Such prohibitions were extended to the Crown of Aragon by the Council of Tarragona in 1243, which laid it down that "both clerics and laymen should avoid a forbidden and damnable association with Jews in receiving medicines or the

---

[79] His wife (by 1334), Bona Domna, was the sister of two physicians, Mosse de Sala of Perpignan and Abraham de Sala of Puigcerdà.

[80] Pere (C 229/292v–293), Joan (C 1299/176), and (as king) Alfons (RP 305/70, 73v). For biographical detail, see *Jewish Encyclopedia* (New York, 1907), II:599–600. Grau i Monserrat, "Metges jueus," pp. 30–1, touches on only a tiny fraction of the documentation in the ACA concerning Abraham des Castlar, which deserves to be studied systematically.

[81] This is raised as a possibility by Jordan, *French Monarchy*, p. 237.

[82] Romano, "Juifs," p. 176.

[83] Tractenberg, *Devil and the Jews*, chapter 7, discusses the recurrent theme of the Jew as poisoner but does not show that it much antedates the thirteenth century.

[84] "Otrosi defendemos que ningunt cristiano non reciba melecinamiento nin purga que sea fecha por mano de judio; pero bien la puede recibir por consejo de algunt judio sabidor, solamente que sea fecha por mano de cristiano que conosca et entienda las cosas que son en ella": *Siete partidas*, 3:673.

[85] Grayzel, *Church and the Jews*, pp. 74–5, 318–19, 332–3, 336–7.

like."[86] By the end of the thirteenth century it was well understood that no Christian in King Jaume's realms was supposed to have anything to do with a Jewish physician, and fear of poison was the ostensible reason.

In fact, however, such prohibitions had few observable social consequences in the Crown of Aragon of the early fourteenth century. Jews might be forbidden to sell drugs (though even to this there were exceptions),[87] but Jewish physicians were able to treat Christian patients with no difficulty, and did so routinely. Not even churchmen felt compunction about using their services. One striking testimony to the ubiquity of Jewish medicine in Christian society is a privilege issued in 1301 by Jaume II to Omar [Tauell], *fisicus*, at the request of the *doctor conventus* of the Franciscans of Valencia, "seeing that you . . . have labored faithfully in your art to assist the Franciscans of the city of Valencia and work to serve them daily."[88] And what was true of the religious life was equally true of the secular world, at every level of society: Christian patients do not seem to have selected their physicians by their religion.[89] A zealous Arnau de Vilanova exhorted his patron Jaume II to forbid Jews to treat Christians in his realms, but in vain.[90]

---

[86] "Item quod tam clerici quam layci in percipiendis medicinis et consimilibus prohibitam et dampnatum iudeorum familiaritatem evitent": Pons Guri, "Constitucions conciliars," 47:117. The prohibition was made more explicit three years later: "Quod nullus clericus sive laycus in eius infirmitatibus judeum in medicum advocet seu medicinam recipiat ab eodem." Pons Guri assigns this text (ibid., 48:301) to a council of 1309–12, but one of his witnesses attributes it to a "sexta synodo," as does an earlier witness not used by him – ACV, perg. 2399 (Olmos, *Pergaminos*, doc. 913), of 4 Dec. 1300 – and it seems likely that this is the sixth Tarragona council of Pere d'Albalat, held in 1246. The injunction can be found repeated in a Leridan synod under Guillem de Montcada (1257–82) reported by Sainz de Baranda, *España Sagrada*, p. 179.

[87] At first there were simply restrictions on which drugs they might sell – *c.* 1310 the Barcelona authorities prohibited them from dealing in realgar, the archetypical poison of the day (see below, chapter 5 at n. 104) – but eventually there were attempts to eliminate their practice altogether: Vidal Xaham, Jewish apothecary of Barcelona, was permitted to stay in business despite a recent ordinance that "nullus judeus uteretur . . . officio apothecarie" there (letter of 3 non. July 1325; CRD Jaume II judios 106).

[88] "Attendentes te . . . de arte tua in serviciis religiosorum fratrum minorum civitatis Valencie fideliter laborasse et quia eis servire cotidie conaris": C 196/296; Régné, *History*, doc. 2750. Another example is Abraham Halleva, who was physician to the Augustinians of Zaragoza in 1325 (document of 27 Nov. 1330; C 482/40). Abraham is known in Zaragoza 1317–38, except for a brief (1329–30) move to Borja. He was still serving the Augustinians in 1332 (Rius Serra, "Aportaciones," pp. 347–8, doc. 12).

[89] Bertomeu Mathoses of Valencia, for example, called on both a Christian (Bertomeu de Casaldoria) and a Jewish (Omar Tauell) physician to prescribe drugs for his household, as we know from the suit brought against Bertomeu by the (Christian) apothecary, Berenguer de Farfanya, who had filled the prescriptions – twenty-six of them, at a total cost of 178 *sous* 4 *deners* – but had never been paid (ARV, Just. Civil 26, 30 May 1330).

[90] Arnau urged the king, "ordinarets que jeu tant com en sa error perseverara no gos en pena de cors et daver medicar negu crestia, et si crestia lo requer, sia punit en certa quantitat." I quote from the letter, "Seynor: vos sots tengut," as published by Menéndez y Pelayo, *Heterodoxos*, p. 276. Arnau was more successful in convincing Jaume's brother, Frederic III of Sicily, to prohibit Jews from treating Christians; Frederic's *constitutiones* for Sicily of 1310, which acknowledged Arnau's incentive, did just that (*AA*, II:698). Nearly simultaneously (1304/6) the

Indeed, the laws tending to segregate Jews were not infrequently overridden in the interest of their wider medical practice, sometimes at the request of their prospective Christian patients.[91] In 1315 (and again in 1320) Jaume II ordered that

> since master Vidal Rouen, a Jewish physician of Barcelona, must by virtue of his profession visit many inhabitants of the said city and its surroundings, and must see to many things in treating the patients whom he has in his care, and since many other people have to show him the urines of the sick and to ask his advice,

no restrictions were to be placed on access to his house in the Jewish quarter.[92] In similar fashion the kings routinely allowed Jews to move their practice from one city to another.[93]

It was not merely their Christian patients but their Christian colleagues, too, who admired Jewish practitioners. A letter of 1326 to the queen from one of her servitors, Pere Folquet, called it to her attention that "there is a Jew in Barcelona named Benvenist Izmel . . . who is the best doctor there is in these parts, as master Joan [Amell] and master Pere Gavet can tell you," and warned her that Benvenist was thinking of moving his residence to Vilafranca del Penedès.[94] For two eminent learned physicians like Joan Amell and Pere Gavet to speak in these terms about a Jewish practitioner implies that religious differences could be overlooked even when professional jealousy might encourage insistence upon them.

counts of Provence forbade Christians to consult Jewish physicians (Barthélemy, *Médecins*, p. 14). See also the views put by Arnau into Frederic's mouth in Arnau's *Interpretatio de visionibus in somniis* (Menendez y Pelayo, *Heterodoxos*, p. 235). Without emphasizing the difference between Aragon and Castile, Schipperges, "Sonderstellung," pp. 208–11, cites Castilian conciliar legislation forbidding Christians to frequent Jewish physicians, but calls attention to Joan I of Catalonia-Aragon who excluded physicians from legislation forbidding Christians to treat with Jews.

[91] In 1309 the *probi homines* of Zaragoza requested that the king allow two Jews – Millis, a physician, and Mosse, a surgeon – to come practice their arts in that city, a request granted by the king (C 205/226v).

[92] "Cum magister Vitalis Rouen physicus Judeus Barchinone ex officio suo plures habeat in dicta civitate et eius convicinio visitare infirmos et plura gerere et procurare ad opus infirmorum quos tenet in cura sua et alios pluras gentes habebunt ei hostendere hurinas infirmorum et requirere ab ei consilium pro eiusdem": the letter, of 29 April 1320 (C 383/26–27v), recapitulates and confirms various privileges granted to Vidal as early as 1309. He was still alive in 1322 (C 222/79v–80), but had died by Jan. 1324.

[93] At the request of men of the county of Ribagorça, Pere III allowed Vidal, *fisicus* of Barbastro, to move his domicile to that county so as to remedy the lack of practitioners there, despite the laws holding him in his original city (letter of 5 Aug. 1338; C 864/85); likewise he allowed Omar Tauell's nephew Ambra to move from Valencia to Xèrica, at its lord's request (1 Nov. 1342; C 874/24v).

[94] "Que aci ha en Barchinona un juheu, qui ha nom Benvenist Izmel . . . qui es lo pus excellent metge, qui sia en aquestas partides, e aço sab mestre Johan et mestre Pere Gavet": quoted in part by Baer, *Juden*, pp. 172–3, doc. 149, and by Cardoner Planas, "Benvenist Samuel," p. 332. Benvenist Izmel already enjoyed a lifetime grant of 650 *sous* annually from Guillem de Entença for medical service, a grant which both Jaume II and Alfons III protected after Guillem's death (29 May 1327, C 190/161v; 20 Oct. 1328, CRD Alfons III 585, 586).

What undoubtedly helped make Jewish medicine seem so attractive to Christians, potential clients and colleagues alike, was its reputation for medical learning, part of a remarkably intense intellectual tradition. A system of schooling in the *aljama*, from primary instruction to the yeshivah, made this learning possible. While education was centered upon the Talmud and Jewish law, secular subjects were still studied privately in both the Spanish communities and the Languedocian ones (notably at Narbonne and Montpellier) with which their Catalan counterparts in particular had had many ties. The attraction of such secular studies is revealed in the long debate that culminated in 1305 in the prohibition by Rabbi Solomon ibn Adret of Barcelona of the study by any "member of our community under the age of twenty-five [of the] works of the Greeks on natural science or metaphysics . . . lest these sciences entice them and draw their hearts away from the Law of Israel."[95] One consequence of the expulsion of the Jews from France in 1306 was the strengthening of the philosophically minded element in Catalan communities like Gerona and Barcelona and the intensification there of this debate.[96] Medicine, however, was not seriously affected. Ibn Adret specifically exempted medical science from the decree, inasmuch as it was sanctioned by the Torah, and indeed the study of Greco-Arabic medical literature – read both in Arabic and in Hebrew translation – flourished within the *aljamas* at the beginning of the fourteenth century.[97] When the philosopher-translator Kalonymos ben Kalonymos of Arles stopped in Catalonia in 1322 on his trip back from Rome, he dedicated his *Eben Bohan* (*Touchstone*) to ten learned friends living there, among whom he numbered the Besalú physicians Bendit des Logar and Abraham des Castlar.[98] Abraham himself composed Hebrew medical treatises: the most successful, his *Aleh Refu'ah* (*Green Leaf*) on fevers, was completed in 1326.[99]

Hence Christians perceived Jews as possessed of an array of knowledge lacking or imperfectly available in the schools; a particular interest taken by Christian physicians in Jewish knowledge is often apparent. For example, before establishing himself at Gerona, Armengaud Blaise had made a name for himself

---

[95] Neuman, *Jews in Spain*, II:131; Baer, *Jews*, I:301–4, with another translation.

[96] García-Ballester, Ferre, and Feliu, "Jewish Appreciation," p. 88.

[97] To be sure, the reputation of some schools was greater than that of others. Çulema de Quatorze of Calatayud chose to travel to Xàtiva in the kingdom of Valencia to study medicine rather than stay at home in Aragon, in Calatayud or even Zaragoza, the Aragonese capital (Sept. 1347; C 645/141r–v).

[98] Renan, "Ecrivains," p. 105; and Grau i Monserrat, "Metges jueus," who identifies Bendit with the physician Bendit des Logar found in Besalú 1310–24. (If this is the same Bendit invited to come to the Crown of Aragon in 1288 [above, n. 76], he was of course not a refugee from the exile like Abraham.) Bendit's level of learning is suggested by the fact that he was on a voyage to Montpellier in 1321 to consult physicians there on the illness of the viscount of Castellnou when he was seized by the seneschal of Carcassonne as part of the new French exile of the Jews; Jaume II had to intercede for his release (letter of 15 July 1321; C 173/195).

[99] Renan, "Ecrivains," p. 645. Assis, "Juifs de France," p. 317, cites three manuscripts of the work.

at Montpellier in the 1290s as the translator of a number of medical and scientific works originally written in Arabic. Some of these works, however, had earlier been translated into Hebrew by Moses ibn Tibbon, and it seems likely that Armengaud produced most of these Latin translations in association with Moses' nephew Jacob ben Machir ibn Tibbon (known as Prophatius in the West) – the latter translating the Hebrew into the vernacular, while Armengaud rendered the vernacular meaning into Latin.[100] Or we may recall the example of Guillaume de Béziers, who on arriving at Lerida in 1301 to teach medicine asked King Jaume to give him access to "certain medical books in Arabic that the Jews possess."[101] It is not difficult to understand why Pere Gavet would have been ready to credit the skills of a Jewish physician like Benvenist Izmel, even without direct knowledge of his practice.

But we ought not to suppose that Christian practitioners were generally ranked as inferior to Jews. During the course of the fourteenth century a number of Jewish physicians came to feel that the new scholastic medicine of the Christian university had advantages that their tradition could not provide, and this led to the translation of several typical university productions from Latin into Hebrew by 1400.[102] Moreover, even before this shift of outlook, the choice of a physician by patients of *any* religion had really been determined primarily by personal considerations. There was in general little to distinguish practice by Christians from that by Jews, and there were no barriers preventing Jews from being treated by Christians if they so desired.[103] In 1324 a Jewish woman complained to the bailiff of Huesca that her son had been struck in the head during a fight, and that other Jews wanted his (Jewish) surgeon to make sure he died; she begged the bailiff, successfully, to find her son a Christian surgeon instead.[104] In one instance, indeed, an *aljama* even attempted to contract a Christian physician to supply medical care to the entire Jewish community.[105]

---

[100] The evidence is summarized by Blue, "Ermengaud Blasi," pp. 37–51.

[101] RL, II:13–14, doc. 16 (of 11 Sept. 1302). See below, chapter 3.

[102] García-Ballester, Ferre, and Feliu, "Jewish Appreciation." In his will of 1346 a Jewish *physicus et cirurgicus* of Perelada, Durand de Sant Ponç, bequeathed two medical books to a friend, an Abulcasis and an Averroes: "unum videlicet vocatum ebrayce zaravi . . . et qui vocatur in latino albucahi, et alium vocatum in ebrayce evanrrost et in latino averohis" (AHPG/CE 215/20). By this time the two learned traditions had so far interpenetrated that we cannot be sure whether master Durand owned Hebrew or Latin versions of these texts.

[103] Examples are plentiful: the Jew of Gerona cared for by Guillem Guerau, surgeon of Besalú, in 1321 (C 369/102v–103); the Jews of Calatayud treated by Pedro Cellerer, physician of Daroca, in 1316 (C 355/87); the Jew of Gerona treated by Ramon de Podio, physician of the same city, in 1348 (AHPG, Notari 4–5/26v).

[104] ACA pergaminos Jaume II 4071, of 30 May 1324.

[105] Ramon de Tesarach, master of arts and of medicine, agreed that for ten pounds yearly "prestabo vobis et omnibus et singulis judeis tam masculis quam feminis dicte aljame [of Castelló d'Empúries] . . . quotienscumque necessarium fuerit et fuerim requisitus . . . consilium super infirmitatibus vestris et ipsorum tam super dietis flebotomiis quam in omnibus aliis necessariis que officio meo incumbunt et iudicabo orinas et videbo et visitabo infirmos et alia omnia faciam et complebo que facere teneor Christianis habitatoribus ville C. iuxta . . . tenorem . . . inde

To set against the many indications of the normality of Jewish practice we have one somewhat contradictory piece of evidence. It is the incomplete report of a lawsuit in Valencia in early 1314, brought by the physician Ismel Abencrespi against Pere Gilabert: Ismel accused Pere of having refused to pay the 100 *sous* agreed on for curing him of epilepsy. In replying, Pere answered in part that "he should not have to pay any fee to the said Ismel, since the church has declared that no Jew should treat any Christian for any illness." (How the case came out we unfortunately do not know.)[106] This text certainly shows that there was public awareness in the Crown of Aragon of the ecclesiastical prohibition but not, I think, that it was taken with much seriousness. Pere Gilabert's knowledge of it had not prevented him from contracting with Ismel in the first place, and the latter's willingness to undertake the case suggests that attempts like Pere's to evade payment were not commonplace (or at least not likely to be successful). In any case, of course, Pere had – perhaps deliberately – misstated the church's ruling: technically, the council had prohibited Christians from using Jews as physicians rather than Jews from attending Christian patients.

Twenty years later, in the 1330s, the church at last took note of its old rule. We will look more closely later at the reasons why it might have tried at that moment to supervise Jewish access to Christian patients. Here we need only say that there was never any question of rigidly enforcing the conciliar legislation of 1243 and forbidding Christians to see Jewish physicians; on the contrary, the church's new policy explicitly permitted Jews to practice among Christians, as long as they worked in association with some Christian practitioner, even an apothecary. The perceived need for medical care was so great, and the role played in this by Jewish physicians so significant, that Christian society was never able to afford to restrict the Jews' activity to their own communities.

Towards relative abundance

We are now in a position to try to respond to the questions with which this chapter opened. To begin with, how do the level and distribution of medical practitioners in the early fourteenth-century Crown of Aragon measure up against the corresponding figures from other European societies? Recent data

confectum inter me et consules dicte ville": the contract, of 15 Jan. 1347, was canceled two years later by mutual agreement (AHPG/CE 221/24v). On contracts, and on Ramon, see further below, chapter 6.

A comparable contractual relationship, but with individuals rather than with the community, was entered into by a Christian physician of Manresa (Ramon Marini, active 1293–1303), who contracted to provide medical care for a year to two Jewish households in exchange for 50 *sous* from each (AHCM, Liber V Judeorum, 18 kls. Dec. 1297; quoted by Miró i Borràs, "Salaris," and in abbreviated form by Rafat Selga, "Aspectos," p. 97).

[106] "No seria tengut de pagar salari alcu al dit Ismel per so con verdat es per lesgleya que nengun juheu no gos curar nengu Xrestia de nenguna malaltia": ARV, Just. Val. 15, 8 id. Feb. 1313/14.

Table 2.10. *Practitioners active in Barcelona and Valencia, 1330s*

	1333		1338	
	PS (per 10K)	A (per 10K)	PS (per 10K)	A (per 10K)
Barcelona	21 (7)	25 (8.3)	12 (4)	25 (8.3)
Valencia	22 (7.3)	24 (8)	20 (6.7)	14 (4.7)

on English, French, and Italian activity in this period, although not perfectly comparable with the data from Spain, make it clear that in spite of Jaume II's concern his realm was at least as well provided with medical care as its neighbors. Indeed, the Spanish information reveals the extent to which some of these other studies with more restricted data bases have underestimated the number of medical practitioners active in their respective societies.

Katharine Park's study of medicine in Renaissance Florence takes its origin with the plague of 1348, and is based on a systematic examination of the detailed municipal records that survive from the second half of the century; hence its figures cannot be compared directly with those of Aragon, fifty years earlier. She does, however, cite the chronicler Villani's estimate of the pre-plague medical population of the city, judge it sound, and use it as a benchmark for the levels after 1348: in the Florence of 1338, Villani wrote, "the association of lawyers had some eighty members; the notaries, some six hundred; physicians and surgeons, some sixty; shops of apothecaries, some hundred" – this in a city population that Park estimates at 120,000.[107] This results in an estimate of 5 *medici* (physicians and surgeons combined) and 8.3 apothecaries per 10,000 population. When we compare these figures for the Florence of 1338 with the minimum levels established above for Barcelona and Valencia in sample years from the 1330s, we find that the Spanish cities had come to enjoy at least as high a level of medical services as the Tuscan capital (table 2.10).

At the other end of the urban scale, the town of Manosque in Provence (sixty kilometers from Marseille) has been closely studied by Joseph Shatzmiller. For the years 1285–1340 he has found an average of six practitioners (Christians and Jews, barbers as well as physicians and surgeons) at work simultaneously in this community of perhaps 4,000 people, a level that held essentially stable throughout the period in question.[108] In size Manosque is comparable to the

[107] Park, *Doctors*, pp. 55, 57.
[108] Shatzmiller, *Médecine et justice*, pp. 8–19. Shatzmiller infers from the eight practitioners he found practicing in Manosque in 1314–15, 1321, and 1338 that eight or nine is a more accurate level than the average found for the entire period he studied (p. 18); it seems to me, however, to be safer to argue from the average. His figures are not all easy to confirm from the data he gives: thus he says that a "Guillelmus Rasoris" was practicing surgery in Manosque 1314–17 (p. 10), but the one document given referring to this practitioner is dated 1304 (pp. 93–4).

Table 2.11. *Physicians identified as active in twenty-year periods*

	Paris		Barcelona		Valencia	
	No.	Per 10K	No.	Per 10K	No.	Per 10K
1290–1309	42	2.1	15	5	12	4
1310–1329	84	4.2	20	6.7	20	6.7
1330–1349	99	5.0	24	8	21	7

Catalan town of Manresa, where steady growth brought practitioners to almost twice that density by 1330: eleven practitioners based in a town of 4,000 or so but, as in Manosque,[109] treating a much more numerous clientele drawn from the surrounding countryside. Again, Catalan communities prove to have been well off in comparison with what we know of the rest of Europe.[110]

If we move from local to national surveys of the medical occupations in the Middle Ages, it becomes much less easy to draw useful comparisons with the data from the Crown of Aragon. Such surveys have recently been made for both France and England, but each was produced by assembling information taken from other printed sources, and neither purports to approach systematic coverage or completeness. The more thorough of these surveys, the analysis of the *milieu médical* in medieval France offered by Danielle Jacquart, uses the various references accumulated by Ernest Wickersheimer from the scholarly literature of his day (1936), with additions of her own from the scholarship of the subsequent forty-five years, to draw a general portrait of the medical world as it developed in France from 1100 to 1500; she has not tried to examine the structure of medical activity on a year-by-year basis, but she has counted the physicians identifiable as active in Paris during successive twenty-year intervals (see table 2.11).[111] For the period 1310–29 she has gone on to provide a fuller account of practitioners by occupation. Her numbers are much higher, in absolute terms, than the corresponding figures for Barcelona and Valencia in the same twenty-year period, but when allowance is made for the much larger population of Paris (perhaps as high as 200,000 in 1328), the Spanish cities reveal a generally greater density of health care (see table 2.12).[112] The contrast cannot be understood as proving that the Crown of Aragon actually had more medical practitioners than France, since the French calculations have been based

[109] Shatzmiller, *Médecine et justice*, p. 18.

[110] Wolff, "Recherches," concentrates on the period 1350–1450; he finds 30–35 practitioners (exclusive of apothecaries) active in Toulouse in 1405, which then had perhaps 20,000 inhabitants; this ratio is comparable to or a little lower than what we obtained for Barcelona in the 1320s.

[111] Jacquart, *Milieu médical*, p. 244.

[112] Ibid., p. 246. I have included Jacquart's 15 *mires* with the physicians.

Table 2.12. *Occupations of practitioners active 1310–29*

	Physicians		Surgeons		Barbers	
	No.	Per 10K	No.	Per 10K	No.	Per 10K
Paris	84	4.2	28	1.4	97	4.9
Barcelona	20	6.7	20	6.7	28	9.3
Valencia	20	6.7	23	7.7	63	21

on only a sampling of evidence; rather, it gives a measure of how limited that sample may have been – and how far from random.[113] The apparent dearth of Parisian surgeons and barbers, relative to Valencia or Barcelona, probably means only that French historians have tended to pay more attention to physicians than to the other health occupations.

It is entirely plausible, therefore, that our figures indicate a likely base level for medical assistance everywhere in the pre-plague West – a level that, in the larger urban centers, was already approaching early modern levels and was perhaps not too different from what one might observe today in Spanish towns of comparable size.[114] More particularly, our evidence for the Crown of Aragon reveals to us in detail a specific society in which there was a ready market for health care, and which encouraged a steady expansion of the pool of health practitioners; if the economic difficulties of the 1330s led to a retrenchment, it seems to have occurred only in the largest cities. It is thus a regional picture that is consistent with our account of King Jaume II's experiences with medical practitioners, and it suggests that, like their king, his subjects – at least in cities and towns – were becoming able to find health care more easily when they wanted it.

---

[113] Similar results can be obtained by analyzing the data recently published for England, which are evidently based on an even more limited sample of evidence; they reveal only one active practitioner per 73,000 population in England as a whole during a twenty-year period at mid-century, less than one-tenth the value I calculate for the Crown of Aragon in a comparable span of time. I derive this English ratio from the figures of Gottfried, "English Medical Practitioners," table 1 (estimating the English population at that time, conservatively, as four million). I use this account, where Gottfried's figures are conveniently assembled, though his subsequent book, *Doctors and Medicine*, pp. 249ff., slightly revised the earlier counts (he increased his number of practitioners included by 5 percent, but agreed that "the general trends remain the same"). His book must be used with extreme caution, not only for its statistics; see the reviews in *Med. Hist.* 31 (1987), 360–2; *Bull. Hist. Med.* 61 (1987), 455–70; *Soc. Hist. Med.* 1 (1988), 93–5; *Speculum* 64 (1989), 168–71. The materials published by Jenks, "Fachkräfte," and by Getz, "Archives," give a further indication of how many more English medical practitioners must await discovery.

[114] At their peak in the 1320s, Barcelona and Valencia had at least one practitioner for every 500 inhabitants. Pelling and Webster, "Medical Practitioners," p. 235, find a ratio of 1:400 in sixteenth-century English centers like London and Norwich; they comment, "it is evident that early modern western society called for a high level of medical assistance from outside the limits of the family." Apparently the trend goes back at least to the later Middle Ages.

3

The success of medical learning

In his great *Llibre de contemplació*, written in Mallorca about 1272, when he was forty, the Catalan genius Ramon Llull included among other topics a chapter, "How we ought to be wary of what doctors do."[1] Meant to contrast the physician as healer of the body with the priest as healer of the soul, it inevitably depicted the former in an unfavorable light – but Llull's criticisms would have lost their force if the picture that he presented of practitioner ignorance had not been widely accepted. Physicians today cannot recognize diseases, he objected, and they don't know how to treat them, as disagreements among physicians prove; instead, they prescribe at random. At the outset of a case they profess to mastery, only to abandon treatment when they find they cannot cure. More people are killed than are healed by physicians, he concluded, and the best cure is to treat yourself.

Furthermore, the ignorance of physicians is matched by their dishonesty:

> for they boast that they understand an illness when they don't; and they drag illnesses out so that they can get more money from the sick; they prescribe syrups and electuaries and other things for the sick because they share in the profits that the apothecaries make on what they sell to their patients. Every day we see that when the physician's cure goes wrong, he blames it on the patient, saying that he hasn't followed the right diet or didn't tell the truth about his illness. It is they who should be blamed for the mistakes they make, yet they blame the patient, who doesn't deserve it. Physicians who first of all understand the illness, *they* . . . can treat it; but every day we see physicians treating their patients haphazardly because they *don't* understand the illness.[2]

---

[1] Llull, *Libre de contemplació en Déu*, II.115: "Com hom se pren guarda de so que fan los metges"; pp. 76–82.

[2] "Car ells se gaben de conèxer la malautía, la qual non conexen; e ells alonguen . . . als malautes lurs malautíes per tal que major loguer najen; els donen . . . als malautes exarobs e letovaris e altres coses, per tal car han lur part in lo guany que fan los especiayres en los coses que venen als malalties. Tot dia veem . . . quels metges qui obren per feica, que con han errada lur metgía sempre sen tornen sobre lo malaute, e reprenenlo e dienli que ell no esta en dieta ni nols diu

Llull's complaints were thus directed, not at the practice of medicine, but at those who practiced without appreciating that their craft had a scientific basis.

By the 1270s Llull was by no means alone in his belief that medical science was of practical advantage. At some level of lay consciousness, a general European feeling that academic training makes for a better physician goes back almost to the earliest years of medical faculties within the new universities. Gui de Sora, as legate of Pope Gregory IX, announced to the Montpellier region in 1239 that often *medici* who rushed quickly into practice were incompetent, ignorant of the rationale for treatment, and killed rather than cured; and that therefore, under pain of excommunication, no one would henceforth be allowed to practice medicine before being examined and approved by two masters selected from the Montpellier faculty by the bishop of Maguelonne; then the candidate might receive a license from the bishop and the examiners.[3] Eight years before, in the Constitutions of Melfi, Emperor Frederic II had enacted a very similar law for Sicily: there, no one claiming the title of *medicus* was to practice unless he should come to the king with letters from the masters of Salerno testifying to his trustworthiness and sufficient knowledge (*sciencia*); then he might receive the royal license.[4]

The policy laid down by the legate for thirteenth-century Montpellier had particular implications for later developments in the Crown of Aragon, because King Jaume I was, by inheritance from his mother Maria, seigneur of the city.[5] Jaume reiterated the rule in his own name in 1272, at the urging of his physician Bernat Calcadell – himself a Montpellier master – at just the moment when Llull was complaining of the lack of knowledgeable medical practitioners.[6] At Jaume's death in 1276 the city passed into the hands of the cadet branch of the family, the kings of Mallorca, who continued the policy of requiring a knowledge of academic medicine for all practitioners in Montpellier and its surroundings. By the end of the century at least two towns in Catalonia had enacted similar rules: Cervera (situated halfway between Lerida and Barcelona) in 1291, and Valls (north of Tarragona) in 1299. In the latter community, the

veritat de la malautía. On, com ells deuríen esser blasmats e represes de la errada que han feta en lo malaute, e ells blasmen e reprenen lo malaute qui mal no mer. Los metges fisicians qui conexen primerament la malaltía en que pecca, aquells . . . poden tractar de la malaltía. Mas tot dia veem que los metges obren en hom a aventura, per so car no han conexensa de malaltía": ibid., p. 78.

3 *Cartulaire*, pp. 185–6, doc. 4.

4 Kristeller, *Studi*, p. 62, n. 118.

5 The Sicilian model, too, could have influenced later developments in the Crown of Aragon: medical learning was still the rule in Sicily when Aragonese forces under Pere II entered the island after the Sicilian Vespers of 1282.

6 On Bernat, see Wickersheimer, *Dictionnaire*, [I] p. 73. He was a master at Montpellier by 1260, and was described as "clericus et fisicus noster" on 7 June 1274, when the king granted him permission to buy houses in Montpellier without paying *laudimium* (C 19/131).

regulations insisted that no one should be allowed to administer a potion who had not learned the "sciencia de medicina," and in 1319 they were made still more explicit: "No man or woman . . . shall practice the art of medicine as a *metge de fisica* in the town or district of Valls without having been examined there before the town court and council."[7] Having populations of 1,500 or so, Cervera and Valls were no more than middle-sized, and neither is likely to have had more than one academically trained physician, if that; the regulations seem to reflect a public perception of the advantages of a learned and scientific medicine rather than the efforts of local practitioners lobbying to maintain an existing monopoly.

However, these rules remained ideals and nothing more. Not surprisingly, there is no evidence from Cervera, Valls, or anywhere else in the Crown of Aragon before the 1330s that such regulations designed to control the access to medical practice were actually enforced. As we have already seen, medical care was not always easy to find in the kingdom in the early years of the century, and no community could afford to be terribly particular about its health-care providers. When the pressure to obtain medical services was so great that apothecaries were granted the right to act as physicians, when towns had to try to bind practitioners contractually not to move elsewhere, there could be no thought of insisting that potential physicians routinely submit to some sort of examination – no matter how many people were coming to feel, like Llull, that the best medical care required a thorough scientific understanding of the subject.[8]

To be sure, one provision of the *fueros* of Monzón (1289) has traditionally been understood as an early attempt to legislate such a policy for all Catalonia. The relevant rubrics read:

> 17. Likewise we ordain and decree that no lawyer [*savi en dret*] shall take part in inquisitions or trials or judgments in any court unless he has been examined by the councilors of the town together with other lawyers; and those who are examined shall swear that they will act faithfully in trials and in the other cases heard by the king's vicar [*veguer*] or by the bailiff and the said councilors of the town.

---

[7] From 1299 – "No sia null hum ne nuylla fembra, crestiá o crestiana, jueu o juhya, sarray o sarrayna, de qualque condició sia, qui no aja appresa scientia de medicina, qui gos donar a persones malautes, metzina, ne algun beuratge en loch de mediçina, per tal cor el gran periyl de mort a aquel quiu pren neu reeb, e condempnació de la anima daquel o daquela quiu dona": Carreras y Candi, "Ordinacions," 12:202. From 1319 – "No sía nuyl hom ni nulla fembra, estrayn ni privat, crestiá ni jueu ho sarray, qui gos úsar en nulla manera, el loch ni el terme de Vayls, doffici de metge de fesica, ne de art de medicina, tro que sia examinat o examinada el dit loch, en presencia de la cort e dels jurats. Ne encara, com examinats seran, no gosen usar sens licencia de la cort e dels jurats, la qual licencia ayen auer en escrit, segelat ab lo segeyl dels jurats": ibid., 12:291.

[8] Similarly, I know of no evidence that the requirement of the Castilian *Fuero real* (c. 1255) that all practicing physicians be approved by their towns was ever applied in the thirteenth century. For the provision, see Ruíz Moreno, *Medicina*, p. 21.

18. Likewise we ordain and decree that the same thing be done with physicians and surgeons.[9]

However, a general test of qualifications may not have been the original intent of this legislation; rather, these provisions (and the two that followed them, concerning notaries and scribes, which historians seem never to quote in this connection) may have been aimed *en bloc* at controlling the competence of participants in court cases – a matter which, at least as far as medical testimony goes, was becoming particularly important in the 1280s.[10] The *fueros* do not address the matter of professional activity independent of a narrowly judicial context. Still, it is certainly reasonable to understand this rubric as springing from a growing belief that it was possible to tell competent physicians from bad, a belief later made concrete in the local provisions of Cervera and Valls (provisions which would be harder to understand if the *cortes* of Monzón had already established the same principle). By the 1330s, as we shall see, this belief was so widespread that the king would appeal to the *constitutiones Cathalonie* as requiring the universal examination of physicians and surgeons – perhaps, like modern historians, reading back into Monzón a more general law than had originally been intended.

If qualification by examination was still the exception, then, how did people normally establish themselves as physicians or surgeons? We will find that the years 1285–1335 were a transitional period in which medicine was taking firm shape as a secular occupation, developing concurrently with a social awareness of the benefits of health care and with a perception that learned or scientific medicine was most desirable. In the first decades of this period we can recognize many different routes by which individuals became accepted as physicians (or surgeons). Eventually, however, as medical learning became more widely disseminated, and schooling in a medical faculty became more frequent, these

---

[9] 17. Item ordonam e statuïm que algun savi en dret no ús en alguna cort de inquisicions, ne de advocacions, ne de jutjaments entrò serà examinat per los prohòmens de cascum loch ensemps ab los altres savis en dret; e equells qui seran elets, juren que se hauran feelment en advocacions e en les altres coses en poder del veguer o del batle e dels dits prohòmens d'aquell loch.
18. Item ordonam e statuïm que allò mateix se faça en los metges e cirugians.

I quote the text provided by Jorge Rubió Balaguer, in La Torre, *Documentos*, p. [3], who believes that this established a general requirement for medical examinations; another who assumes this is Cardoner i Planas, *Història*, p. 93.

[10] The ensuing rubrics are:

19. Item que allo mateix se faça en los notaris publics.
20. Item ordonam e statuim que tots jutges delegats per lo veger o per lo batle pusquen elegir scrivans publichs aquells ques volran en les causes o plets a ells comanats.

I follow the text in ACA, Generalitat, Codices, vol. III (a collection of "Usatges i Constitucions" assembled in the second decade of the fifteenth century), ff. 40ra, 28rb. On the inchoate state of the *constitucions* before their authoritative collection about 1418, see Pons i Guri, "Constitucions de Catalunya," pp. 68–9. For the new importance of medical testimony in the 1280s and thereafter, see below, chapter 7.

routes began to draw together. By the 1330s it had become widely agreed that a certain level of academic preparation guaranteed a physician's competence, and that people who lacked such training might be required to prove that they were equally well prepared; the legislation of that decade first provided an explicit definition of what it was that a physician must know in order to be allowed to practice, and mechanisms for enforcing that definition. Though it was at first enforced only irregularly and capriciously, it had created a role for a medical profession – in the Crown of Aragon, at least.

From clerical to lay practitioners

When Ramon Llull was writing his *Llibre de contemplació*, many of the clergy were still providing medical as well as spiritual care to the populace, as they had done (in the absence of lay physicians) during much of the earlier Middle Ages. But the two functions were beginning to draw apart, as society began to hope for special expertise from its secular ministers of health; Llull remarked sadly, "I marvel, Lord, that people are so blind and stupid as to put more trust in those who heal the body, and to give them more credence, than those who heal the soul."[11] In the 1270s it was still meaningful to contrast the healing (physical as well as spiritual) offered by the church out of understanding and love with that promised by those lay physicians who based it on ignorance and self-interest. But Llull belonged to the last generation in the Crown of Aragon when clerics could be generally imagined to possess medical skill; in his day their importance to medicine was already starting to diminish, and by the 1330s it was essentially at an end. The growing emphasis upon a trained medical corps would make their practice unnecessary.[12]

In Llull's lifetime (he died in 1316) we can still identify several clerics whose lives show how varied a fusion of ecclesiastical and medical careers had once been possible:

(a) Brother Alberto, a Franciscan of the province of Aragon, turns up first in 1291, preparing medicines for the infante Pere, the brother of Jaume II, but he

---

[11] "Molt me do gran maravella, Sènyer, de les gens con son tan orbes ni tan pegues que més se fien en los metges dels cors e més los tenen per vertaders que los metges de la anima": Llull, *Libre de contemplació*, p. 78.

[12] Only 1 percent of the Christian physicians I have identified in the Crown of Aragon can be shown to have been clerics. This is a much lower percentage than scholars have found in other societies, but regional peculiarities make an unqualified comparison of little value. Thus, 14 percent of the physicians counted by Jacquart in France 1300–50 are clerics, and her figure for the next half-century declines only slightly; but many of these men were French regent masters of medicine who held ecclesiastical benefices while teaching at Paris or Montpellier, a type of cleric-physician that does not appear among my practitioners (Jacquart, *Milieu médical*, pp. 363, 383, 157). Ussery (*Chaucer's Physician*, pp. 28–31) concludes that the cleric-physician was common in later fourteenth-century England; on the other hand, Naso (*Medici*, pp. 226–7) finds a greatly diminished role for the clergy in medicine in late medieval Piedmont.

had apparently previously attended the late Alfons II. Fifteen years later Alberto was still to be found serving the royal family, now as *phisicus* to Queen Blanca. When in 1307 the minister general of the order commanded Brother Alberto to travel to Castile or Leon to treat the noble lady Juana Alfonsi for five months, the king and queen each begged that he be allowed to stay in Aragon "pro conservatione sanitatis nostre." He last appears in 1310, caring for the health of the king's nephew, the lord of Vizcaya, and that of his wife.[13]

(b) Ramon de Vilalta is identified as a *fisicus* of Lerida in 1302, called in June to attend the king. In 1314 he was appointed royal *fisicus*, this time identified more precisely as a canon of Lerida "skilled in the art of medicine," and by April 1315 he is found named canon of Seu d'Urgell as well as of Lerida, and rector of Balaguer. These ecclesiastical responsibilities did not put an end to his activity as a physician, and he soon took on a leading medical role in his relatively remote region: he had already provided medical care to the count of Urgell (d. 1314), and went on to attend his son-in-law and successor in the county, the infante Alfons.[14]

(c) Roger, rector of Vallbona and chaplain to the infante Jaume, was ordered by his patron in 1315 to assist Domènech de Aladren, who had asked for a surgeon to treat his son's leg; Roger had earlier given surgical care to the infante's late mother Blanca. During 1316 and 1317 Roger continued to act as surgeon to the infante, who let some of his retainers travel to Vallbona to be treated there. By July 1318 he had died, leaving a remarkable surgical library and collection of tools.[15]

Such case studies suggest that the relationship between the church and medicine in 1300 was markedly different from what it is usually taken to be. It is easy, when reading surveys of the history of medieval medicine, to form the impression that by the end of the thirteenth century conciliar decrees had wholly prohibited the clergy from practicing medicine and especially (since it could entail the shedding of blood) surgery. Darrel Amundsen has recently gone back to the canon law itself to make clear what was and what was not prohibited, and

---

[13] C 86/24v; RP 620/142v; C 290/8; C 140/73v, 107r–v. Professor Jill Webster reports (personal communication) that he seems to be spoken of as dead in Oct. 1309 (C 289/134), yet his attendance on the king's nephew is apparently commanded in C 289/171v, dated 29 Sept. 1310.

[14] C 120/90; González Hurtebise, *Libros de tesorería*, p. 56, doc. 204; C 211/231v, 346/32v–33, 418/33v; RP 556/92v. The last reference I have found to him alive is dated 5 Feb. 1320 (C 364/39). This is perhaps the same Ramon de Vilalta who is recorded as physician in Puigcerdà, 1298–1301 (AHCP, Ramon de Caborriu Liber firmitatis 1298–9, 14 kls. Aug. 1298; Ramon de Coguls Liber extraneorum 1300–1, 2 kls. Mar. 1300/01).

[15] C 353/82, 298/112v, 362/40. Roger's death is reported 30 July 1318 (C 357/172); more details on his estate are in C 357/173v, 362/104, 165/51v. His nephew, master Nicholas the Englishman, requested payment of his inheritance 12 April 1319 (C 359/24); his books were given to the king's surgeon, Bernat Serra, 30 July 1319 (C 245/152; published in MF, II:205, doc. 283). On Roger's library, and Bernat, see below, p. 94.

he has argued that the restrictions were far less sweeping than is generally assumed.[16] By one part of the *Decretales* of Gregory IX (1234), regular clergy – that is, monks and canons regular – were forbidden to leave their cloisters to study medicine, though the text says nothing about their practice of the art. The *Super specula* of Honorius III (1219), also incorporated into the *Decretales*, extended the prohibition of medical studies (but not practice) to priests, deacons, and other beneficed clergy; subdeacons and clerics in minor orders were apparently not affected by the provision. Eventually the *Liber sextus* promulgated by Boniface VIII in 1298 softened the restrictions of the *Decretales*: it permitted parochial clergy (priests and deacons) to study medicine, and provided a means of dispensation to permit regular clergy to do so also. The *Decretales* also included the often-cited canon of the Fourth Lateran Council prohibiting the practice of surgery; but Amundsen has shown that the provision applied only to secular clergy in major orders, and only to their practice of "that part of surgery involving burning or cutting," leaving them canonically free to treat wounds, fractures, sores, and so forth. Thus, to summarize, in 1300 secular clergy in minor orders could study or practice medicine or surgery freely; some of those in major orders could study medicine, all could practice it, and all could practice many aspects of surgery. Monks and canons regular could now receive permission to absent themselves for medical study and could practice medicine or (if they were not in major orders) even surgery.

Amundsen's analysis is of the texts of canon law, and he has urged its supplementation by prosopographical studies. The three cases summarized here generally conform to his analysis. Alberto, the Franciscan, is found not studying medicine (which would have been canonically questionable) but practicing it; Ramon de Vilalta, canon and rector, is likewise unaffected by canon law in his practice of medicine. Even Roger, the rector of Vallbona with a surgical practice, was on canonically safe ground so long as he did not use the cautery or shed blood. All told, I have found archival testimony from the half-century before 1335 to the secular medical activity of six monks or clerics in major orders – four beneficed priests, one Benedictine monk of Sant Cugat (just north of Barcelona), and another man in an unidentified order – besides the three I have already mentioned. None of the testimony reveals a contravention of canon law as explicated by Amundsen.[17]

Why then did the medical role of the clergy diminish after 1300, if not because of ecclesiastical prohibitions? Certainly the lay public did not regard clerical

---

[16] Amundsen, "Medieval Canon Law."

[17] In the one case where a question of canonical legality might have arisen, Pere de Font, *ebdomadarius* in Sant Esteve de Palautordera, who was also a bachelor of medicine, sought and received permission from the bishop of Barcelona to return to a *studium* to carry his schooling further (ADB, Collationes 4, f. 18v; 27 April 1331). I know nothing more about Pere's career, in medicine or in the church.

practice as inherently unqualified or incompetent: as we have seen, clerical practitioners could build up a considerable public reputation among lay doctors and patients alike, not only locally but – as in the case of Brother Alberto – throughout the peninsula. In 1326, when at least twenty other physicians or surgeons were practicing in Barcelona, the city councilors begged that Brother Bertomeu des Pujol be allowed to come back to his order's convent in that city, for "he had had the treatment of many patients who say they were helped by his medical care."[18] Such clerics' lay associates in health care spoke no less respectfully of their skills.[19] As late as the 1340s the occasional priest famous for his medical knowledge may still be found consulting with *phisici* or *cirurgici* from the secular world – the prior of Solsona, who in 1348 joined Montpellier-trained Guerau de Sant Dionis and Bernat de Figuerola in treating the final illness of the infante Jaume d'Urgell, is a case in point.[20]

What was apparently responsible for the virtual disappearance of clerics as medical practitioners was neither canonical prohibition nor public mistrust but their displacement by a gradually increasing pool of secular physicians and surgeons. A heightened public perception that health care was desirable and in short supply, and a willingness to pay for it, were encouraging laymen to move into the medical occupations, all the more since entrance to them was still uncontrolled; no doubt some individuals simply called themselves *phisici* and hoped thereby to attract patients. Still, some degree of prior training already conferred a competitive advantage on a few would-be practitioners: insofar as the medical marketplace of the time offered them a choice, patients tended when possible to consult physicians in whose competence and technical knowledge they had reason to believe.

One indication of competence was membership in a local dynasty of practitioners. In some towns, generation after generation of a family would follow the same occupation, often for a remarkably long time – fathers teaching sons and bringing them into their practice, thus imparting to them not only skills but some measure of authority and reputation. The physician-surgeon Jacme d'Avinyó was in practice in Valencia by 1295; he had associated his son Jacme with himself by 1309, and it seems to be the son who is named as *phisicus* in documents of 1331 and 1338.[21] A "Jacme d'Avinyó *medicus*" appears again in

[18] "Cum per nonnullos quos . . . in diversis casibus morborum tenuit in cura, et qui ex eius medicinalibus operationibus dicunt se iuvamenta sensisse." La Torre, *Documentos*, p. [14]. The name of the order has been obliterated by water damage.

[19] See, for example, the praise for the care given by Brother Alberto to the infantes, expressed to the king by the apothecary Guillem Jordà (CRD Jaume II sin fecha 754).

[20] The "Prior Celsone" had been associated with Bernat de Figuerola in another medical case earlier in the same year (AHCM 178, document of 9 kls. Feb. 1348). On the treatment of Jaume d'Urgell, see further below, chapter 5.

[21] McVaugh, "Royal Surgeons." The father is the "Avinyó" consulted on the infanta Isabel's dental problems in 1313 (*AA*, I:346).

Valencia in 1352,[22] and this may or may not be the same as the Jacme d'Avinyó who was physician to the Valencian hospital of En Clapers in 1374–82, or the one still practicing in 1400.[23] Moreover, as a family became famous for its role in a health occupation, it evidently became profitable for several members to enter the craft in the same generation: during the half-century after 1285, no fewer than six members of the Vaquer family were practicing (some simultaneously) as barbers in the tiny Catalan town of Perelada (136 hearths in 1365).[24]

Family tradition thus undoubtedly acted to maintain or expand the pool of secular practitioners, but so did what has been called "occupational endogamy," the custom of marrying one's daughter to a man who practiced or would adopt one's own occupation. Such ties were by no means rare, especially among barbers' and apothecaries' families:[25] Bernat de Calidis, for example, apothecary of Barcelona (active 1330–8), divided his estate into thirds among the daughter of his dead son, Pere; his daughter Sança (m. Pere de Berga, apothecary of Barcelona 1321–38); and his other daughter, Gueraula (m. Francesc de Armentera, apothecary of Barcelona 1314–46).[26] For another example: the ça Riera family furnished the most successful surgeons of Gerona – we have already noted the king's dependence on one of them, Berenguer ça Riera, for medical as well as surgical counsel – but it was linked by marriage with the Moragues family, which had settled in Valencia and was producing surgeons

---

[22] On 8 Nov. 1352 "Jaime Aviñón, médico de Montpellier," bought (through a procurator) a house in Valencia: Olmos y Canalda, *Pergaminos*, doc. 2478.

[23] Rubio Vela, *Pobreza*, p. 122; Rubio Vela, *Peste negra*, p. 131.

[24] Bernat, 1284–1324; Jaume son of Pere, 1298; Jaume son of Guillem, 1300–2; Jaume son of Jaume, 1307; Pere, 1308–46; Guillem, 1310–26 (unfortunately, not enough information survives to construct a complete family tree). Another example is the Gensor family of Valencia, which produced a remarkable number of barbers in the thirteenth and early fourteenth centuries, only some of whom can be fitted into the following table of relationships (dates are those of documented practice):

Pere d' Aranya (1293–8)
|
Maria - - - Folquet Gensor (1299–1314)
|
Bernat Gensor (1314–21)   Guillem Gensor (1305–34)
|
Guillem Gensor (1325–36)

Many of these relationships can be established from the will of Maria, daughter of Pere d'Aranya, in ACV, perg. 4131 (Olmos y Canalda, *Pergaminos*, doc. 1479), of 14 March 1322, and perg. 1698 (ibid., doc. 1480), of 23 March. Other members of the family who cannot be placed on this chart are Miquel Gensor (barber of Valencia, 1318–36) and Ramon Gensor (barber there 1325–8).

[25] Certainly this practice seems to me to be less rare in the Crown of Aragon than Judith Brown believes it to have been in early modern (seventeenth-century) Florence ("Women's Place," pp. 211, 366). I suspect, however, that such marriages should be seen as a technique for establishing occupational solidarity in a competitive environment, rather than as evidence for the training of daughters in their fathers' occupation.

[26] Barcelona, Arxiu Parroquial de Sant Just, will of 1 Oct. 1338.

there. The ça Riera clan continued to be a surgical dynasty in Gerona throughout the fourteenth century.[27]

In such family settings, occupational training was undoubtedly carried on in an informal apprenticeship that passed insensibly into an associated or independent practice. We can probably infer the wider existence of informal apprenticeships, outside the immediate family circle, but not infrequently we find contracts drawn up to define more strictly the terms of training. It is worth emphasizing, however, that contracts for medical or surgical training are like contracts for other crafts, in that they never refer to the specific qualifications that apprentices would eventually possess. Their masters might occasionally have an academic degree, but learning was not necessarily part of the standard to which they themselves would be held: Paris-educated Pere Gavet, for example, merely undertook to teach Joan Cuto of Mallorca the art of medicine "as well as you are able to learn it."[28]

Yet another route besides these of family training and apprenticeship suggests how unimportant formal qualifications or certifications actually were for entry into medical practice. Concerned for the availability of medical care in his realms, Jaume II was, as we have seen, constantly trying to ensure the presence of practitioners who could serve him and his family as well as the public. In a variety of ways he did his best to entice foreign physicians and surgeons to move to his kingdom to settle and practice among his subjects – and he does not appear to have been concerned about their expertise, issuing permits without any verification of their credentials at all; he trusted instead to reputation or to a candidate's own self-assessment. Many permits were granted to Jews, perhaps because intolerance kept them constantly on the move: the royal safe-conduct given in 1325 to Mayer, a Jewish physician and surgeon of Perpignan, took him at his own valuation, though its tone is mildly non-committal:

> since he is as we hear skilled in the art of physic and surgery and other matters, and has humbly requested that we allow him to use his skill in the art in the kingdom of Aragon in treating those who believe he can do them some good, we permit him to come and treat anyone who desires it.[29]

But Christians, too, were encouraged and admitted to practice on their own say-so – like Pierre Ysnard of Grasse in 1323, "skilled in the art of surgery, who plans to move his residence to our realms and there practice the art of surgery for

---

[27] Guilleré, "Une famille."

[28] "Docebo vos scienciam medicine prout eam melius adiscere poteris": letter of 27 June 1329; ACB, manual de Bernat de Vilarrúbia, July–Sept. 1329, ff. 25v–26.

[29] "Sit ut accepimus in arte fisice et cirurgice et aliis officiis peritus, et nobis humiliter suplicaverit ut nobis placere dignetur ut in regno Aragonum artis et officiorum pericia possit uti in eos qui ipsius artem seu periciam sibi crediderunt posse prodesse": letter of 24 May 1325 (C 373/192v). Mayer had been granted a nearly identical permit 30 Sept. 1317 (C 356/60v).

our benefit and that of our subjects," to whom Jaume gave a permit allowing him to practice freely (*uti libere arte cirurgie predicte*).[30]

In only one – exceptional – case do we find the king granting permission to practice on the basis of written credentials. In Naples in April 1299, in the middle of the Sicilian campaign, Jaume issued a license to practice medicine to the Neapolitan physician Leonardo da Príncipe, who "has been certified as adequate and praiseworthy in the art of medicine by numerous testimonials from various medical masters of Naples, which he has shown to us."[31] Almost certainly, however, these testimonials were volunteered by Leonardo rather than demanded by the king. The form of Leonardo's credentials suggests that the Arabic *ijāzah* – a formal certification by a teacher that the bearer had read and studied with him and was qualified to teach and practice – may have continued to exist in southern Italy side by side with the procedures laid down by the Constitutions of Melfi;[32] in Sicily, unlike the Crown of Aragon, an Islamic learned tradition had been able to maintain itself within a Christian society. We have no evidence from Jaume II's own realms that letters testimonial were ever used as a means of certifying professional competence.

The spread of academic medical training

Though King Jaume may not have shown much concern for qualifications when he permitted practitioners to move into his kingdom, he had firm opinions as to what kind of medicine was desirable; Jaume II was a devoted patron of academic medicine in preference to mere empirical skill, and he did his best to raise the level of formal medical training in his realms. In 1291, when he began to reign in Aragon, academically formed physicians were rare, very much the exception rather than the standard or rule. In France, where medical education was available both at Paris and at Montpellier, Danielle Jacquart has been able to identify only forty-four medical graduates produced by these *studia* during the second half of the thirteenth century.[33] The faculties themselves were small: Montpellier apparently had only eleven medical masters in 1313, with perhaps

---

[30] Letter of 15 Oct. 1323 (C 180/190v–191).

[31] "Notum facimus . . . quod magister Leonardus de Principe fisicus civis Neapolitanus . . . ad nostram accedens presenciam per plures testimoniales litteras diversorum magistrorum in arte medicine de Neapoli quas nostri culmini presentavit ad eandem artem medicine sufficienter et laudabiliter extitit approbatus, propter quod de ipsius providencia et legalibus confisi . . . donavimus ei licenciam artem medicine ubique in civitatibus terris et locis nostro dominioni subiectis ac fideliter exercendi": letter of 29 April 1299 (C 113/153).

[32] The form of Leonardo's certification – apparently a collection of testimonials from a number of different masters – was not the usual license granted in the kingdom of Naples, which was an official document signed by one or two masters asserting that the licensee had been examined and found competent to practice. See Calvanico, *Fonti*, which itemizes over two thousand such licenses from the period 1290–1335 alone.

[33] Jacquart, *Milieu médical*, p. 365.

no more than five students beginning (which is not to say concluding) a course of medical study in any one year; in 1332 there were just seventeen *bacallarii in medicina* and twelve other *scolares* in the faculty available to sign an agreement.[34]

Precisely because it was uncommon, it is impressive to find Jaume II convinced of the advantages of a learned, book-oriented medicine and even surgery.[35] Throughout his life, as we have seen, he sought to acquire medical writings (in Latin or in Catalan), but even more importantly he was a major patron of learned practitioners. Down to about 1325, many of the physicians in the kingdom who can be identified as products of a medical faculty came at his request. Not surprisingly, they had virtually always been trained at Montpellier: it was the nearest school with a medical faculty,[36] and had been famous for more than a century; besides, Mallorcan-ruled Montpellier was in a sense a Catalan city. University learning was not merely a last hope in desperate cases – as suggested by the several royal summonses to the best Montpellier could offer, to Jean d'Alès (1302) and Jordan de Turre (1318, 1335)[37] – but something the king sought to have always available for routine care and counsel. From virtually the beginning of his reign, he chose – summoned – Montpellier-trained academics to be his principal household physicians: Arnau de Vilanova, Armengaud Blaise, Joan Amell.[38] Their permanent attachment to the court ensured that Jaume could count on all that modern medical learning had to offer.

---

[34] *Cartulaire*, I:287–8, 232.

[35] In early 1320 Jaume asked Pere Gavet, who had been trained in Paris (below, n. 61), for the latter's copy of a new Parisian book on surgery (Lanfranc? Henri de Mondeville?) – "nobis, sicut vos bene scitis, placeat habere huiusmodi nova opera" – so that he could read it and, if necessary, make himself a copy. The text is published in MF, II:235, doc. 315 (26 Feb. 1320), where the missing words appear (after inspection of the original) to be "facta est."

[36] The *studium* at Toulouse was closer than that at Montpellier, but it had not been given a medical faculty when it was set up in 1229; at the beginning of the fourteenth century, a moment when many Toulouse practitioners were ill-qualified, the *studium* was apparently seeking to institute one (Smith, *University of Toulouse*, p. 74; Wolff, "Recherches," p. 128). An enumeration of its faculties in 1311 does not include medicine, but another one two years later does (Fournier, *Statuts*, I:475). Rashdall, *Universities*, II:169 n. 3, suggests that medicine was not an important faculty at Toulouse before the fifteenth century.

Lynn Thorndike called attention to a fifteenth-century document that challenges this view of the Toulouse *studium*, a letter from a master of arts and medicine in Valencia, Pere Fagarola, giving advice to his sons studying at Toulouse and dated "1315" (*University Records*, pp. 154–60). Thorndike himself acknowledged that the copyist had first written "1415," and I believe that the later date is the correct one. No physician named Pere Fagarola has appeared after a systematic search of the Valencian documents from the first part of the fourteenth century, whereas (as again Thorndike noted) it *is* a medical family at the century's end.

[37] Above, chapter 1, pp. 11, 23, 34.

[38] I have so far found no proof that Amell studied at Montpellier, but it seems highly probable, given his origins. When Jaume II followed Armengaud Blaise's suggestion and invited Joan Amell to court, he addressed him as "magistro Johanni Aymelii de Bromio magistro et doctori in medicina" (letter of 24 May 1306; published in MF, II:22, doc. 36, where *afecciose* should read *afectuose*). He used the same phrase at least once again, 11 Sept. 1315: "Cum dilectus phisicus maior noster J. Amelii de Bromio medicine professor . . . accedat . . . ad Tholosanas partes pro

After 1325 we can identify a somewhat greater number of academic physicians practicing in the kingdom. The identifications are made possible by their tendency to insist upon their graduate status in legal documents: all practitioners normally prefixed "magister" to their names,[39] but those who also suffixed terms like "professor in medicinali sciencia" or "magister in medicina" were advertising their special claims to learning. This new generation of learned physicians includes several men who claimed, not a master's degree, but a preliminary one – "bacallarius" or "licenciatus" (table 3.1).[40] Such titles are

parentibus visitandis . . . " (C 156/240). We can interpret this, I believe, by linking it with Amell's claim to be of noble birth (above, chapter 1, n. 31). Among the nobles of the *baillie* of Castelnaudary who swore faith to Philippe III of France in 1271 was an "Amelius de Bromio" (Dossat, *Saisimentum*, p. 212). This must certainly be Joan Amell's close kinsman; hence the physician came originally from Bram (*département* of the Aude), between Toulouse and Montpellier, though closer to the former. He could not have received his medical degree yet from Toulouse, so Montpellier would have been for him as for everyone else in southern France or Catalonia the logical spot to study, and training there would explain the acquaintance with Armengaud that led to his being recommended to the king.

The question of Amell's origins is not yet fully resolved, however: in another letter he is referred to as "magister Joh. Amelii de Sancto Aniano" (3 Dec. 1313; C 210/117v), and his natural son Ramon is labeled similarly 10 Dec. 1339 (C 867/234v–235); what this refers to I have not yet discovered.

[39] The simple title "magister" had no particular academic significance in the Crown of Aragon and might be given to almost any occupation: e.g., a stone-cutter (C 93/244), a bowman (C 194/290), a veterinary (C 268/15v), or a glass-maker (AHPG/CE 48/27v).

[40] I list below the practitioners I have identified who assumed an academic title, together with the earliest year in which the title is given. I have not included in this list those individuals who are known only as masters at Montpellier or Lerida (Jordan de Turre, Guillaume de Béziers, Jaume d'Agramunt) and had no independent practice documented in the Crown of Aragon.

1300–9:	Bernat de Berriac, *magister in medicina* 1309
	Joan Amell, *magister in arte medicine* 1307
1310–19:	Alfonso de Burgos, *magister in medicina* 1311
	Bernat de Girona, *licenciatus* 1311
	Henricus Teutonicus, *medicinalis sciencie professor* 1310
	Gaufridus [= Rubeus?], *professor medicina* 1313
	Pere Gavet, *magister in arte et medicina* 1318
1320–9:	Guerau de Sant Dionis, *magister in medicina* 1322
	Guillem Salva, *bacallarius* 1329
	Maurat Vitalis, *professor in medicina* 1326
1330–9:	Berenguer ça Coma, *magister in medicina* 1332
	Berenguer de Torroella, *bacallarius* [1330s]
	Pere de Font, *bacallarius* 1331
	Pere Oliver, *bacallarius* 1334
1340–9:	Andreas sa Bench, *bacallarius* 1341
	Arnau ça Riera, *magister in medicina* 1344
	Berenguer de Prat, *bacallarius* 1342
	Bernat de Lemena, *bacallarius* 1349
	Joan Alacris, *licenciatus* 1346
	Michael Arlovino, *bacallarius* 1346
	Pere Ros, *magister in medicina* 1347
	Ramon Tesarach, *magister in arte et medicina* 1346

Berenguer Eymerich may have been a student at Montpellier in the 'teens (above, chapter 2, n. 46), but he never claimed a degree. It is curious and perhaps significant that the only

Table 3.1. *Academic medical titles assumed in the Crown of Aragon*

	1300s	1310s	1320s	1330s	1340s
Bacallarius			1	3	4
Licenciatus		1			1
Magister etc.	2	4	2	1	2

virtually unheard of in the first decades of the century, when the master's title was what mattered. By the second quarter of the century, on the other hand, *any* medical education was perceived to be worth advertising.

Still, the failure to claim a degree need not imply a lack of medical education. Bernat de Berriac appears in documents from Vic and Castelló d'Empúries from 1301 to 1308 with no hint that (as we know from other sources) he had almost met Montpellier's requirements for the mastership; then in 1309, having completed the requirements, he immediately assumed his new title.[41] Cases like his make it plain that at least a limited degree of medical education must have been more widely diffused than a simple count of academic degrees would suggest, especially for the first part of the century.

The career of one man in particular, Pedro Cellerer, shows the depth and extent of learned medical culture that can lie hidden behind the mere label, "phisicus." Pedro first appears in practice in July 1310 at Daroca, at the barren edge of Aragon, from which he was called hastily to attend Jaume II in Teruel, 100 kilometers to the south.[42] Teruel can have had few if any resident physicians, for the king simultaneously summoned to his side two doctors from Valencia, another from Barcelona, and one more from Xèrica. Within a few years the town councilors of Teruel had decided to meet this need, and promised Pedro a salary of 300 *sous* if he would move there and practice medicine – but, as he complained to the king in November 1316, though he had stayed there a year he had only been given a part of the salary agreed upon.[43] Daroca, where he had vineyards and other property (some of it held as the dowry of his wife Rama), remained throughout these early years his home and base, though in his practice he traveled throughout Aragon. Then in 1317 he moved from Daroca and settled in Calatayud, forty kilometers to the northwest, with a contract from the town that kept him nominally resident there for the rest of his life.[44]

individual who claimed a lower degree before 1325, Bernat de Girona, is also the only person I have found to have been ordered expelled from the kingdom for incompetent practice (ARV, Just. Val. 13, 3 id. Aug. 1312; C 241/86, letter of 28 Nov. 1313).

[41] McVaugh, "Bernat de Berriacho," pp. 241–2.
[42] Letter of 26 July 1310 (C 297/242v–243); RP 273/56v.
[43] Document of 22 Nov. 1316 (C 159/108v–109).
[44] The move to Calatayud can be dated from a letter of 6 July 1317 (C 162/294v).

In 1316, however, Pedro had begun what would be twenty years of intermittent medical service to the king's children when he attended the infante
Jaume and was taken formally under his protection.[45] Four years later he appears
briefly as physician to the infanta Maria,[46] and then in 1321 he began to act as
physician to the infante Joan, the twenty-year-old archbishop of Toledo;[47] Pedro
kept this position until Joan died in 1334. Brief visits to care for Joan (who was
translated to Tarragona in 1328), to advise on the health of his sister the infanta
Constança, or to treat his other sister, Blanca, in Sigena, could be accommodated
to Pedro's responsibilities to Calatayud, but on at least two occasions when
Pedro was needed to attend the archbishop the town councilors had to be asked
to release him temporarily from his promise to reside in the town. Apparently his
absences were not held against him, for in 1332 the council freed him and his
family of all taxes in consideration of his contribution to the health of the
community, a privilege confirmed to him by King Pere III in 1337 and reconfirmed after Pedro's death to his daughter Maria, in 1350.[48]

Attention has recently been called to a manuscript of Arnau de Vilanova's
Speculum medicine whose colophon was glossed to identify Arnau's birthplace
as Villanueva de Jiloca, seven kilometers southeast of Daroca in Aragon; the
gloss concludes, "his disciple was master Pedro Cellerer of Daroca."[49] This
casual reference conforms so well with our independent knowledge of Pedro's
career that it must be taken seriously, and indeed it helps us understand why
he was taken up by the royal family: it was presumably at Arnau de Vilanova's
recommendation. Indeed, two works attributed to Arnau, the *Antidotarium* and
the *De venenis*, now appear from internal evidence to have been completed
or compiled by Pedro Cellerer while he was practicing in Daroca.[50] We can
probably conclude that Pedro had been Arnau's disciple at Montpellier, where
the latter had taught 1291–1300 (and perhaps 1305–8); it does not seem likely
that Pedro would have had the opportunity to study with Arnau (who died in
1311) outside the setting of a medical faculty – that is, as an apprentice. But
because in legal documents he is never given a title such as "magister in
medicina" or "doctor" or "professor in medicinali sciencia," it is reasonable to
suppose that Pedro never actually completed a course of study to incept as a
master, though he may well have reached the level of *bacallarius* or *licenciatus*.

Here then we have a physician who, degree or no, carried academic medicine
into one of the more remote and barren corners of the Crown of Aragon, who
seems indeed to have considered himself a representative of learning more
generally. Shortly after settling in Calatayud, Pedro made a gift to the town of

[45] Letter of 7 March 1316 (C 354/79v).   [46] Letter of 24 Oct. 1320 (C 218/143r–v).
[47] Letter of 28 Sept. 1321 (C 246/276).
[48] Letters of 30 April 1337 and 6 March 1350 (C 861/229r–v and 890/142r–v).
[49] "Cuius discipulus fuit magister P. Cellerarius Darocensis": Benton, "Birthplace," p. 249.
[50] Arnau de Vilanova, *De dosi tyriacalium*, p. 66.

books and money with which to establish an endowment that could support students in medicine and theology.[51] Pedro's history is a vivid demonstration that learned medical culture, a reasonably thorough acquaintance with basic academic theory, was more widespread throughout the Crown of Aragon than our direct testimonies to the presence of medical training there would suggest.

The increased supply of academically trained physicians that seems to characterize the Crown of Aragon after the 1320s was apparently facilitated by Jaume II's foundation of a *studium generale* to serve his realms, one designed in part to make medical training available there as a supplement to Montpellier. "No university," as Hastings Rashdall remarked, "was more entirely the creation of a monarch's will."[52] After receiving authorization from Pope Boniface VIII to establish such a school, to which the pope promised all the privileges of the University of Toulouse, the king settled on Lerida in western Catalonia as its seat, a town where for a decade there had been agitation for a *studium*.[53] The charter of 1 September 1300 that established the new university explained that "our faithful subjects will no longer have to seek foreign lands to pursue the sciences," and provided for faculties in canon and civil law, medicine, philosophy, and arts; it promised the Leridan *studium* a monopoly on instruction in these subjects within the Crown of Aragon.[54] The new school was already functioning to a limited extent by the end of that month, when it elected its first rector, but there is reason to think that serious instruction there began only with the next academic year (running from St. Luke's Day, 18 October, to St. John's Day, 24 June). Jaume wrote a series of letters in July 1301 that in effect attempted to create a nuclear faculty: he invited Arnau de Costa to teach canon law, Pere Domènech to teach grammar, Ramon des Vilar to teach civil law, Ramon Mor de Castiello to act as banker to the students, and Jaume de Salmona to operate as the university bookseller ("stacionariam peciarum et librorum medicinalium et librorum iuris canonici et civilis").[55] No invitation to a medical master has yet turned up, but one was presumably sent to Guillaume Gaubert de Béziers, then a master at Montpellier, who was teaching in Lerida by November 1301.

In the first years of the *studium*'s existence Guillaume was its only medical master. He took up his responsibilities with seriousness and energy. Shortly after his arrival he gave notice of his desire to check the school's standard texts

---

[51] RL, II:37, doc. 42. Not all those who received the assistance valued learning as highly as Pedro; the town complained to the king in 1328 about a recipient who instead of studying was wandering about, squandering the income and scattering the books he had sworn to keep (ibid., I:81, 93–4; docs. 69, 76).

[52] Rashdall, *Universities*, II:92.

[53] Lladonosa Pujol, *Lérida medieval*, I:105; and see Rashdall, *Universities*, II:92 n. 1, who traces such agitation back to 1229.

[54] For a general account of what follows, see McVaugh and García Ballester, "Medical Faculty."

[55] Published by Gaya Massot, "Provisión de cátedras," pp. 281–4.

against the Arabic originals from which they had been translated or derived, and Jaume II was happy to help: at Guillaume's request, the king commanded in 1302 that

> because certain Arabic medical books belonging to Jews in our realms are needed to correct these medical texts . . . we command that whatever medical works written in Arabic may be required by this master shall be turned over to him by these Jews until he has had them translated or has used them to correct the other texts.[56]

How many students Guillaume actually had, however, we do not know. In early 1304, when a royal command sent him off on a trip to Montpellier, the councilors complained of his absence from the *studium* and insisted that he should at least summon a bachelor from Montpellier who could give his lectures in his absence,[57] so there were presumably at least some individuals there beginning their studies – but the school was certainly not large enough to support a master by student fees. By statute, Guillaume could receive no more than 20 *sous* from each student to whom he awarded the degree of master, and his students were still far from that stage; it was urgent, therefore, that the councilors meet their financial obligations to him, but as increasingly he was drawn away from Lerida by his attendance on the king, they resisted doing so. The situation was exacerbated by the interest of the bishop and chapter of Lerida in wresting control of the *studium* from the town, and between 1305 and 1310 the school seems to have closed; certainly Guillaume de Béziers left Lerida and by 1306 had returned to France.

The cessation of the *studium* at Lerida evidently encouraged Barcelona to think that the monopoly on higher education granted the Leridans by Jaume II was no longer in force. In November 1309 the bishop of Barcelona attempted to fill the void by decreeing the establishment of a *studium* where the liberal arts and "certain other permitted sciences and faculties" could be taught, apparently in order to unify administratively the diverse schools of arts in the city.[58] The language of the bishop's letter did not challenge the Leridan monopoly directly, since it did not specifically mention higher faculties like medicine or law, but by conferring the rectorship of the new *studium* on a medical master, Bernat de Berriac, the bishop seemed to be hinting at the possibility of creating a *studium generale* in Barcelona. The bishop's plan, in fact, had been instigated by Bernat, who after many years of practice in Catalonia had just completed his degree at Montpellier and seems to have been ambitious to return to an academic career.[59]

---

[56] RL, II:13–14, doc. 16.

[57] "Faceret ibidem venire infra certum tempus de Montepessulano unum bachallarium qui in eiusdem absencia lecciones suas continuaret": letter of 13 Feb. 1304 (C 235/18).

[58] Perarnau, "L'"Ordinacio'."

[59] McVaugh, "Bernat de Berriacho," p. 243.

In July 1310 the Barcelonan councilors announced to the king their plans to hire two masters who would lecture on law in the city; this was a still more open threat to the privilege granted to Lerida, and the larger and more cosmopolitan Barcelona might well have nurtured a university more successfully than the smaller inland town.[60] But soon thereafter the Lerida *studium* reopened, forestalling further institutional developments (although individual masters did continue to give instruction in fields beyond the liberal arts in Barcelona during the fourteenth century); indeed, Jaume II's formal restatement of the Leridan monopoly on education (in 1311) may have been called forth by the menace of competition from the Catalan capital.

The reopening of the *studium* was accompanied by a series of compromises that ended by again giving the town control over the university, and new invitations to come to Lerida to teach were sent out by Jaume II in July 1311. The king first asked the Paris-trained Pere Gavet to lecture on medicine, and then two months later approached the Montpellier master Bernard de Bonahora with the same request.[61] There is no evidence that anyone actually gave medical instruction there, however, until the year 1315–16, when Pere Gavet appears at the school. The town councilors seem almost immediately to have been dissatisfied with Gavet's performance in the *studium* (perhaps because, like Guillaume de Béziers before him, he was repeatedly called away to attend the royal family);[62] in 1317 they began to resist payment of his salary and the next year looked about for a lecturer with whom to replace him. Jaume II had to intervene several times with the town in 1318 and 1319 to try to force it to pay Gavet his back salary and allow him to lecture there as long as he chose. It was not a relationship with which Gavet could have been very happy, and by 1322 he had left Lerida and its *studium* for Barcelona, where for twenty years he was established as the city's leading representative of the world of medical learning.

The pool of academic physicians in Catalonia was still so small in the early 1320s, despite the king's efforts, that Lerida was unable to replace Pere Gavet with a fully accredited master. His successor was Pere Colom, who complained

---

[60] La Torre, *Documentos*, pp. [8–9], doc. 5. See Gaya Massot, "Por qué se retardó."

[61] The letters of invitation (C 208/20v) have been published by Gaya Massot, "Provisión de cátedras," p. 287. On Pere, see La Torre, *Documentos*, pp. [13–14]. The invitation to him may have come because he was originally from the Lerida region: in his will of 1345 (ACB perg. Div. A 2545) of 4 June 1345 he refers to many relatives in the Leridan diocese – his brother's son in Tabach, his sister's children in Torrebesses, and an apothecary cousin in Lerida itself. Pere's training at Paris is established by ADB, Not. Comm. 5/197: "Parisius licenciatus in septem artibus et in sciencia medicine professor." Bernard de Bonahora can be fixed at Montpellier 1313–20 (Wickersheimer, *Dictionnaire*, [I] p. 72). Luke Demaitre has suggested plausibly that Bernard is to be identified with the Bernard de Bona Fortuna whose commentary on the *Viaticum* is known in two manuscripts – both names would be translations of the French "bonheur" (see Wack, *Lovesickness*, p. 129).

[62] To the queen in Tarragona in February 1316 (C 300/100v–101), to the king in Montblanc in July 1316 (C 243/138v).

to the king in November 1324 that more than a year before the town councilors had promised him an annual salary of 600 *sous* to teach medicine in the *studium*, provided that he passed an examination for the master's degree within a fixed period. Now, he continued, the town was refusing to pay his salary because he had failed to take his degree – yet he had sought the necessary examination, and had failed to undergo it only because masters Joan Amell and Pere Gavet had never had the free time to come to Lerida to examine him.[63] In 1327 he was still trying to extract 900 *sous* in back pay from the town council.[64] Thus the Leridan *studium* had had in effect to settle for a medical student to teach other medical students, and there were not enough masters in Catalonia to assure him an examination at need.

The history of medical teaching at Lerida in the first quarter of the fourteenth century does not encourage us to believe that it could have contributed significantly to a growing practitioner population in the Crown of Aragon. Yet during the next fifteen years it was somehow transformed: a master's license granted there in 1344 to Arnau ça Riera, the third generation in a family of Geronan practitioners, reveals that by this time the Leridan *studium* had not just one but two medical masters – a Catalan, Jaume d'Agramunt, and an Englishman, Walter de Wrobruge. Arnau ça Riera had begun his medical studies at Montpellier in the late 1320s, when Lerida was still weak, but chose to return to complete the formalities in the Catalan *studium*, whose faculty showed new signs of intellectual achievement – nothing is known of Walter de Wrobruge (of Roborough?), but Jaume d'Agramunt finished a vernacular *Regiment de preservació de pestilència* in April 1348 (intended to protect his fellow citizens against the approaching plague) that drew on Avicenna and Rhazes, Galen and Hippocrates, and was carefully constructed upon a foundation of contemporary scholastic medicine.[65] Furthermore, there are indications in the language of Arnau's license that the Leridan faculty was now insisting that their discipline had the status of *sciencia*, true knowledge based on assured principles – an assertion that in more famous schools like Montpellier or Bologna had already helped claim greater intellectual authority and social prestige for the academically trained physician.[66]

Although we have no further evidence about Lerida in the 1330s and 1340s, what we do have is certainly consistent with what we have already inferred on other grounds: that in the twenty-five years before mid-century the prestige of medical learning was on the increase in the Crown of Aragon, as was the number of physicians there who could claim at least some training in a medical

---

[63] McVaugh and García Ballester, "Medical Faculty," pp. 16–18, doc. 1.
[64] Ibid., pp. 18–19, doc. 2.
[65] An edition was published in 1971 by Veny i Clar; Jon Arrizabalaga has in press a study of the work's content.
[66] McVaugh and García Ballester, "Medical Faculty," p. 9.

faculty.[67] It is not unreasonable to understand these developments as to some extent the consequence of Jaume II's interest in supporting and promoting academic medicine.

The diffusion of medical literature

The town of Vic lies sixty kilometers north of Barcelona. It is the center of a fertile plain at 500 meters' altitude, ringed by mountains, a relatively isolated community which from the late ninth century was free of Muslim incursions and became an early focus of Catalan intellectual and religious activity.[68] But by 1300 this isolation was less advantageous; its intellectual lustre had faded, and it was not attractive to academic physicians, who occasionally came to town only to move on quickly.[69] At the beginning of the fourteenth century it had perhaps four thousand inhabitants and one major physician, Guillem Galaubi, who had lived there since at least 1297 and died there in 1324.[70] There is no reason to think that Guillem, who chose to remain in Vic, had had extensive training in the thirteenth-century schools – he never claimed any sort of academic status – yet when he drew up his will he mentioned owning two books, a *librum de sententiis* and an "Evincena," the latter presumably part or all of Avicenna's encyclopedic *Canon*.[71]

Guillem's will is a further indication that even physicians who could not boast any sort of university degree tried to absorb or at least associate themselves with the new learned medicine. A certain number of these would have had at best an education in a local school of grammar, but there must have been a number who had had arts training, and some in this second group could have begun their medical education and then dropped out before they received their first degree – Ramon Ardey practiced medicine in Vic in the 1330s but could call himself only "bacallarius in artibus."[72] It is remarkable in how many small Catalan and Aragonese towns the teaching of grammar was given over to medical practitioners in this period: in Manresa to "magister Raymundus" in 1294; in Vic to João of Portugal before 1316; in Castelló d'Empúries to "magister Bremundus"

---

[67] The sophisticated learning represented at Lerida by the end of the century is suggested by the writings of its medical master Antoni Ricart: see Dureau-Lapeyssonnie, "L'œuvre."

[68] Freedman, *Diocese of Vic*, treats its history in the eleventh and twelfth centuries.

[69] Like Bernat de Berriac, who came to Vic in 1306 and left the next year; McVaugh, "Bernat de Berriacho," p. 241.

[70] The first evidence is from ACFV 59, 28 Jan. 1313, where a document refers to a debt to him contracted by the bishop and chapter of Vic on 8 July 1297; he was apparently originally from Saint Paul de Fenouilledes (Sant Pau de Fenollet), today in France (ACFV 38–III). He must have married his wife Saurina late, for her will was drawn up 8 Feb. 1368 (ACFV 3522/424).

[71] ACFV 244/44r–v (21 Dec. 1324): "Item dimitto fratribus minoribus Vicen. unum librum meum de sententiis . . . Item recognosco quod debeo P. de Surigeres ducentos sexaginta et quinque sol. ratione libri vocati Evincena."

[72] ACFV 225, 3 non. Oct. 1334.

in 1322, and to Ludovicus de Turri in 1323; in Besalú to "magister Petrus" in 1323; in Barbastro to Fernando de San Facundo before 1333.[73] These physicians (none of whom ever claimed a specific academic degree) did not generally stay long in their positions,[74] and perhaps we should understand them as men with an incomplete academic training who were using their skills in elementary education while hoping to launch into medical practice; they were one of the few visible representatives of the learned world in town.[75]

There were thus many physicians and even surgeons in the Crown of Aragon able to profit from technical medical literature, and insofar as that literature was available, a learned medicine could spread among the practitioner population independent of formal academic training. But how available was it? Luis García Ballester has called attention to the presence of collections of medical texts in the cathedral libraries of late-medieval Castile,[76] and similar materials were surely present in the Crown of Aragon. The Catalan cathedrals still preserve a number of medical codices: typically, they are fourteenth-century copies of texts and commentaries from the thirteenth-century curriculum.[77] Monasteries, too,

---

[73] Raymundus (perhaps Ramon Marini: below, n. 93) in AHCM, Llibres de consell 1, 11 kls. Dec. 1294; João of Portugal, ACFV 64, non. Oct. 1316; Petrus, AHCO, B–3, 5v (28 April 1323); Ludovicus de Turri, AHPG/CE 113/37v (23 Aug. 1323); Fernando de San Facundo, C 569/9 (1 June 1333). Bremundus (named as a physician AHPG/CE 113/42) hired an apothecary to act as his school's beadle, "as is done in the schools of Perpignan, Narbonne, and Montpellier" (AHPG/CE 40/22; 7 Oct. 1322). Petrus and João of Portugal had both subcontracted the grammar school out to someone else.

Physicians were still running the grammar schools of Cervera in the second half of the century (1355; 1373–7; 1398–1411); see Durán y Sanpere and Gómez Gabarnet, "Escuelas."

[74] An exception is Ramon Ferrer in Manresa 1322–34, but he was a surgeon rather than a physician.

[75] This pattern is suggested by the career of Pere Oliver of Perelada, who apparently had his bachelor's degree in medicine by 1334 (AHPG/P 53/130v); in 1341–2 we find him sharing the teaching responsibilities in the local *scolas gramaticales*, but he gave up the post in 1344, and when he appears next, during the 1348 plague, it is as Perelada's municipal physician (AHPG/P 70/125). As more representative of a generalized learning, consider the grant of a boy by his parents as a servant to a *medicus* for ten years in exchange for room, board, and the assurance of "docendo sibi literas" (AHPT 3826/67; 30 Aug. 1317).

[76] García-Ballester, "Medical Science," esp. pp. 190–5. This does not always distinguish between materials which are in the cathedral libraries today and those which were demonstrably there in the thirteenth century.

[77] Seu d'Urgell 2052 (13c) contains Isaac *De febribus, De dietis universalibus, De dietis particularibus*; Constantine's *Viaticum*; Gilles de Corbeil, *De pulsibus*; Hippocrates' *Regimen acutorum*.

Tortosa 234 (13c) includes an *antidotarium*; Platearius, *Herbolarius*; *Practica Bartholomei*; *Liber de gradibus* of Constantine; Galen, *De succedaneis*; Isaac, *Dietis particularibus*; *Antidotarium Nicolai* with Platearius' commentary. See also MS Tortosa 144, ff. 90v–95, containing Constantine's surgery. The collection is described by Bayerri Bertomeu, *Codices medievales*.

Gerona, Arxiu Capitular 75 (14c): glosses (by "Giles") on the *Viaticum*, Isaac *De febribus* and *De dietis universalibus*, and the *Regimen acutorum*; the *Astronomia Ypocratis*; Gerard of Montpellier, *De modo medendi*; Arnau de Vilanova, *De flebotomia* and *Medicationis parabole* (notes on f. 80v show assimilation of Arnau's peculiar techniques for calculating a medicine's qualitative strength).

Gerona, Arx. Cap. 76 (14c): glosses on Isaac *De dietis universalibus* and on Hippocrates'

held medical works in their libraries, which the laity sometimes made free with.[78]

A more solid index to the availability of books comes from our knowledge of personal libraries, libraries revealed when executors inventoried an estate. Even though a detailed account of their contents is not always given, there is enough evidence to make it clear that academically trained physicians often possessed sizable numbers of books. Maurat Vitalis of Castelló d'Empúries, master of medicine from Montpellier, died in 1346 and left twenty-two books "tam medicinales quam naturales quam etiam gramaticales" to his son Pere.[79] The widow of Guerau de Sant Dionis of Gerona, also a university master, sold his books in 1349 to a *bacallarius de medicina* from Montpellier, Bernat de Lemena, for more than 350 *sous*.[80]

The earliest important practitioner-inventory that has survived from the Crown of Aragon is that of the possessions of Arnau de Vilanova, drawn up shortly after his death in 1311. The enumeration of his books – over a hundred of them, of which perhaps thirty are medical or scientific – suggests the types of medical literature then available in our region.[81] There is represented there, first, the Salernitan and Constantinian literature that had been the staple of medieval study down to the middle of the thirteenth century: Gariopontus' *Passionarius*, Isaac's *Liber febrium*, the *De urinis* of Gilles de Corbeil. Then there are the new translations from the Arabic of the late twelfth and thirteenth centuries which were coming to constitute a new medical curriculum, mostly works of Galen (*De interioribus*, *De differenciis febrium*) but also including Avicenna's *Cantica* in its recent translation by Armengaud Blaise. Finally, there are the attempts of contemporary scholastic medicine to digest and develop the Greco-Arabic sources. Arnau's library evidently contained treatises and commentaries by other authors of his generation – Bernard Gordon's *Lilium medicine* seems to be there[82] – but not surprisingly his own contributions to this genre are particularly well represented: commentaries on Hippocratic aphorisms ("Ars longa," "In

---

Prognostics and *Aphorisms*; Platearius' commentary on the *Antidotarium Nicolai*; Gilles de Corbeil, *De pulsibus*.

Gerona, Arx. Cap. 80 (14c): Rhazes' *Almansor* and Ricardus Anglicus' *De medicinis repressivis*, with some Catalan notes in a fourteenth-century hand.

It is noteworthy that the Catalan libraries occasionally contain the scholastic commentaries that García Ballester did not find in Castile.

[78] Pere de Vilanova, the *medicus monasterii* at Poblet (Cistercian), asked for protection from the king's retinue for his books and medicines: C 887/36v (1 Aug. 1346). This man was perhaps the nephew of Arnau de Vilanova: see Santi, *Arnau de Vilanova*, p. 51.

[79] His will is in AHPG/CE 215/9 (21 Jan. 1346); the inventory made on 6 Feb. (ff. 10v–11), after his death, gives the number of books but no titles.

[80] AHPG, Notari 3–1, 3 Dec. 1349, where the buyer acknowledges that that sum remains to be paid.

[81] A résumé is given by Carreras Artau, "Llibreria"; the basic text is published by Chabás, "Inventario," which I have emended in some respects after examining the original (ACV, pergaminos 7430; Olmos, *Pergaminos*, doc. 1410). See also d'Alós, "De la marmessoria."

[82] McVaugh, "Nota," p. 332.

morbis minus"), theoretical writings (his *Speculum medicine, Aphorismi de gradibus, De intentione medicorum*),[83] and clinical compendia for the guidance of his royal and ecclesiastical patrons (*Medicationis parabole, Regimen sanitatis ad regem Aragonum, Practica summaria*).[84] Arnau was unusually ambitious for learning, certainly, yet other medical libraries of the time reveal, on a smaller scale, exactly the same combination of Greek and Arabic texts, practical compendia, and recent European scholarship.[85]

This list is not merely of interest as showing the sort of library one man might accumulate; it implies something, too, about the potential for circulation of books in the Crown of Aragon. Arnau's executor put some of his medical books on sale in Valencia, and they brought in modest sums: 30 *sous* for his *chef d'œuvre*, the *Speculum medicine*; 15 *sous* each for the *Cantica* and *De interioribus*; 6 *sous* for the *Liber febrium*; and only 2 *sous* for *De differenciis febrium*. These prices seem low, but they are not utterly out of keeping with the little we know about the value of medical books in Catalonia.[86] Indeed, some people there perceived the market for medical books to be so poor that they preferred to ship them to Montpellier to be sold.[87] Yet this meant that medical writings were within the means of practitioners who wished to acquire them.

To be sure, men who had not spent years in a *studium* had fewer opportunities to collect books, and their libraries are consequently smaller than Arnau's; but even so they show the same range of interests, while often testifying to an interest in learning that is not just narrowly medical. The books pledged with an apothecary, Bernat Quer, in tiny Besalú in 1325 included Johannitius, Gilbertus Anglicus, Bernard Gordon's *Lilium medicine*, Walter Agilon, Rhazes' *Almansor*, a volume of Galen's writings, and the surgical textbook of Teodorico Borgognoni.[88] Pere d'Arenys bought and sold books of many kinds during his

---

[83] Chabás' item 38 should read "Item unus liber de gradibus medicine" (he could not make out the last two words); his item 39 misreads "institutione" for the inventory's "intentione" [intñtõe]).

[84] For a survey of this material, genuine and otherwise, see Paniagua, *Arnau de Vilanova*, esp. pp. 46–64.

[85] Another extraordinarily rich medical library is that of Sanç del Miracle of Valencia, itemized in his will of 4 kls. June 1351 (ARV, protocolos 2959): it included, among other works, Avicenna's *Canon* (with commentaries), Averroes' *Colliget*, Avenzoar, Aristotle's *De animalibus*, many works of Galen – and the *City of God*.

[86] D'Alós, "Marmessoria," pp. 303–4. Compare these prices with the few other instances where we have concrete information: four medical books pawned for 170 *sous*, then sold outright for 210 *sous* (below, n. 89); two unidentified books – one on medicine, the other on surgery – pawned for 44 *sous* in 1309 (AHPG/CE 26/18v); the *Canon* sold at auction for 300 *sous* (below, n. 93). Not surprisingly, bigger books seem to have cost more (Arnau's *Speculum* runs to nearly forty folios in sixteenth-century editions).

[87] In his will, setting out his executors' responsibilities, the physician Gundissalinus Petri noted, "verum cum libri artis seu sciencie mee in civitate Barchinone invendibiles sint, rogo et supplico quod ipsos libros . . . non . . . hostendant in ipsa civitate set in quodam cofro clauso ad montem pesulanum mittant et ibi eos vendant seu vendi faciant prout melius poterunt": ACB, manual de Bernat de Vilarrúbia, wills 1308– , ff. 147–8 (21 June 1334).

[88] Grau i Monserrat, "Medicine a Besalú," pp. 108–10.

documented years (1297–1308) in Castelló d'Empúries; at his death his estate contained at least four medical works, including Mesue, Jean de Saint-Amand, and "Gilabert."[89] Pere Franch (active at Santa Coloma de Queralt 1317–29) left, among other items, Platearius' commentary on the *Antidotarium Nicolai*; a Hippocrates; Isaac on fevers; an unspecified Galen; and a work on urines and pulse.[90] Pere d'Arenys' library was sold as a unit (through a Geronan apothecary) in 1319 to Pere Bos of Castelló for 210 *sous*; Pere Franch's was passed on intact to his son when the boy reached his majority in 1340, and it was then apparently dispersed. Such proofs of dissemination or recirculation are reinforced, more summarily, by the many surviving accounts of unidentified medical libraries or books passed on to new owners by sale, bequest, or theft,[91] while even accounts of the loss of medical manuscripts help convince us of their wide distribution.[92]

Two authors are particularly prominent in the medical literature known to have circulated in the kingdom. One is Avicenna, whose name is often used, by metonymy, for an unidentified book – almost surely his encyclopedic *Canon*, which is also identified by name a number of times.[93] This work was evidently widely accepted as the most useful guide and reference to medical practice. King Jaume II's enthusiasm for the book is a measure of its public reputation: he

---

[89] This statement assumes that the "Petrus de Aregnis phisicus" found in Castelló 1297–1308 and there dealing in books (e.g., an "Innocent," 6 kls. May 1301 [AHPG/CE 75]) is to be identified with the "Petrus de Bel Soleyl de Arenis phisicus quondam" whose books, named above, were bought by Pere Bos (16 Nov. 1319; AHPG/CE 98/50v). Simply as an indication of circulation, it is interesting to recognize that the book entitled "Jean de Saint-Amand" must be a Parisian work no more than fifty years old, and probably much less.

[90] The document (AHPT 3845, loose leaf) is incomplete. "Hec bona habuerunt March. Denam et Bng. Continyach. Confitentur Bn. Olz. etc. quod habuerunt ab ipso hec bona infra scripta que fuerunt magistri Petri Franch quondam, videlicet unum librum de paper medicine cum postibus, item unum librum cum coperta vermilia, que incipit liber iste quem legendum proponimus etc., item alterum librum vocatum arts dipocras, item alterum librum vocatum febres disach, alterum librum de galie, item alterum librum dorines et de pols, item unum librum de natures, item sextum librum degratalium, item unum librum vocatum istituta, item librum vo." (The contents are summarized by Segura, "Aplech," p. 175.) A document on the reverse of this sheet bears the date 4 non. Sept. 1332. Pere Franch was in Santa Coloma by 1317 (AHPT 3826/67, where he acquires a servant to whom he promises to teach his letters); his will was drawn up 13 May 1328 (AHPT 3836/47r–v). The fate of the library is described in AHPT 3860/23 (21 April 1340).

[91] Arnau Amell, surgeon of Carcassonne, dying in Castelló in 1331 ordered his books to be sold there to redeem captives (AHPG/CE 150/21v; 28 June 1331); Thomas Anglesii of Lerida was robbed in 1330 of an unnamed medical book (RL, I:110, doc. 83); Bertomeu de Bonells left medical books worth 1,000 *sous* which were part of his daughter Agnes' dowry (AHCV, misc. loose sheets xiv, kls. Nov. 1349).

[92] Bernard Marini lost books in a shipwreck (C 294/65v–66, 15 Aug. 1302); Ulrich of Germany lost a book to water damage when his mule fell in the river (C 149/128; 27 March 1312).

[93] In addition to those mentioned elsewhere: "una Avicena" was pawned by a *fisigo* of Zaragoza 12 May 1346 (AHPZ, manual de Miguel de Almenara, f. 11v); the *Canon* left by Ramon Marini *phisicus* of Manresa 1297–1303 was exposed for sale in Barcelona in 1304 and auctioned for 300 *sous* (AHCM 33, 2 kls. Nov. 1304).

himself owned a copy, and he bought others for the use of his medical staff.[94] The *Canon*'s popularity was already established in medical schools in the 1290s. In that decade Arnau de Vilanova wrote scornfully of his colleagues' worship of "their god Avicenna": "they boast of poring over his huge volume . . . and chatter on and on in his name as though they have forgotten the text itself, or as if it were enough for them to see or read or show off the great bulk of the volume on their shelves."[95] Elsewhere Arnau emphasized his independence of Avicenna by arguing that the *Canon* had misunderstood the solid truth of Galenic doctrine, and the curriculum he helped design in 1309 for Montpellier stressed the reading of Galenic texts with only an incidental role for the *Canon*.[96] Nevertheless, Arnau was far from lacking in respect for Avicennan medicine. We cannot show that the *Canon* was a part of his library – the only Avicennan work there is Armengaud's translation of the *Cantica* – but we *can* show that Arnau drew on the *Canon* (usually without acknowledgment) for ideas which he elaborated in his own theoretical works of the 1290s. His *De intentione medicorum* makes regular use of Avicennan examples and language in defending a medical instrumentalism;[97] his translation of Avicenna's *De viribus cordis* evidently brought home to him the importance of *forma specifica*, a concept that played a central role in his doctrine of pharmacological activity.[98] Neither the theoretically nor the clinically oriented practitioner could afford to neglect the *Canon*.

The other author of obvious popularity was Teodorico Borgognoni, the disciple and perhaps son of the innovative Bolognese surgeon Ugo of Lucca. Teodorico entered the Dominican order and under Innocent IV was appointed first papal penitentiary, then bishop of Bitonto (1261), and finally bishop of Cervia (1266); nevertheless, much of his career was spent in Bologna, teaching medicine and surgery. While at the papal court he served as chaplain to another Dominican, Andrés Albalat, for whom he drew up a rough account of his

---

[94] The king gave his copy as a pledge to his surgeon Berenguer ça Riera, who promptly pawned it for 500 *sous*; Jaume found the money to reclaim it two years later. He subsequently paid for personal copies for both Berenguer and Martí de Calça Roja (McVaugh, "Royal Surgeons"; and above, chapter 1, n. 39).

[95] "In cuius magno volumine se studere gloriantur . . . et . . . eciam ipsi sepissime garriunt auctoritate illius: unde videntur immemores documenti, aut videtur quod reputent se contentos si videre aut legere possint et in magnis cathedris sarcinam voluminis ostentare": Arnau de Vilanova, *De consideracionibus*, p. 196. The sarcastic reference to Avicenna as "eorum deus" is on p. 245.

[96] For treatments of Arnau's view of Avicenna (and Arabic medicine in general), see Paniagua, "L'Arabisme," and García Ballester, "Arnau de Vilanova," esp. pp. 141–5.

[97] McVaugh, "Medical Certitude," pp. 75–9.

[98] The properties governed by specific form, wrote Arnau, had been discovered by divine inspiration rather than human reason, "sicut scribit Avicenna super tiriaca et metridato in tractatu de viribus cordis et medicinis": Arnau de Vilanova, *Repetitio*, f. 278va. On the doctrine, see also below, chapter 7 at n. 36.

master Ugo's teaching as modified by his own practice. Andrés carried this version off to Spain when he was named bishop of Valencia in 1248, but he subsequently asked Teodorico to send him a corrected text; the latter, now known as Teodorico's *Chirurgia*, was completed after 1264.[99] The work is distinguished not only by its practical and empirical cast, but by its obvious interest in embedding surgical treatment in a framework of Galenic doctrine, drawn in large measure from Avicenna's *Canon*. Perhaps partly because two versions had become available in Valencia by 1270, the *Chirurgia* soon circulated widely in the Crown of Aragon and enjoyed a particular esteem among the surgeons of the region. One anecdote is especially telling: planning for his old age, a surgeon from Foix agreed to teach a Geronan surgeon all he knew about their common craft in exchange for food and clothing, and also to turn over immediately to the younger man all his books – with the exception of "uno Tedricho," which he insisted on retaining himself until he died.[100]

A further measure of the *Chirurgia*'s popularity in northeastern Spain is its remarkably rapid translation into Catalan, at a moment when vernacular medical translation was still unusual anywhere in Europe. A Catalan version had been produced by 1305, apparently by the Valencian surgeon Guillem de Correger (perhaps in Montpellier),[101] and a copy of this version was in the possession of

[99] Karl, "Théodoric de l'ordre des prêcheurs," pp. 151–2. A two-volume English translation by Eldridge Campbell and James Colton is available as *The Surgery of Theodoric* (New York, 1955–60).

[100] AHPG/CE, 24/22 (2 June 1305).

[101] The study by Contreras, "Difusión," presents much useful information but needs development and correction. Contreras has concluded that the two complete manuscripts of the Catalan version (one in Paris and one in Graz), which appear to be ascribed to two different authors, contain different translations, but a comparison of the excerpts he transcribes from them (pp. 56–7) suggests to me that it is basically a single Catalan version that is in question; so does the edition (from both MSS) of the translation of Teodorico's prologue given in Karl, "Theodoric der Katalane," 262–6. By looking more closely at the text of the two ascriptions we can imagine what may have happened. The Graz colophon reads, "Aquest libre fo fenit en Maylorcha en l'any de M.CCC.X., esmanat per maestre Bernat, metge del senyor Rey de Malorques" (Perarnau, "Hypotesi," 280), while the translator's introduction to the Paris version describes him as "G[uillem] Correger de Mayorcha aprenent en la art de cirurgia." Now Guillem Correger is a known historical figure, a surgeon who left the Crown of Aragon in 1302 to study surgery (C 125/96v), almost certainly at Montpellier (in the kingdom of Mallorca); he is not heard of again in Aragonese territories until 1308. (On Guillem and his apparent role in the attempt to make surgery a more "learned" art, see McVaugh, "Royal Surgeons.") It seems reasonable to conclude that Guillem's text was finished at some point before 1310 and then reworked – "esmanat" – by "master Bernat" (who Pernarnau speculates may be the physician Bernat de Berrica), thus creating the two versions that now survive.

A parchment dated 6 id. Jan. 1304 (= 8 Jan. 1305; ACB perg. Div. C [e] 804) refers to "quendam librum medicine sive cirurgie in papiro scriptum" of sixty-five leaves, "et incipit sic: Es contengut en lo primer capitol los menbres de que es major tener; et finit in ultima carta: la sobre scrita cura sapies que es molt profitosa e bona." If a comparison of these passages with the Catalan Teodorico should show that they are from that work (and I know of no other Catalan-language surgery at this early period),we would have to acknowledge that Guillem's translation had already been completed by 1304.

the Crown's Templars as early as 1307.[102] Another had arrived in Castelló d'Empúries before 1326 and was owned by an apothecary, Bernat de Llampaies, who had sufficient medical expertise to be contracted by the town to give medical prognoses to its citizens.[103] Arnau de Vilanova and the surgeon Bernat Serra are two other practitioners known to have owned copies of Teodorico's work.[104] To find a text situating surgical practice in Galenic doctrine in the hands not only of surgeons but of physicians and apothecaries as well reveals the extent to which a learned medical culture was becoming the common property of practitioners at many different levels.

In fact, one of the most impressive Catalan medical libraries for which an inventory survives is not a physician's but a surgeon's – the library of the Bernat Serra just mentioned, whose family came from the region of Vic but who had established himself in practice in Barcelona by 1317, soon entered royal service, and died there in 1338.[105] Early in his career as surgeon to Jaume II Bernat asked the king for the books of the rector of Vallbona, Roger, who had just died, and who had also been a practicing surgeon (above, p. 73). Roger's books probably constituted the core of Bernat's collection, which included, first, every one of the works of the new Italian surgery of the previous 150 years, together with the principal Arab authorities: the texts of Roland, Teodorico, Roger, Bruno, and Lanfranc, and the glosses of the Four Masters, as well as Abulcasis and Rhazes. But it also included an astonishing set of medical treatises that is as extensive and varied as can be found in any contemporary physician's library: Constantine's *Viaticum*, Hippocrates' *Aphorisms*, Rhazes' *Almansor*, Jesus Haly's *De oculis*, Serapion's *Aggregator*, Galen's *Megategni*, Macer's *De viribus herbarum* – bringing together encyclopedic and specialized literature, preventive and therapeutic, traditional authorities and recent translations (the *Aggregator* had

---

[102] A record of the Templars' copy was made in that year when the order's possessions passed into the hands of Jaume II (Villanueva, *Viage literario*, p. 200); it was still in the king's possession in 1323 (Martorell, "Inventari," p. 562). It began "En nom de Deu comença lo Tedrich" and ended "val mes que d'altre e pebre un poch."

[103] Bernat was already established in Castelló as an apothecary in 1294 (AHPG/CE 74; 9 kls. Oct. 1294), and soon had a working relation with a local physician, to whom he promised to refer all his customers (AHPG/CE 16/28; 3 Feb. 1296). His agreement with the town read: "quamdiu residenciam fecero in villa Castilionis bene et legaliter pro posse meo videbo et iudicabo omnes urinas que mihi apportabuntur" (AHPG/CE 113/34; c. 17 Aug. 1323). After Bernat's death, his son gave a kinsman "quendam librum vocatum Tederich," beginning "En nom de la santa et denopartida trinitat" and ending "quant hom ne levera lespatula": AHPG/CE 122/37 (28 Oct. 1326).

[104] Arnau – who had grown up in Valencia during Andrés Albalat's episcopacy – owned a copy of the Latin *Chirurgia*: a partial list of his books in ACV, pergaminos 9402, includes "Cirurgia tederici in pergameno et latino scriptus" (d'Alós, "Marmessoria," p. 304; in Chabás, "Inventario," the same work appears [#70] without indication of idiom). Bernat Serra of Barcelona also owned at least one copy of the work, but whether in Latin or Catalan is uncertain: Carreras Valls, "Bernat Serra," pp. 21–2.

[105] McVaugh, "Royal Surgeons."

been translated only by the 1290s).[106] Whatever the relative roles of Roger and Bernat in assembling this collection, one and perhaps both must have been imbued with this culture of medical learning that was coming to permeate not just medicine but surgery too in the early fourteenth century.

Towards regulation of medical practice

Given what we have already detected – an increase in the number of academically trained medical practitioners in the Crown of Aragon, especially pronounced after 1330 – it is perhaps not surprising that procedures were announced in the 1330s that formally recognized such training as a qualifying standard. These procedures were now on a national scale and had an evident effect in the larger cities. Both Catalonia and Valencia introduced at this time what amounts to a system of licensing for physicians, one that presupposed several years' study in a faculty of medicine (or its equivalent). Their attempts to implement such medical supervision prepared the way for the eventual establishment of health professions in the kingdom.

In Valencia the innovation appears abruptly in the *furs* promulgated by Alfons III in 1329–30, whose chapter "De metges" sets out seven provisions regulating medical behavior.[107] Three of these have to do with concrete aspects of day-to-day professional activity: the requirement that surgeons provide expert testimony when asked for it by a competent authority; the insistence that every practitioner, physician or surgeon, take an annual oath not to treat a gravely ill patient if the patient has not already confessed; and the requirement that medical recipes be drawn up in "Romance," naming the different ingredients not in Latin but in Catalan to render them more easily understandable by apothecaries. But the other four provisions define the route leading through examination to practice, whether for physicians, surgeons, or indeed barbers. The fundamental part of this legislation comes at the beginning:

> We command and ordain that the justiciar and the *jurats* elect, every year, three days before Christmas, two leading physicians who shall be the examiners of all the practitioners of physic who have recently come to practice in the city or in the towns of the kingdom; and those whom they find competent, and who have followed the art of medicine for at least four years in a *studium generale*, shall be admitted to practice the said art, and if not they shall not be admitted. And if they practice without the said examination and license, they shall be liable to a fine of 100 gold *morabatíns* for each occasion, of which a third part shall go to the court, a third to the town, and a third to the accuser.

---

106 AHPB, manual de Pere Folqueres, May–Sept. 1338, pp. 134–41; publ. in Carreras Valls, "Bernat Serra."

107 Some of what follows is developed more fully in García-Ballester, McVaugh, and Rubio-Vela, *Medical Licensing.*

Those who wished to practice surgery had also to undergo examination by the medical tribunal, although they were not required to have had medical studies, and this requirement of supervision via examination was further extended to barbers who hoped to practice medicine or surgery: "no barber shall practice medicine or surgery if he has not been examined by the examiners of practitioners and found competent." As for the physicians who at the moment when the new provisions were approved were already practicing medicine or surgery, they were required to prove their suitability before the examiners, and those who did not pass the tests were to be disqualified.[108]

The fourteenth-century records of the Valencian council list the medical examiners virtually without interruption after 1336. Those elected for the first four years on record –

1336	Bertomeu Casaldòria (phys.)
	Pere Correger (surg.)
1337	Berenguer Eymerich (phys.)
	Francesc ça Bruguera (surg.)
1338	Bertomeu Casaldòria (phys.)
	Jacme d'Avinyó (phys.-surg.)
1339	Berenguer Eymerich (phys.)
	Pere Correger (surg.)

– manifest what seems originally to have been a conscious plan: to select one physician and one surgeon each year, preferably ones who had long been in practice; they could be re-elected to the office.[109] From the years before 1336 – that is, for the first seven years after the issuance of the *furs* – there survives no municipal list of examiners, but materials of other sorts from that earlier period make it apparent that the *furs* were already in effect and that examiners were available to judge the qualifications of would-be practitioners. Such materials also suggest that the *furs* were from the outset less prescriptive than they might now seem – that is, that they indicated an ideal that was not often enforced.

The case of Ramon sa Lena, for example, indicates that outside the capital, medical care of any sort was so scarce that the new legislation could be perceived as a threat to public health. Ramon had been an apothecary in Borriana (on the

---

[108] The 1329 regulations bear a strong generic resemblance to the ordinances of Valls from 1299 and 1319: compare the Valencian text in *Medical Licensing*, pp. 59–60, with the fragments from the Valls documents cited above, n. 7.

[109] Bertomeu Casaldòria evidently had some medical reputation when he was called to care for Ruggerio II di Loria in 1321 and 1323 (C 172/172v, 223/284v); he was named examiner again in 1343. Francesc ça Bruguera appears in Valencia as "medicus" in 1311 and 1317, but is usually called "cirurgicus" after 1320; he was named examiner again in 1346. On Pere Correger, see McVaugh, "Royal Surgeons"; he was in practice by 1318 and was named examiner again in 1342. All were still living in 1347. On Jaume d'Avinyó and Berenguer Eymerich, see above, p. 75 and chapter 2 n. 46.

coast, forty kilometers north of Valencia) since at least 1328, but in the absence of any other practitioners he had also provided medical care to the public, and in 1332 he was accused of violating the recent *furs*. Absolved by the justiciar of Valencia, he nevertheless appealed to the king for positive endorsement of his medical activity – asking, in effect, for a license. His appeal was supported enthusiastically by one of his patients, Guilabert de Centelles, lord of Nules (five kilometers outside Borriana), who pointed out to the king that the local population had no one else to attend to their medical needs and without Ramon would have to travel to Valencia for care; on these grounds the king agreed that Ramon should be allowed to practice freely.[110] This scarcely encourages us to think that – at least in the countryside – the provisions of the Valencian *furs* were looked on approvingly, or had much effect.

The suit brought against master Jacme Lama in 1334 suggests the very different context of medical care in the city of Valencia proper. Jacme was perhaps the son of "maestre Lama," the latter a physician of Valencia active between 1279 and 1304 who treated both Pere II and Jaume II. The notary Miquel de Roures accused Jacme of having practiced medicine in Valencia for about three years without having been examined and licensed by the municipal examiners or having studied medicine for four years in a *studium generale*; of having split fees with apothecaries; and of having written prescriptions in Latin – all contrary to the provisions of 1329. The report of the charges also preserves Jacme Lama's defense: he pleaded (1) that clerical orders removed him from civil jurisdiction, and (2) that Miquel de Roures was not a proper plaintiff, since he was not directly affected by the case and moreover himself stood accused of a crime (theft). Unfortunately we do not know how the case was resolved, but it is clear that it did not end by excluding Jacme from the practice of medicine, for he was still being described as "metge" in June 1335 and indeed as late as 1347.[111] There is no suggestion that the other physicians of the city found him unqualified; as he himself emphasized, his accuser de Roures had no professional concern with the case, and in fact other evidence hints that the accusation had been made simply as an episode in a family vendetta. This seems to be the only fourteenth-century complaint against someone for contravening the provision "De metges," nor is there even proof of a municipal license having been issued on the basis of an examination before 1378, when one was granted to a Jew, Içach Çaroxel·la.[112] All in all, the evidence does not suggest that the legislation of 1329 was of immediate impact in the city any more than it was in the countryside.

In Catalonia there was apparently no new legislation corresponding to the Valencian *furs*. Even so, it is plain that practice was evolving in the 1330s along

---

[110] García-Ballester, McVaugh, and Rubio-Vela, *Medical Licensing*, pp. 19–20.

[111] Ibid., pp. 22–3.   [112] Ibid., pp. 68–71.

a variety of lines towards at least local control of medicine and licensing. It is plausible that the Valencian example was the stimulus behind events and that it encouraged both ecclesiastical and secular authorities in Catalonia to revive their earlier concern for medical regulation.

The church in Catalonia had forbidden Christians to take medicines from Jews, for fear of poison, for nearly a century, but there is no evidence that it had ever tried to enforce this. In the early 1330s, however, this tolerant attitude ended abruptly, and Jewish physicians of Barcelona began to appeal to the bishop for permission to practice under supervision. The first to do so, Vidal Habib, was told in May 1332 by Bishop Ponç that, since inquiries from physicians about his person and learning had shown him to be competent and skilled in the art of medicine, he might offer medical treatment to Christian patients (and Christians might seek him out for care) so long as he associated himself with another, Christian, physician.[113] Towards the end of 1333 Vidal sought relegitimation of his practice, this time attaching a copy of a letter of accreditation that the physician Pere Gavet had drawn up for the king's vicar in Barcelona. Gavet mentioned his own preparation in an academic *studium* and testified to his examination of Vidal carried out jointly with another Barcelona physician, Francesc de Pla; the two had agreed that Vidal might be licensed to practice. Gavet stipulated, however, that whenever Vidal wished to administer a laxative medicine he should first seek the advice of another experienced physician, and he added (with the self-assurance of his training) the further requirement that Vidal should study medical texts for two years more. The bishop thereupon renewed his authorization of Vidal's practice, broadening Gavet's stipulations to include the requirement of 1332 that Vidal associate with a Christian physician whenever he treated Christian patients.[114] In February 1334 Bishop Ponç granted a similar authorization to another Barcelona Jew, Samuel Gratiani, whose medical skill had been vouched for by a Christian apothecary in the city, Pere Janer; Samuel was assured that he might see and treat Christian patients, notwithstanding any contrary laws, so long as he was accompanied by his apothecary sponsor.[115] In both these cases the Valencian theme of qualification by examination was introduced, but the bishop's real concern was that Christians oversee Jewish medical practice on Christian patients,

---

[113] ADB, Notularium Communium 5/69v (20 May 1332).

[114] Ibid., 5/197r–v (11 Oct. 1333).

[115] Ibid., 5/232 (18 Feb. 1334). Pere Janer has been briefly mentioned by Jordi González, "Viejos papeles 1334–1344–1354" and "Viejos papeles 1312–1316–1339–1336" (though I do not believe the material presented in the second article refers to the apothecary). But there is much additional information in the royal archives: he was an apothecary by at least 1325, apothecary to the queen by 1333, and her chamberlain by 1340. He was still alive in 1349, when he was made *collector questiarum aljame Gerunde*. His association with Samuel Gratiani went back to at least 1329: AHPG, Notari 4–3/143v.

and such a provision continued to be incorporated into subsequent episcopal licenses.[116]

Simultaneously, secular authority in Catalonia was awakening to its own supposed precedent for controlling medical authority, that offered by the *fueros* of Monzón (1289). In mid-September 1334 the infante Pere responded to a complaint from the physicians of Cervera about the town's many incompetent medical practitioners, and agreed that the town might require an examination of anyone wishing to practice there unless he already had at least a bachelor's degree in medicine. The infante cited the *constitutiones Cathalonie* in support of his action, exempting from examination not just academics but any other practitioners comparably qualified. He made exactly the same response to a similar request from the *medici* of Barcelona a month later.[117] In the new regulatory atmosphere, Pere was perhaps reading more into the Monzón provision than had been intended; his statement that training in a *studium generale* exempts a physician from the need for an examination has no counterpart in the earlier legislation, and instead echoes a new feature of the Valencian *furs*.

Again it was Jewish practitioners who perceived a threat and who moved immediately to evade possible restrictions by appealing for licenses to a higher authority, this time the monarchy. David Abrahe of Cervera sought out Pere Gavet for examination and certification, and his certification was confirmed by the infante Pere on 3 October 1334.[118] Three weeks later Vidal de Castellfollit asked for an exemption from the requirement on the grounds that he had been treating the sick of Cervera for a long time, and he was granted it by the infante; at the same time, three other Jews – Samuel Gratiani (he who had already been licensed by the bishop in February), Vidal Bonaffos, and Juceff Bonaffos – were given the same exemption with regard to their medical practice in Barcelona.[119]

It was exclusively Jews who reacted defensively to the new royal insistence on regulation; does this mean that they had been the intended target of royal as well as of episcopal action? Do *both* series of events reveal a general suspicion of medical practice by Jews in particular, perhaps made explicit when the level of Christian practice seemed high enough that Jewish physicians need no longer be automatically tolerated? Without more direct evidence it is impossible to say: it may simply be that the Jews' consciousness of their tenuous status as practitioners in Christian society, reinforced by a new episcopal severity, led them to

---

[116] See, for example, Hillgarth and Silano, *Register Notule Communium 14*, p. 200, doc. 554 (of 1347).

[117] La Torre, *Documentos*, pp. [19–20], doc. 13.

[118] Published by Rius, 'Més documents," p. 140, doc. 10. It may be that Pere Gavet's letter to the royal vicar accrediting Vidal Habib (above, at n. 114) reveals a still earlier stage of Jewish appeals to royal authority for license to practice.

[119] C 576/81, 81v, 82v–83, 83.

take the royal insistence on licensing with particular seriousness. The fact that no Christian physician rushed to ask the king for either an examination or an exemption is not good evidence either way. Many Christians, after all, could automatically have been exempted by a period of university study, and as we have already seen there is some reason to believe that a not inconsiderable number of practitioners had had at least a limited amount of such study by this time. Jews, on the other hand, were excluded from the Christian *studia*, and one went so far as to complain to the king about the unfairness of imposing an arbitrary tribunal upon a people who were prevented from obtaining the university degrees that would allow them to bypass its judgment.[120] Furthermore, at least one Jewish physician evidently believed that two different issues were involved: Jucef Bonaffos, licensed by the king in 1334 to practice *legaliter et bene*, felt it necessary thirteen years later to get episcopal sanction for his practice as well.[121]

Whatever the original motive for instituting examinations, it was no more than three or four years before most of the Catalan towns of reasonable size had a qualifying system in place and were applying it to some candidates of both religions. The need for municipal examinations was reaffirmed for Cervera in September 1337 and for Barcelona in May 1338 because of the supposed presence in both cities of unexamined practitioners, "tam Christiani quam Judei," as Barcelona's letter put it.[122] The citizens of Montblanc complained to the king in 1339 about ignorant practitioners who were injuring or killing their patients; the result was a royal command to the vicar and bailiff in Montblanc formally to prohibit anyone from practicing medicine or surgery there "until he be examined and approved in accordance with the *constitutiones* [of Catalonia]."[123] Other towns, however, like Tortosa,

---

[120] In 1346, Jaffudanus Abenvives of Valencia complained that although he had studied medicine for a long time and had asked to be examined for a license, the examiners had refused, saying that, according to the *furs*, no one could be licensed who had not studied in a *studium generale* for four years. He told the king that it seemed unreasonable "quod Judei, qui studium generali non habent, si reperti fuerint sufficientes in dicta arte sive sciencia medicine, ad praticandum . . . non admittantur – potisime cum tempore quo forus predictus fuerit ordinatus et postea eciam Judei fuerunt recepti et admissi si sufficientes erant reperti in arte predicte ad praticandum" (C 640/92v–93). Park, *Doctors*, pp. 72–4, shows that in Italy by mid-century Jews might attend lectures in a medical faculty, though they could not receive degrees; the same was true at Montpellier by the second half of the century (García-Ballester, Ferre, and Feliu, "Jewish Appreciation," pp. 95–7).

[121] The bishop allowed him to accept Christian patients without the latter being subject to ecclesiastical censure so long as he practiced in association with a Christian apothecary: Hillgarth and Silano, *Register Notule Communium 14*, p. 200, doc. 554.

[122] In Cervera, a *iurisperitus* and a surgeon, Bertomeu Domènech, were given authority to proceed against offenders; a further investigation was ordered in March 1338 (Rius, "Més documents," pp. 149, 151–2; docs. 29, 35). The letter to Barcelona is dated 2 May 1338 (C 1055/4); the first recorded examination from Barcelona dates from October of that year (see below, chapter 4).

[123] "Donec examinata et approbata fuerit iuxta constituciones predictas": C 603/137v.

apparently simply implemented the new system without asking for permission to do so.[124]

While the royal letters reaffirmed the right of the Catalan municipalities to examine aspiring physicians, they did not require them to do so, and the towns' power to examine had the potential for use as a selective and variously motivated instrument of individual or even religious control. It may be significant that Jewish practitioners from Cervera and Barcelona continued during the 1330s and 1340s to seek qualification outside the system, submitting to an examination by an independent physician – usually Pere Gavet – in order to gain a royal license to practice, rather than submit to a municipal panel. Certainly in some cases an insistence on fulfillment of the regulation was a manifestation of competitive jealousies. In April 1338 Ramon Roquer of Socarrats, near Olot, complained to King Pere that "he had practiced the art of surgery for a long time, and although he was a layman and unlettered, he owned good books and had good cures to his credit, as was well known in his district; but now some surgeons envious of him have maliciously caused royal officials to order him not to practice surgery until he has been examined *per medicos*."[125]

In the westernmost part of the realm, Aragon, where medical care was scarce enough that carpenters might be contracted to cure cases of bladder stone, the need to regulate practice was bound to seem less urgent to consumers than it was in Valencia and Catalonia.[126] Here it was occupational jealousy, reinforced by sensitivity to the activity of a sizable Jewish minority and fired by particular circumstances, that was responsible for the introduction of regulation – or so a curious episode would seem to suggest. In 1324 we find Teruel's physician, Alfonso de Burgos, at the center of controversy, accused of eating meat in Lent and on Fridays, of having married no fewer than three wives, and of other unnamed "enormities." Though nothing more is heard of these charges for ten years, others were raised against him; he was often blamed with defaulting on debts (in one case, of failing to return books to the Franciscan convent), and he continued to be the intermittent object of much local hostility and animosity. On more than one occasion mobs attacked him and his house, and at one point

---

[124] The procedure appears abruptly in the Tortosa council meeting of 17 May 1343: "Provehiren los dites consellers que sobre la examinacio que faedora es den R. de Vilalbii e dels altres metges estans en la ciutat trameten los procuradors a maestre Gerau metge qui esta a Sent Matheu que vingua a la ciutat e a nescio de la ciutat per la dita examinacio faedora ensempses ab maestre Francesch licenciat segons ques diu en medicina e cirurgia la qual examinacio sia feyta ab sagrament" (AMT, Provisions 2/47v). Arrangements for another examination were made on 12 June 1346 (AMT, Provisions 3/63v).

[125] Quoted in García-Ballester, McVaugh, and Rubio-Vela, *Medical Licensing*, p. 9, n. 23.

[126] For the carpenter, ANZ, manual de Domingo de Figuera 1326, fols. 57v–58 (of 25 April). Another indication that some inhabitants of Zaragoza perceived a continuing shortage of dependable physicians is the appeal to Pere III from three different people at the same time – his aunt Violant, her husband Lope de Luna, lord of Sogorb, and the archbishop of Zaragoza – that he send his physician Alazar Avinardut to that city to care for them (C 1059/92).

King Alfons III had hurriedly to withdraw his protection from the physician temporarily, for fear of the scandal it might arouse in Teruel. What was behind this animosity finally emerges in the spring of 1333, when we find Alfonso cited before the archbishop of Zaragoza to respond to complaints from "certain people who accuse you of returning to the vomit of perfidious Judaism, of committing heresies and awful, terrible crimes": Alfonso, though a married cleric, was a converted Jew. He enjoyed another two years of liberty, but in the fall of 1335 he was arrested once again, accused of bigamy and other crimes, and executed.[127]

What has this to do with occupational jealousies? It happens that by 1330 Teruel had acquired a second Christian physician, Guido – and that it was this Guido who in 1333 had brought the charges of "heresy and many other foul crimes" that two years later would result in Alfonso's death.[128] May we not imagine that Guido was seizing the opportunity to eliminate a competitor in Teruel, using whatever weapons were at hand? The new talk of licensing must have suggested to him that there might be subtler weapons to use in the future, for it was this same Guido who, two years after Alfonso's disappearance from the scene, complained of unqualified wandering practitioners in Teruel and persuaded Pere III to extend municipal regulation of medical practice to that city – the first such instance in Aragon.[129]

However mixed the underlying motives may have been, a new sensitivity to the issue of professional qualification was certainly abroad in all parts of the Crown of Aragon in the 1330s – yet there were limits to public willingness to restrict medical practice. Pere III put them into words in 1340, responding to a citizen of tiny Pallerols (some fifteen kilometers east of Cervera) who had been accused of unlicensed practice:

> We find that he has cured men, women, and animals of his village and nearby towns of broken arms and heads and other things of little danger, not as a *medicus* or pretending to be one [*non fingens se esse medicum*], and without receiving any fees, merely out of a love of God and friendship or neighborliness.[130]

---

[127] On the 1333 summons, C 578/121v; on his trial and death in 1335, C 579/161v, 170, 173. His death is established in C 489/191v.

[128] "A requisicion de maestre Guido et del official de Teruel fue prise[?] maestre Alfonso acusado de heresi et de muytos et diversos et leydos crimenes et delitos": C 578/127–128, At the end of 1330, Guido had complained to the king that the city of Teruel had promised him 400 *sous* yearly for six years if he would serve as their physician but had not yet paid him any money (C 441/24v; 8 Dec. 1330).

[129] López de Meneses, "Documentos culturales," pp. 671–2, doc. 3.

[130] "Quia ut pro parte ipsius suplicantis percepimus ipse non ut medicus nec fingens se esse medicum fecerit aliquas curas absque aliquo salario aliquibus hominibus et feminis ac creaturis dicti loci de Paylorols et quibusdam aliorum locorum eidem circumvicinorum amore dei ac racione amicicie et vicinatus scilicet de fracturis capitis seu brachii aut aliorum modici ponderis seu periculi, et propterea pro parte eiusdem fuerit nobis humiliter supplicatum ut cum dictum

The king accepted the argument put forward by the village empiric: regulation of practice should really be aimed only at those who professed to be *medici* and who charged a fee for their services, especially if they treated grave illnesses or injuries. Village healers or neighbors who provided free advice or home remedies for minor health problems posed neither an economic nor a medical danger and could continue to practice as they had always done.

We evidently should not understand the new Valencian and Catalonian regulations as meant to put into effect a system of licensing based on a uniform level of professional expertise. Even though we may not be able to decide to what extent they were aimed at a selective social, rather than an exclusively medical, control, we must still acknowledge that they left largely unaffected the traditional patterns of medical qualification and practice, and that municipal authority retained the right to decide whether it wished to insist on a particular standard of knowledge among its practitioners, while the king could always exempt a candidate from the requirement of an examination. But we must acknowledge, too, that these regulations finally made explicit a cultural ideal that had been gaining strength in the Crown of Aragon for more than thirty years: that academic training, at some level, was unchallengeable testimony to a physician's competence. In this respect they laid the foundation for future codes of professional licensing.

The status of women's practice

The participation of women in medieval health care is a widely discussed subject for which relatively little factual information has yet been made available. In two recent studies Monica Green has examined carefully the received historical interpretation and the bases on which it rests.[131] Women in the Middle Ages are often supposed to have practiced solely as midwives, limited to treating problems of female health – gynecology and obstetrics – but enjoying a monopoly within that sphere until at least the seventeenth century. Green has shown that this model is open to question on many grounds, raising the possibilities that for much of the Middle Ages women – more of them than has usually been supposed – had, not a narrowly gynecological practice, but one involving the medical and surgical care of men and women alike; and, conversely, that male as well as female practitioners cared for the health of women. Her suggestions are confirmed, broadly speaking, from what we can learn about the Crown of Aragon in the early fourteenth century.

---

privilegium non se extendat nisi ad illos qui sunt medici et fingunt se esse medicos et decipiunt parentes ut possint extorquere peccuniam ab eisdem . . . nos . . . dicimus et mandamus quatenus . . . uti permitatis libere dicta arte absque tamen salario": (C 608/56r–v; 12 Sept. 1340).

[131] Green, "Women's Medical Practice"; Green, "Problems."

We may begin by acknowledging that women gave informal care, like men but perhaps more often. Among learned physicians like Arnau de Vilanova, women – "old women," *vetule* – often symbolized those rustics and illiterates who offered empirical remedies with no known basis in traditional theory, which had to be verified before they could be passed on.[132] Women can be found providing basic medical advice in the countryside, or nursing care in the home.[133] Remarkably little evidence survives to prove their role as midwives – the meticulous household accounts for Jaume II reveal the services of wet-nurses but not of *obstetrices* for his ten children[134] – but there is reason to think that at this date midwifery was still relatively new as a specialized craft, capable of being sustained financially only in towns of a certain size, and we can assume that women assisted at deliveries without claiming an occupational title.[135]

How widely women engaged in some kind of medical practice as a more or less formal occupation is much more difficult to decide. As Green has emphasized, searches through medieval documentation for specific occupational labels (like *phisicus* or *cirurgicus*) almost automatically overlook women, who normally were not treated as exercising an occupation in their own right.[136] A woman might work side by side with her artisan husband, but only he would display the occupational title in legal records while he lived, though one sometimes finds a widow continuing alone in that joint occupation after her husband's death and assuming the occupational label herself. In the Crown of Aragon, this practice is amply attested for apothecaries. When Guillem Duran, an apothecary of Puigcerdà, died about 1313, his widow Sibilia first hired another apothecary to run the shop for a year but then operated it herself together with her sons – Pere until he died about 1322, then Ramon until at least 1344; in legal documents she spoke of it variously as "our" or even "my" shop.[137] Barbering, however, was an occupation in which women evidently did not help or follow their husbands:

---

[132] Agrimi and Crisciani, "Medici e 'vetulae'."

[133] Green, "Problems," explains the problematic character of the term "nursing"; it seems to me still valid for those regularly charged with (and paid for) caring for sick members of the royal household as they convalesced (see, e.g., C 1296/8 and C 1297/215r–v).

[134] Nevertheless, midwives must surely have been present at the births, as they were at the birth of Jaume's grandson Pere in 1319; Pere III, *Crònica*, I.40 (in Soldevila, *Cròniques*, p. 1017).

[135] Green, "Women's Medical Practice," p. 454; Green, "Problems." I agree with her that we cannot assume that the women called on to make determinations of virginity (typically called "mujeres dignas de fe" [CRD Jaume II sin fecha 1369] or simply "matronas" [C 141/53r–v]) were actually midwives.

[136] Green, "Problems."

[137] AHCP, Mateu d'Oliana Liber firmitatis 1315–16, f. 15v; Bernat Blanch Liber extraneorum 1329–30, 4 id. Feb. 1329/30; Guillem Bernat de Santfeliu Liber extraneorum 1336–7, 4 id. April 1335. Similarly, after Balagarius de Farfanya *especier* died in Valencia in 1312, his wife Elicsenda assumed the business and indeed the label of "apothecaria" (C 373/114v, 13 May 1325, makes it clear that she is her late husband's successor by speaking of her as "Balagaria apothecaria"!). Their son Berenguer was eventually associated with her and succeeded to the enterprise after her death: ARV, Just. Val. 26, 3 kls. June 1330.

there are several instances known of widows instead renting their late husband's shop and tools to a man (sometimes a kinsman) who takes over the business.[138]

With regard to medical or surgical practice by women the case is less clear-cut, and regional differences may complicate matters. For the kingdom of Valencia, the position of women practitioners is illuminated only by the *furs* of 1329, since there is almost no direct evidence of their medical role in the kingdom before the second half of the century. After laying it down that anyone wishing to practice medicine had to undergo an examination if he had not had four years' training in a *studium generale*, the *furs* commanded that "no woman shall practice medicine or give potions [*dar bouratges*], under penalty of being whipped through the town; but they may care for little children and other women – to whom, however, they may give no potion."[139] Although the prohibition seems suddenly to be drawing a distinction between men and women as practitioners, the distinction is not quite as sharp or as sudden as it seems. The Valencian *furs* recapitulate earlier regulations from Catalan communities, like Valls, which thirty years before had enacted that "no man or woman . . . who has not mastered the science of medicine shall give the sick any medicine [*metzina*] or potion [*beuvatge*] in lieu of medicine," and had prescribed the same penalty of a public whipping.[140] For it was not just the Jewish physician whose medicines were to be feared. As the Valls regulation understood, even a well-meaning physician, whether man or woman, might not be aware of the dangers with a particular drug: Jaume II, we may remember, refused to take a purge unless his *medicus maior* was at hand to administer it. The Valencian prohibition against giving potions, therefore, was not aimed against women practitioners as women, since the dangers represented by inexpert men should already have been controlled by the law ensuring that medical practitioners possess an academic training or its equivalent. And it was not an idle concern: that very year a woman named Margarita, *arte medicine utendo*, fled Valencia when she was accused of the death of a patient, returning only on condition of never practicing again.[141]

In what it left uncontrolled, the 1329 law actually sanctioned women's practice among women and children. Giving potions was never a major part of any physician's activities, precisely because of the threat it posed; most medical

---

138 Thus, when the *barbitonsor* Andreas Solario of Manresa died, his widow contracted with his uncle Pere, another barber, to run the shop for a share of the profits (AHCM 28, 19 kls. Feb. 1302); when Bernat Guerau was absent from Barcelona, his wife agreed that Martí Danielis could run the shop in exchange for half the income (AHPB, manual de Jaume de Comarmena Oct. 1336–Aug. 1337, f. 70v, of 24 March 1337).

139 García-Ballester, McVaugh, and Rubio-Vela, *Medical Licensing*, p. 60.

140 For the text, see above, n. 7.

141 C 479/243r–v; 13 Oct. 1329. Cf. the case of Barchinona of Campdevànol (near Camprodon in Catalonia) who in 1309 was accused of using "indebitas medicinas," with the understanding that if the charge was not made good she could continue to practice (ACA, varia de Cancillería 257/51v); this attitude is very like that adopted towards the practice of Gueraula de Codines (above, p. 41).

practice involved diagnosis, prognosis, prescription of diet and regimen, and external medication – salves, suffumigations, embrocations, etc. – all of which women could still provide for their patients. But this is not to say that women practitioners did not treat men: perhaps formally the statute excluded them from doing so, but the very fact that it seemed necessary to insist on this point implies that women practitioners were often found treating male patients, and the *furs* of 1329 did not bring this to an end.[142] Moreover, the language of the *furs* – "no ús de medicina" – left surgery open for a woman to practice without hindrance; in this field, of course, book-learning was not yet seen as a prerequisite to practice. It is probably not by chance that the one woman we find practicing unchallenged in Valencia in the first two decades after the *furs* is a surgeon, the Muslim Macahat.

While for Valencia we have almost no direct testimony from the first part of the fourteenth century, and have to infer the status of women practitioners from legislation, in Catalonia we have no legislation but fortunately do possess indisputable evidence of the independent practice of individuals, though we cannot tell whether it followed an association with a practitioner-husband. We know of their practice because in the late 1330s and 1340s a few women were caught up in the new public sensitivity to qualifications, the attempts to screen out the uneducated and incompetent.

(a) Towards the beginning of 1338 Pere III was told of a woman living near the Barcelona monastery of Santa Ana who laid claim to "officio et arte cirurgie" but who was said to be harming her patients, men and women, by her *curas et medicinas ineptas et indiscretas*. The monarch responded, not by forbidding her practice outright, but by ordering that she be subjected to an examination by "masters in the art of surgery"; then, if found incompetent, she should be punished and prevented from practicing further.[143] There is nothing in the document to suggest that it was in itself either unusual or improper for a woman to practice surgery; if she had the necessary skills (in this instance Pere showed some scepticism), she might do so.

(b) A second instance is that of Jacmeta, a woman of Barcelona about whose surgical practice certain other surgeons of the city brought a complaint in 1341. Here the king intervened directly in the suit, commanding his justiciar to take no further action against Jacmeta without royal authorization: "by the testimony of several trustworthy people we understand the said Jacmeta to have comported herself very well in this occupation, and to have cured many who were suffering from serious illnesses."[144] The king made a similar intervention a month later on

---

[142] See the cases cited in García-Ballester, McVaugh, and Rubio-Vela, *Medical Licensing*, pp. 31–2.

[143] C 594/23; 9 Jan. 1338.

[144] "Nosque nonnullorum fidedignorum relatu percepimus ipsam Jacmetam in cura ipsius officii se multum bene habuisse et plures de gravibus infirmitatibus detentos curasse": C 613/33 (28 May 1341).

behalf of Magdalena, another Barcelona woman "who is said to practice the art of surgery and physic."[145] In both instances there is more than a hint of professional jealousy, but nothing demonstrably gender-related; and again, more clearly than before, the king has insisted that women for whose surgical skill there is evidence shall be allowed to practice.

(c) A final case deserving comment concerns the Jew Astruga, wife of master Astruch of Barcelona. In 1342 the royal justiciar discovered that she was practicing surgery without having undergone the prescribed examination and proceeded against her, only to be restrained by the king on the grounds that Astruga was practicing surgery alone, not medicine, and "only on Jews."[146]

Together, these cases appear to show that in Catalonia there was no formal (legal) bar to a woman's practice – of surgery, at least – in the period before the institution of qualifying examinations; that when those examinations were introduced, women were in principle permitted to present themselves for formal qualification; and that some women were accorded the right to practice even after qualifying standards were introduced. They suggest, it seems to me, no systematic animus against women – men can be found involved in exactly similar cases – but they do raise one interesting possibility. All four women whom we have found in practice were surgeons – one reason, indeed, why Astruga was allowed to continue in practice unexamined was that she was practicing surgery rather than medicine. May it not be that women found it more convenient to pursue a career in surgery? were tolerated in that field precisely because, unlike medicine, it did not presume the academic training from which women were debarred?[147]

---

[145] C 613/87, of 27 June 1341. Both Magdalena and Jacmeta were or had been married, but neither husband has yet been shown to have had a medical occupation.

[146] "Dicta judea non utitur nisi practica cirurgie . . . et in personis eciam tantummodo judeorum": C 873/160v (1 July 1342).

[147] Vinyoles, *Barcelonines*, pp. 45–8 (and doc. 39 of 1394), insists on the normalcy and legitimacy of medical practice by women in the second half of the fourteenth century, citing documentation from the reign of Joan I.

4

A spectrum of practice

There is, then, good evidence that medical education was becoming more common in early fourteenth-century Aragon. Academic formation unquestionably produced an elite who possessed a common scientific book-learned culture; furthermore, the wide circulation of medical books in the Crown suggests that this culture could be shared by practitioners who did not have such an education. Yet even so it is hard to believe that a majority of the physicians practicing there before 1350 ever enjoyed direct access to the sources of the new learning – to say nothing about surgeons, apothecaries, and barbers. We might wonder, therefore, whether two types, two levels of medicine and of practitioners were current in the kingdom – one learned and theoretical, the other traditional and empirical – and perhaps two corresponding patient populations. A closer look at the social setting of the health occupations, however, reveals that there were structures promoting intellectual if not professional unity among all types of practitioners, allowing the new learning to spread within and among every level of practice. Down through the 1340s, medical practitioners were in continual association and interactive discourse, of a sort that inevitably yielded a common scientific culture in which all shared – crossing boundaries that might otherwise have been set up by different methods of training and entrance into practice.

Medical cooperation

In the smaller towns physicians (and surgeons) seem to have banded together for social and economic reinforcement, without much regard for status. Between 1320 and 1345 Manresa was served continuously by one physician, Pere de Gostemps (active 1309–45), and two surgeons, Berenguer de Acuta (1306–40) and Pere de Fontanet (1321–45): the town gave each of the three a salary (or at least freedom from taxation) in exchange for his promise not to move away.[1]

---

[1] For Gostemps and Acuta, AHCM, Llibres de Consell 2, 13 kls. Mar. 1322 (contracts for 400 and 100 *sous* respectively); for Fontanet, ibid., 13 kls. Aug. 1335 (enfranchisement).

These three men, over time, found various occasions for association. The surgeons treated cases together.[2] Berenguer regularly invested money with Pere Gostemps.[3] In his will, Berenguer named the two Peres as his executors;[4] Pere de Gostemps in his turn chose Pere de Fontanet as his executor three years later.[5] These three men dominated health care in Manresa and its surroundings, but they did not monopolize it. From time to time other physicians and surgeons settled briefly in Manresa, and had no difficulty in being absorbed into these relations; these newcomers can be found joined with the long-established practitioners in the treatment of particular medical or surgical cases.[6]

In Vic, slightly larger than Manresa, the same tolerance of competitive practice is still to be seen. Berenguer Diache, a surgeon from Caldes de Montbui, often treated patients in Vic, fifty kilometers away, apparently without arousing any resentment among local surgeons.[7] Indeed, practitioners there often collaborated across ostensible boundaries of occupational identity. A particularly striking instance of this is an agreement of 1328 whereby a Vic couple contracted with no fewer than four practitioners collectively to treat their son for a head injury, suffered when he was beaten with a club: the four included two surgeons (Guillem de Soler and Miquel Alger) and, surprisingly, two physicians as well (Martí de Soler and Martí de Comells).[8] Five years later Guillem de Soler and "Martí," surgeon and physician, were associated in the treatment of an *infirmitas*, seemingly a medical problem rather than a wound requiring surgical intervention.[9] In communities like Manresa and Vic there seem to have been no sharp lines defining areas of expertise, and no signs of professional jealousy.

In small towns that attracted relatively few practitioners and whose rural population had little spare cash to pay medical bills, such associations could provide economic security through fee-splitting; by pooling their time and thought in exchange for a division of fees, practitioners could minimize the impact of a run of defaulting clients. Fees could be divided evenly or in some agreed-upon proportion, but everyone would get something.[10] Such arrangements could culminate in the formal establishment of joint practices, in which all

---

[2] AHCM 150, 5 kls. May 1335.
[3] AHCM 101, id. Mar. 1325, an investment of 225 *sous* (one instance of many). He also stood surety for Gostemps for 55 *sous* (AHCM, Liber judeorum 10, 4 kls. Sept. 1328).
[4] AHCM 170, 12 kls. Dec. 1340.
[5] AHCM 194, 3 non. Apr. 1345.
[6] AHCM 150, 9 kls. May 1335: Fontanet and Pere Metge (a surgeon active 1331–45) join in treatment of wounds, dividing the fee of 75 *sous* unequally but sharing two pairs of hens. AHCM, Llibre dels jueus 1341–2, 15 kls. July 1342: Gostemps and Enric de Montdor (physician active 1342–3) associate in treating the fatal illness of a Manresa Jew, dividing the 100 *sous* fee equally.
[7] ACFV 76/[1], *c.* 4 Jan. 1322; ACFV 207, 6 id. Feb. 1324.
[8] ACFV 248, 2 non. June 1328.
[9] ACFV 284, 3 id. Jan. 1333. "Master Martí" could refer to either Martí de Soler (active 1330–47) or Martí de Comells (active 1327–41).
[10] See above, n. 6; and, for barbers, below, p. 124.

fees – not just those for cases treated by the two men together – were divided between the partners. For fifteen years Pere Ritxart and Guillem Arnau practiced surgery together in Santa Coloma de Queralt, until Guillem moved to Cervera in 1344. Their relationship apparently began as a family one – Pere was Guillem's uncle – but they decided to formalize it and put it on a business footing by creating a *societas* in 1333:

> I the said master Pere shall give you one-third of all the money that I make in the said occupation, and of all the goods that are given me, whether gauds and other jewels or animals or weapons (but not including clothes); likewise I master Guillem shall similarly give you one-half of the aforesaid, except for clothes. And we will render a just and legal account, one to the other, whenever one asks the other to do so.[11]

Such an arrangement, of course, provided still more incentive to share knowledge and techniques, since each partner stood to profit from the success of the other.

In the principal cities of the kingdom the situation was slightly different. Because the more ambitious physicians tended to gravitate to the prosperous population centers where they had the prospect of wealthier patients, a city like Barcelona could witness instances of occupational competitiveness. A case in point is the illness of Ruggiero II di Loria, the son of the count-kings' great Italian admiral (who had died in 1305).[12] By 1316 the young Ruggiero had come under the care of Nicolau Andree, a Barcelona physician of considerable experience.[13] Nicolau was unable to cure the boy, yet despite his failure he vigorously resisted all attempts to bring any other physicians into the case, trying to keep his patient to himself. What helped temper this sort of occupational possessiveness was the public's belief in the potential of medicine and

---

[11] "Ego dictus magister Petrus tenear vobis dare de omni lucro quod cum dicto officio facere potero et de omnibus serviciis que michi dederint tam indumentariis et aliis joyes quam animalibus seu armis (exceptis vestibus) terciam partem; similiter et ego dictus magister Guilelmus tenear vobis dare sub dicta forma de predictis medietatem, exceptis vestibus. Et reddemus unus alteri verum iustumque et legale compotum quantumcumque fuerimus unus ab altero requisiti": AHPT 3847/191 (8 Dec. 1333).

[12] I call him Ruggiero II to distinguish him from his older half-brother, Ruggiero I, who died towards the end of 1307 (Jaume II spoke of the latter boy as an epileptic; MF, I:84 n. 3). The younger son, christened Berengario, took the name Ruggiero some time after 1312 and died in mid-December 1324: Fullana Mira, "Casa de Lauria," pp. 89–111. Allusions to his chronic illness are: (a) supplementing the care provided by the physician Nicolau Andree, 11 Oct. 1316 (C 243/184, 184v); (b) Mosse's assertion that he can help the boy, 10 Nov. 1321 (C 172/100); (c) sending Bertomeu Casaldòria to him, 10 Dec. 1321 (C 172/172v); (d) contracting with Casaldòria to provide continuing care for him, 2 June 1323 (C 223/284v; Fullana Mira, p. 108 n. 2); (e) sending Alazar to examine him, 5 June 1323 (C 177/299v).

[13] Nicolau Andree can be traced securely back to June 1301 (ACB, manual de Bernat de Vilarrúbia 1301– , f. 32v), but he was certainly in practice before that. Joan Amell's wife was his first cousin (C 351/231; 7 July 1313). He may have been in late middle age in 1316, for he died in the winter of 1320–1 ("noviter ab hac luce migravit": C 171/114r–v; 28 Feb. 1321).

its willingness to search for what it considered satisfactory care. In young Ruggiero's case, his mother Saurina wrote to Jaume II expressing dissatisfaction with master Nicolau's lack of progress, complaining that "he doesn't want any physician but himself to have a role in Ruggiero's treatment." She wanted the advice of one or two other physicians, and the king quickly agreed, "since it is a great responsibility, and dangerous, for the care of such a person and such an illness to be entrusted to a single physician."[14]

As the king's language ("such a person") suggests, elite urban patients expected more and different service than did a rural clientele, and what is more they were prepared to pay for it. The way in which elite patients' demands generally encouraged communication rather than jealousy among practitioners is exemplified by the patronage of those indefatigable consumers of learned medicine, the royal family. To some extent, of course, the king's demands were unique. From the first decade of the fourteenth century, at least two physicians were always retained in the king's service because the king's person was of particular importance and could not be entrusted to one physician alone, in medieval as in early modern times.[15] But as the exchange over Ruggiero's case shows, other classes too wanted collaborative medical care, and undoubtedly this practice encouraged some degree of consultation and cooperation.[16]

In other respects, too, the behavior of the royal family as it sought medical attention suggests how the concerns of a medically sensitized public trying to identify the best care could foster contact among physicians. For example, in 1322 the infante Alfons asked his father's *phisicus maior*, Joan Amell, to recommend a personal physician, and Amell suggested Bertomeu de Gauders of Valencia. Alfons thereupon invited Bertomeu to join his service, instructing him first to stop at court to be informed by Amell – presumably about Alfons' complexion and state of health.[17] Instances like this one reveal how often physicians who served the royal family had known of and appreciated one

---

14 "Minime velit quod alius phisicus nisi ipse intendat in cura Rogeroni predicti"; "cum multum honerosum et periculosum sit uni soli phisico talem curam et talis persone comitere": letters of 11 Oct. 1316 (C 243/184r–v).

15 It was also a way of ensuring that at least one physician was likely always to be on hand: as Jaume II put it, summoning Joan Amell back to court when Martí de Calça Roja was absent, "utroque carere nolimus" (C 247/302; 29 June 1323). This was formalized in Pere III's *ordenacions* of 1344: "ordenam que en la cort nostra ordinariament sien dos metges instruyts e provats en medecina o phisica qui diligentment insisten per la conservacio de la nostra salut": Pere III, "Ordenacions," p. 76. Comenge y Ferrer, *Medicina en el reino*, pp. 57–8, asserts that in the thirteenth century it was already customary for the royal household to retain two physicians, one surgeon, two barbers, and an apothecary, but he gives no evidence for this.

16 Not only the nobility but the urban aristocracy used collaborative consultations of this sort, as evidenced by Guillem de Laceria, "civis Barchinone," who hired one physician (Bernat ça Llimona) and two surgeons (Pere de Hospitali and Bernat de Pertegaç) to care for his daughter's wounds (C 156/156r–v; 2 Aug. 1315).

17 C 386/124v (22 Sept. 1322). Bertomeu came to the infante from Valencia in spring 1323, and probably went on the Sardinian expedition with him (C 398/127, RP 560/70v).

another's work before they were associated at court, and prove the existence of a network of interrelationships within what may be thought of as a nascent if not yet self-conscious medical community.

The slow but irresistible penetration of learned medicine into the Crown of Aragon must further have strengthened interchange among medical practitioners, university-trained or not, who were trying to assimilate the new knowledge. Those who had actually undergone the experience of the *studium* shared a further bond; besides, if Arnau de Vilanova's teaching is any guide, students trained in a medical faculty had been prepared by their masters to accept consultation and mutual assistance among practitioners as entirely natural.

Arnau's commentary on the Hippocratic aphorism "Vita brevis," as preserved in his *Repetitio* (so-called as a student transcription) of *c.* 1300, introduces his listeners to the quotidian problems of medical practice and illustrates them with examples based on specific situations.[18] It is striking that Arnau almost invariably shows the physician solving such problems, not by unaided reason or by common sense, but by consultation with another practitioner. Perhaps in part this had a pedagogic motive, to convince medical students of the need to take their teachers seriously, but even so his examples must represent the sorts of cooperation and interdependence that could be expected in the early fourteenth century. There is a complete spectrum of such interaction: the physician who takes medicines prescribed by a colleague *pro necessitate sui corporis*; the two physicians associated jointly in a case who disagree as to the proper treatment; the one who treats a patient following the counsel of another; the one who, unable to effect a cure, turns to a colleague and asks him to examine the patient; the one who, afraid to grant a patient's demands, writes to a friend for help and gets a letter back with technical medical advice; the two friends from medical school who in later life correspond on abstract problems of pathology and therapeutics[19] – the last with its counterpart in Arnau's dedication of his own *De amore heroico* to a school friend with whom he had debated this and other themes.[20] The message communicated tacitly by Arnau's *Repetitio* to his students was that cooperation and collaboration among physicians are certainly normal and probably indispensable.

---

[18] The *Repetitio* is printed in the various sixteenth-century editions of Arnau de Vilanova's *Opera* and is also preserved entire in one (fifteenth-century) manuscript, Munich CLM 14245, ff. 13–38v (manuscripts of truncated versions also exist). The Munich text contains long sections missing from the printed one (which is essentially the same in all editions), while the printed text has had inserted into it even longer sections from an unidentified work apparently on metaphysics. I have transcribed the Munich manuscript, and my quotations below are based on that transcription, but insofar as possible I give citations to the same passage as present in the printed editions.

[19] Arnau de Vilanova, *Repetitio*, ff. 280rb–281rb, 278rb–va.

[20] Arnau de Vilanova, *De amore heroico*, p. 43.

Surgeons and medicine

It may seem surprising that many of the cases discussed above show physicians in close, collegial, contact with surgeons, for physicians and surgeons are often supposed to have been incompatible and even antagonistic groups. Henri de Mondeville's *Chirurgia* was begun in 1306, and draws on its author's training in medicine at Montpellier as well as in surgery at Montpellier and at Paris;[21] Mondeville was thus Arnau de Vilanova's younger contemporary at Montpellier, perhaps even his student, and his classic account of the manoeuvering that characterized relations between medicine and surgery is presumably as true of Catalonia as of Languedoc. He describes vividly a world of cut-throat competition between the two, where each was trying to steal patients from the other.[22]

Yet the evidence from the Crown of Aragon suggests that at the beginning of the fourteenth century the two were in fact functioning as something of a single occupational community. The competitiveness described by Mondeville was possible only because the two occupations shared so much common ground; the examples he himself provides make plain that there was often no easy way to decide that a complaint was medical rather than surgical, or vice versa, so that the public did not always pay much attention to the occupational label. When Jaume Ritolphi, justiciar of Vic, fell ill in Berga in 1325, he called in Guillem de Soler, his town's leading surgeon; then, when he did not improve, he turned to Guillem Galaubi, the principal physician in town.[23] The very use of the terms *medicus* and *metge* as indiscriminate labels for physicians and surgeons alike shows how in the popular understanding the two functions overlapped.

Not only in their social role but in the nature of their skills, too, the two occupations were difficult to distinguish. Surgery, like medicine, was beginning to see itself as a text-based, academic subject. Surgeons in the Crown of Aragon were responding eagerly to the view being developed in the Italian tradition of the thirteenth century, from Roger and Bruno to Teodorico and Lanfranc, that surgery was a discipline with an important theoretical component;[24] and, what is more, the Iberians shared the conviction that the best surgical training could be gained, not by mere practical apprenticeship, but in a university setting. In 1302 the Valencia surgeon Guillem Correger, after some years of practice, asked permission of the king to travel out of his domains to study (*audire*) the art of

---

[21] "Parisiis et in Montpessulano operando audiendo et per plures annos legendo cyrurgiam publice utrobique et in solo Montis pessulanensis studio medicinam": Henri de Mondeville, *Chirurgia*, prologue (in Pagel, "Die Chirurgie," 40:263).

[22] On what follows, see McVaugh, "Royal Surgeons."

[23] ACFV 99, 4 kls. Dec. 1326; ACFV 101, 5 kls. Dec. 1326.

[24] Siraisi, *Medieval and Early Renaissance Medicine*, chapter 6.

surgery, pointing out that "de arte ipsa in terra nostra non legatur ad presens."[25] Guillem knew Latin, but surgeons who read only Catalan also proved receptive to conceiving of their art in a theoretical framework. It was the same Guillem Correger who decided to prepare a vernacular translation of Teodorico's surgery because, as he explained, "some surgeons in King Jaume's dominions do not understand the Latin terms; [they] all go more by practice than by theory."[26] The rapid success of the Catalan Teodorico indicates how willing the surgeons would be to give their practice a theoretical footing.

The ties between the Crown of Aragon and the *studium* at Montpellier make it plausible that it was there that Guillem Correger sought his learned surgery. We know that surgical instruction was available at the school from Mondeville's autobiographical remarks, but nothing he says and nothing to be found in other sources reveals how surgery may have been taught. The statutes of the faculty give no indication that it was incorporated into the curriculum there, and Mondeville's own language suggests that instruction in surgery was distinct from medical education and was probably not associated with a degree. Yet Mondeville's text on surgery is suffused with up-to-date scholastic medical learning, far more so even than Teodorico's (whom Mondeville quotes more than anyone except Avicenna and Galen, a fact in itself an index of his priorities).[27] Mondeville explains surgery in terms of a Galenic physiology and pathology, in the characteristic format of the schoolroom. His conviction of the interdependence of learned medicine and surgery was apparently shared in his day by masters on the medical faculty at Montpellier: annotations to the surviving manuscripts of his work give both Guglielmo da Brescia and Bernard Gordon (each associated with the school in the early years of the fourteenth century) credit for convincing Mondeville to undertake his work, and there are passages in Bernard's own writings that suggest that he "was himself quite familiar with several surgical procedures and may have applied them personally."[28] In such an environment it would have been entirely possible for Guillem Correger to get the training he wanted.

As Guillem complained, no such training was then available in Jaume II's realms: even after the establishment of the Leridan *studium* in 1300, medical instruction there was at best intermittent. It is all the more remarkable, therefore, to find reference in 1330 to the teaching of surgery at Lerida. In April 1330 King Jaume wrote to the town councilors there proposing that Guillaume

---

[25] McVaugh, "Royal Surgeons."

[26] "Alcuna partida de los surgians que son en la seyoria del noble en Jacme per la gracia de Deu rey dArago no entenen los vocables latins, cor tots los homens daquestes nostres encontrades obren mes per pratica que per teorica": quoted by Morel-Fatio, *Catalogue*, p. 33.

[27] Mondeville cited Galen 431 times, Avicenna 307, and Teodorico 113; next comes Hippocrates, with 68 references (Nicaise, *Chirurgie*, p. xxxviii).

[28] Demaitre, *Bernard de Gordon*, p. 150.

d'Avignon (recommended by Brother Jaume of the order of Santa Maria de Montesa) be appointed to the lectureship in surgery (*pro lectura artis cirurgie*), paying 400 *sous* yearly, that had been left vacant by the recent death of Bertran de la Torre.[29] If the city of Lerida was prepared to hire a professor of surgery as well as a professor of medicine for its *studium* (as apparently even Montpellier was not), we must acknowledge that by the 1320s not only practitioners but their public understood the subject to have a theoretical component, and believed that in this respect surgeons were no different from physicians in needing an understanding of their practical activity.

Examining the career of a prominent surgeon from the first decade of the fourteenth century will make plain that this expectation was in keeping with the orientation of practitioners. Berenguer ça Riera was a leading figure in a family of Geronan surgeons and had practiced in that city since the 1280s. In the 1290s he began to serve Jaume II, and curiously his recorded contacts with the king were frequently mediated by the world of written learning. He can be found informing the king about books that the monarch might find of use for his health; pressing the king to make a copy of Avicenna available to him; and translating into Catalan, at the queen's request, the *Regimen sanitatis* that Arnau de Vilanova had drawn up for the king. Berenguer read Latin, was well grounded in medical theory, and in his surgical practice followed the approach of Teodorico Borgognoni.[30] When he died in 1310 he would have been acknowledged as the professional peer of any contemporary physician, even of one with an academic preparation.

Yet within two decades the social and occupational setting had begun to change markedly. Academic medical training, once quite rare, was now significantly more common, at least in the cities, where there were also now more people prepared to rate medical learning as a valuable commodity and where specialization was now possible. In this setting, the labels *phisicus* and *cirurgicus* seemed more obviously to denote a difference in preparation, even though most *phisici* in the Crown of Aragon would still have had no academic training. At this point, therefore, a number of young surgeons, often sons of surgeons, decided to identify themselves as physicians. There was still enough technical and intellectual overlap between their domains that for some the change might have involved no more than adopting a new title. Pere Correger of Valencia, evidently Guillem's son, called himself a surgeon in his first years of practice (1318–23), but beginning in 1325 he used the title *fisicus* just as often, and at the height of his career in the service of Alfons III he called himself *fisicus et sirurgicus* (1333).[31] Moreover, at least one young surgeon went so far as to earn formal accreditation as a physician. Arnau ça Riera, Berenguer's son

29 McVaugh and García Ballester, "Medical Faculty," p. 19, doc. 4.
30 McVaugh, "Royal Surgeons."   31 C 456/66v (17 Jan. 1333).

and at least the third generation in a surgical dynasty, attended Montpellier in the late 1320s and attained the status of *bacallarius in medicina*; thereafter he, like Pere, called himself *fisicus* at least as often as *sirurgicus* and was appointed in 1336 to serve Pere III as "phisicus et cirurgicus, peritus in medicinali sciencia." In 1344 Arnau capped his new career by receiving the rank of *magister in medicina* at Lerida.[32]

Arnau is the only surgeon we can yet prove to have opted to qualify in medicine, but there are other university-trained physicians who display a suggestive professional interest in surgery: the translator of Lanfranc's *Surgery* into Catalan, for example, Guillem Salva (1329), had taken at least a preliminary medical degree at Montpellier.[33] In any case, there were many surgeons like Pere Correger in the larger cities who, between 1320 and 1340, adopted the label of "physician" with or without formal justification.[34] Their ability to change fields so easily confirms the existence of a generally held medical culture among physicians and surgeons, and the flexibility of those occupational labels, down through the 1330s.[35]

Apothecaries and medicine

Superficially, apothecaries (*apothecarii, herbolarii*) may seem occupationally more distinct from physicians than do surgeons; actually, both technical and economic necessity bound them tightly together. For the apothecary's apparently simple role of providing the medicines called for by the physician

---

[32] McVaugh and García Ballester, "Medical Faculty."

[33] Guillem Salva is perhaps to be identified with the surgeon Guillem ça Selva who was practicing in Castelló in 1341 (Roca Traver, "Ordenaciones," p. 119) and in Morella in 1344 (C 877/17r–v). His translation was identified by Beaujouan, "Manuscrits médicaux," p. 192. It is contained in MS Madrid, BN 10162, where the Lanfranc begins on f. 1 and refers to Guillem as "licenciat de Montpeller en la art de medicina." It incorporates "addiciones," glosses bringing both medical and surgical authorities (Avicenna and Teodorico) to bear on Lanfranc's text, and apparently some other materials as well: at f. 43 a section beginning "Tot hom qui vol saber lo cors de la luna" appears to be a translation of the Latin astrological tract, "Quicumque cursum lune scire . . ." (TK2 col. 1236). On f. 53 an *explicit* reads: "Aci es acabada la suma de çirurgia la qual a Lemfranch de Milla compone molt utilment ha deu gràcies. La qual mestre Guillem Salva baxeller in mediçina he a profit del molt alt senyor en R. Berenguer comte de les muntanyes de prades aprechs de dos cars amichs seus tresladi de lati en romanc felment he clar. En lany de nostre senyor deu m.ccc.xx.ix al mes de mag" (the infante Ramon Berenguer held that title 1324–41). On f. 76 another *explicit* announces the conclusion of (another?) translation by Guillem, but the Catalan continues (to f. 109v) with more material on medicine, on recipes and *experimenta*, some of which at least draw on Montpellier sources. The whole deserves much closer study than I have been able to give it.

[34] McVaugh, "Royal Surgeons."

[35] Consider the case of the surgeon in Alzira (Valencia) who was told in 1347 that since he had been examined in surgery, and since he would have to have understood medicine in order to be able to treat wounds and the like, he could therefore practice medicine too without taking a separate examination, despite the 1329 *furs* (C 882/144v–145).

was in reality complicated and difficult, and placed considerable responsibility upon him. He dealt in two broad categories of drugs: simples, or individual medicinal plants (sometimes animal and mineral products might also be called for); and compound medicines, drugs made up of a mixture of ingredients, each one performing its own proper function – warming, opening, ripening – in the body, and the whole with perhaps a superadded property, in medicinal theory the *forma specifica*.[36] In neither case was the apothecary's task straightforward. In the case of simples, he had to be able to identify a plant from its technical name – not so hard perhaps as regards the case of native plants that he himself had collected, but vastly more problematic when it involved exotic materials that he had never seen alive, especially since part of his task was to report on the conditions in which the plant had been growing. In the case of compounds, if he was not to trust to a larger apothecary or wholesale supplier and chose to prepare his own, he had to know which ingredients would produce the sought-after effects, alone or in combination, and had to mix them in the correct proportions and manner. In both cases, therefore, an apothecary's job presupposed medical as well as botanical expertise.

A physician who prescribed medicines for a patient thus had three choices: to prepare them himself, to supervise an apothecary's work, or to trust entirely to the apothecary's competence. In several works Arnau de Vilanova held up the first as an ideal, while admitting implicitly that it was usually impossible to maintain. But he warned that if you use an apothecary's services you place great responsibility in his hands. It is now he, not you, who knows whether a simple medicine was gathered from a dry or a wet locality, for example; the different circumstances may critically affect the pharmacological properties of the sample. Hence you should oversee the apothecary's work as far as possible, lest he lead you into error – giving you the wrong medicine, for example, whether by mistake or by design. "Suppose you want to administer hemp agrimony [*eupatorium*] but you do not know what it looks like, and the *herbolarius* brings you wild salvia [*salviam agrestem*]; if you are to avoid a mistake you will have to see how the authorities describe *eupatorium*."[37] Sometimes outright fraud is involved: "In Montpellier they make up a 'licorice juice' out of starch and the marrow of *cassia fistula* and sell it to visitors [*occidentalibus cunctis*], so in order to avoid this fraud it is helpful to use fresh licorice

---

[36] Arnau de Vilanova, *Aphorismi de gradibus*, pp. 17–19.

[37] "Et propter minores introducatur exemplum, verbi gracia: tu vis eupatorium ministrare, nec tamen cognoscis et herbolarius apportat tibi salviam agrestem. Si vis vitare deceptionem considera qualiter eupatorium describunt sapientes. Sic enim invenit quidam medicus in opere suo circa usum eupatorii et spice celtice et multarum aliarum medicinarum": *Repetitio*, f. 280va; MS Munich, CLM 14245, f. 35v. The thirteenth-century *Herbal of Rufinus* confirms that for many people, if not Arnau, *eupatorium* and *salvia agrestis* were one and the same plant (ed. Thorndike; pp. 129, 284).

instead."[38] Compound medicines rouse additional concerns about the accuracy and care with which they were prepared – to illustrate what may happen, Arnau describes a case when a collyrium intended to soothe the eyes instead produced excruciating pain in a patient, and was found to have been prepared by an apothecary who the day before had worn the same clothes while grinding up verdigris.[39] The potential for confusion and danger is such that the physician "should give thanks, in treating patients, for the skill and dependability of a good and honest [*bonus et pius*] apothecary."[40]

For Arnau, one such apothecary was Pere Jutge of Barcelona, with whom he had been associated in medical care since at least 1285 – that is, before his period of teaching at Montpellier.[41] The adjectives *bonus et pius* in Pere's case would have had more than merely medical implications, inasmuch as he and Arnau were close friends linked by religious conviction as well as professional function: Arnau chose Pere as one of his executors, and the scriptorium where Arnau's theological writings were copied seems to have been located in Pere's Barcelona home.[42] But Arnau was not the only Catalan physician to depend on Pere Jutge. Guillaume de Béziers called on him to prepare medicines – electuaries and juleps – for Jaume II,[43] and Pere continued to make up comfits for the royal family until his death in 1316. His frequent close contacts with other Catalan physicians in Barcelona and elsewhere – Martí de Calça Roja, Bernat ça Llimona, Ramon Marini of Manresa, Joan de Salerno of Santa Coloma – show how fully and broadly a respected apothecary could be integrated into a medical community.

Apothecaries, of course, were in themselves another community: the distinctive economic character of their occupation enforced an awareness of one another's activity. The very fact of living and selling in the same area – in Barcelona, on the same street, the *carraria apothecariorum* (today the *carrer de*

---

38 "Palam quod componunt in Montepessulano succum liquiritie ex amido et medulla cassiefistule quem vendunt occidentalibus cunctis, ad quam fraudem evitandam salubriter ponitur pro ea liquiritia recens": Arnau de Vilanova, *Antidotarium*, f. 244rb.

39 "Compertum est etiam quod colirium suaviter dolorum mitigativum oculorum tritum ab apothecario induto veste qua die precedente indutus triverat viride eris immissum oculo patientem cruciabat": ibid. Arnau tells the same story in *Repetitio*, f. 281rb.

40 "Ipsum felicitat in sanando peritia ac fidelitas apothecarii boni et pii": ibid. Not surprisingly, therefore, one can occasionally even find apothecaries being taught their trade by physicians – what the different herbs are, and how to prepare electuaries: AHCP, Bernat Blanch Liber firmitatis 1289–90, f. 51 (31 March 1290).

41 Inferred from RP 620/37v, where Alfons II pays the debts of the late abbot of Montearagón, including, close together, sums owed to Arnau de Vilanova, Pere Jutge, and two other physicians, presumably for medical care.

42 On Pere, see Perarnau, *L' "Alia informatio,"* pp. 113–14, and Batlle i Gallart, "Apotecaris," pp. 101–2.

43 One such order is reported in C 258/95v, of 18 March 1303; another is quoted by Sorní and Suñé, "Boticario," pp. 11–13, extracting a letter of April 1304 also published by MF, II:339–40, doc. 463.

la Llibreteria[44] – though it fostered competition, also facilitated the creation of a common occupational culture. Moreover, apothecaries were compelled to depend on each other in ways that physicians, for example, were not. The trade depended on supplying the public with drugs that could not be grown locally, and hence local apothecaries were often forced to turn to bigger merchants for their supplies. At any moment there were one or two Barcelona retailers who had established themselves as distributors to provincial apothecaries, who in turn might resell drugs to apothecaries in even smaller towns. Until 1316 Pere Jutge fulfilled this function, supplying drugs to apothecaries in Gerona and else-where.[45] Subsequently still more important in this role, for the two decades before his death in 1339, was Pere de Berga: Pere (assisted by his brother Bernat) was at the heart of the apothecaries' network within the city of Barcelona, representing the trade in the municipal *consell* (*jurat* in 1321, 1325, 1332, 1333, and 1338) and linked by marriage to other Barcelonan families in the same trade (son-in-law to one apothecary, Bernat de Calidis, and brother-in-law to another, Francesc de Armentera). He was also linked professionally to apothecaries throughout Catalonia, supplying them with their drugs: his clients can be found in Castelló d'Empúries (1324), Cervera (1331), Santa Coloma de Queralt (1333), Puigcerdà (1337), Manresa (before 1339), and even Zaragoza (1332).[46]

The need to supervise an apothecary's production of medicines was neither new nor peculiar to the Crown of Aragon. One solution that had gained favor was the acceptance of one particular *antidotarium* or dispensatory as a standard. The collection that had emerged as a general choice was the so-called *Antidotarium Nicolai*, a compilation of recipes for compound medicines that was already circulating in the first half of the thirteenth century. By the 1270s it was a school text for the medical faculty at Paris, and within a few more years its use was being imposed on apothecaries in some European cities. The *Antidotarium Nicolai* described the preparation of compounds in amounts up to two pounds, and many of its recipes incorporated indefinite quantities ("quod sufficit") of honey or sugar – these materials, introduced into pharmacy by the Arabs, had a certain preservative power, and compounds made up in bulk according to the formulas of the *Antidotarium Nicolai* would thus keep and could be doled out little by

---

[44] Sorní and Suñé, "Barcelona. Baja edad media," p. 145; Batlle i Gallart, "Apotecaris," pp. 97–8.
[45] C 158/137v, 230v (13 Dec. 1315 and 26 Jan. 1316), complaining of the unwillingness of Geronan apothecaries to pay what they owe for the goods they have bought.
[46] AHPG/CE 43 bis/114v–115 (25 Sept. 1324); AHCC, manual de Jaume Ferrer, Llibres 1349–50, ff. 23–4 (15 May 1350); AHPT 3847/88v (11 Aug. 1333); AHCP, Guillem Bernat de Santfeliu Liber debitorum 1337–8, 6 non. July 1337; AHCM 187, 16 kls. Oct. 1343; ANZ, manual de Miguel Perez de Tauste, 1332(II)/88r–v (7 April 1332).
  Another illustration is furnished by Ramon de Sant-Medir, an apothecary of Gerona who supplied drugs to apothecaries throughout that diocese – to La Bisbal (AHPG, Notari 5–40, 18 kls. Dec. 1337), Banyoles (AHPG, Notari 5–23/86; 29 Nov. 1341), and Camprodon (AHPG,

little.[47] This made it possible for physicians to oversee the production of drugs once or twice a year rather than every time they were needed, and this sort of control is already incorporated into the medical legislation of Frederic II of Sicily from the 1230s, even though there is no proof that the *Antidotarium Nicolai* provided the particular standard to be followed in that kingdom.

Library lists and inventories indicate that the *Antidotarium Nicolai* was penetrating the Crown of Aragon in the early fourteenth century, though it is not always possible definitely to distinguish it from other *antidotaria* that were also circulating. As we have already noted, the work is found (together with other similar texts) in fourteenth-century manuscripts now in Catalan cathedrals;[48] the one pre-plague inventory of an apothecary known from the kingdom, that of Arnau Torrella of Valencia (active 1320–9), lists fifty or so simple and compound medicines found at his shop, and, at the end, "un libre de paper apellat antidotari."[49] But we ought not to imagine the genre as of interest merely to apothecaries narrowly defined, for *antidotaria*, like apothecaries, were part of a more general medical culture. After all, the *Antidotarium Nicolai* was incorporated into the Paris medical curriculum, and perhaps the most successful composition of the Paris master Jean de Saint-Amand (fl. 1260–90?) was his commentary on this very work – which may have been among the books bought by the physician Pere Bos of Castelló d'Empúries in 1319.[50] The one original composition of Armengaud Blaise that survives is a *Tabula antidotarii* that gives summary accounts of seventy-three compound medicines – their ingredients, function, dose, and manner of administration – sixty-two of which can be found in the *Antidotarium Nicolai*.[51] Arnau de Vilanova himself began to write an *Antidotarium*, starting by describing for his medical readers the problems they would confront in identifying and preparing medicines; the second half of the work, with the list of compounds, appears to have been compiled by his disciple Pedro Cellerer by drawing heavily on the *Antidotarium Nicolai*.[52] The surgeon Bernat Serra had an *antidotarium* in his

Notari 5–128, 2 non. Aug. 1347). In turn, provincial apothecaries resold to others still further away: Guillem Martorell of Manresa bought from a supplier in Barcelona (AHCM 187, 16 kls. Oct. 1343) and resold in more remote towns like Tremp (AHCM 63, id. Oct. 1317).

    Catalan wholesaling of drugs probably extended to customers as far away as Toulouse in this period, though I have no direct testimony to this; Wolff, *Commerce et marchands*, pp. 145–6, 215–17, emphasizes the importance of this trade in the second half of the fourteenth century.

[47] Goltz, *Mittelalterliche Pharmazie*; some of her findings are briefly summarized by Hunt, *Popular Medicine*, pp. 13–15.

[48] Above, p. 88, n. 77.

[49] ARV, protocolos 2205/51 (inventory of 19 Sept. 1329).

[50] Above, p. 91.

[51] Above, chapter 1. One manuscript of the work actually refers to it as a "compendium super Antidotarium Nicolai," and it may be that the shorter title should be understood as *Tabula antidotarii [Nicolai]*; see Daems, "Ermengald Blasius' Tabellen."

[52] The genuineness of the first half is supported by its repetition of the Arnaldian anecdote mentioned in n. 39 above.

library of medical and surgical texts, for surgeons too needed to understand pharmacy.[53]

The availability of *antidotaria* and the preparation of compound medicines in bulk did not, however, eliminate the need of constant close association between physicians and apothecaries. Practitioners could not always be sure that the standard remedies would be sufficient: sometimes it was necessary to design a new medicine adapted to the patient's age, gender, and condition. Naturally it was not always possible to anticipate such a need for a new medicine, but the physician should try to do so in order to plan with his apothecary and ensure its availability at the proper moment: "the compounding [of medicines] involves, in order, the cleaning, powdering, measuring out, mixture, and coction [of the ingredients] – and with regard to coction [the physician] should forewarn his helpers, the apothecaries, and agree with them upon a time [when the drug will be ready], lest for lack of warning they prepare them later than they ought."[54]

This is no doubt an important reason why physicians so often set out on calls accompanied by apothecaries. In 1321 the king's sickly son Joan, then archbishop of Toledo, was ill in Castile; his own physician Pedro Cellerer looked after him, his father's physician Martí de Calça Roja was consulted by mail for his knowledge of the infante's complexion, but Bernat de la Grassa (active 1321–33), physician of Valencia, was also summoned to treat the young archbishop.[55] Bernat prudently took with him his own apothecary, Jacme Espanyol (active 1320–34), whom he evidently continued to think of as a dependable man – *bonus et pius*: ten years later Jacme appears as Bernat's procurator, appointed to collect monies owing to the physician.[56]

It must have been a temptation to both parties to formalize this interdependence, in the manner suggested by a surviving contract:

> I master Pere Ritxart, surgeon, of Santa Coloma [de Queralt], promise you Ramon Roqueta, apothecary of the said town, that for five years to come I will get or cause to be gotten anything that has to be bought in my practice from your shop and

53 "Quendam alium librum vocatum Anthidotari scriptum in pergamentis cum cohoperta nigra": Carreras Valls, "Bernat Serra," p. 21.
54 "In preparacione vero debent attendi per ordinem mundacio, pulverisacio, dispensacio, remollicio, coccio – circa quorum decoccionem informare debet ministros, ut apothecarios, et horas et tempora eis determinare, ne defectum precepti tardius preparent quam debent": Arnau de Vilanova, *Repetitio*, f. 280va; MS Munich, CLM 14245, f. 35v.
55 For Pedro and Martí, see C 246/276 (29 Sept. 1321); for Bernat's visit, C 246/294 (5 Nov. 1321).
56 In April 1321 Bernat and Jacme had brought a complaint against an apothecary of Narbonne who, they claimed, had stolen money, rings, and a sword from them; they could not immediately follow up the case, however, because of the summons to the infante (ARV, Just. Val., 36/107r–v). Their later association is established in ARV, Just. Civil 36/31 (8 March 1331).

For another example of close collaboration between an apothecary and a *medicus*: Jaume d'Avinyó (surgeon) and Ramon Llimons (apothecary), traveling together from Valencia to the king at Borriol: C 298/99–100, expenses of April 1312, and RP 275/96.

nowhere else, so long as I remain in Santa Coloma, and I will bring you business insofar as it pertains to my art of surgery, to the best of my ability, so long as you are faithful [*legalis*] to me in things pertaining to my profession.

I the said Ramon Roqueta promise to be faithful [*fidelis et legalis*] to you. Both swear and do homage mutually with mouth and hands.[57]

Ramon (active 1333–48) seems to have just arrived in Santa Coloma, so the arrangement secured him a livelihood.[58]

To the public, indeed, the economic connection between physician and apothecary had long seemed both conspicuous and dangerous. Suspicions of the relationship are manifest, for example, in municipal contracts that require a physician to swear that "he will have no ties [*partem nec communionem*] with any apothecary,"[59] and in municipal attempts to regulate apothecaries correspondingly.[60] The Valencian *furs* of 1329 address an only slightly different side of the economics, fee-splitting, by laying it down that "no physician shall share in the fees of apothecaries, and each year they shall swear an oath . . . promising to set apothecaries' fees moderately."[61] But there were more than economic reasons why the two might swear faith in this way, for, as Arnau suggests, a dependable apothecary was the physician's other self, a semi-autonomous agent of his mind and will. And the public saw the apothecary in the same light, as, ideally, "a scientific worker and practitioner, experienced in an art that serves medicine just as the body's members serve the

---

[57] "Mag. Petrus Rixart medicus in serurgia habitator Sancte Columbe ex certa sciencia firma atque solempni sa.. promito vobis R. Roqueta ypothecario dicti loci et vestris quod hinc ad quinque annos etc. ego quicquid officio meo fuerit necessarium quod emi habeat accipiam et accipi faciam in vestro operatorio dum sim in loco Sancti Columbe et non in alio, et aportabo et procurabo vobis comanda . . . vestro officio de omni hoc quod officio meo pertinant secundum artem meam cirurgie iuxta posse meum, et prout ita tamen quod poteris vos legalis sitis michi in rebus necessariis meo officio. Et ego dictus R. Roqueta promito vobis esse fidelis et legalis. Ambo iurant et faciunt homagium ore et manibus adinvicem" (AHPT 3847/191; 8 Dec. 1333). Another example is between Bernat de Llampaies and Martí de Rivalta in Castelló, where the apothecary (Bernat) promises more explicitly to direct all patients to his partner: AHPG/CE 16/28 (3 Feb. 1296).

[58] He was apparently from Cervera, and married the daughter of a recently deceased physician of Santa Coloma shortly after he arrived.

[59] The quotation is from a contract of 1307 in Castelló d'Empúries. As early as 1243 the statutes of Avignon prohibited such associations between apothecaries and physicians, including arrangements designed to force the sick to patronize a particular apothecary (Barthélemy, *Médecins*, p. 11), and Ramon Llull warned of such practices in the 1270s (above, chapter 3). Cf. Diepgen, *Theologie*, pp. 44-5.

[60] The city of Lerida was already by 1330 requiring its apothecaries individually to swear to the "stabilimenta civitatis facta supra facto apothecariorum" (AML 769/32); the individual *stabilimenta* are not listed there, but by 1351 at the latest they included the promise not to make any private arrangements with physicians (AML 775/14). Dulieu, *Pharmacie*, pp. 20–1, summarizes the terms of the oath sworn by Montpellier apothecaries from the thirteenth century; and see also Naso, *Medici*, pp. 148–9, though her examples are all from the fifteenth.

[61] García-Ballester, McVaugh, and Rubio-Vela, *Medical Licensing*, p. 60.

head."[62] It is not surprising therefore that we can find apothecaries who, like surgeons, were able to cross the blurry occupational line and set themselves up as physicians in name as well as fact.[63]

Barbers

It would seem implausible that barbers should have had a significant place in a learned medical culture. Only a portion of their activity was even loosely medical in character, and what there was – bloodletting, and perhaps in rare cases some dentistry – required manual dexterity rather than a knowledge of pathology or even physiology. The learning necessary for their craft was so slight that the *fueros* of Monzón do not anticipate the need for them to demonstrate it before a court. Yet the historical evidence suggests that barbers recognized the growing opportunities for medical practitioners in fourteenth-century society and therefore made medical care a greater and greater part of their public character – some, indeed, changing their occupational identification into the bargain. By the 1340s barbers had become much more fully a part of medical life than they had been a generation before.

Evidence of many kinds seems to suggest that this process had begun in the 1330s, as barbers began to assume the role of surgeons.[64] It can be seen, for example, in the new occupational labels being adopted by individual practitioners like Guillem de Tortosa of Valencia, barber in 1320 but surgeon in 1335;[65] or Pere Nadal of Gerona, calling himself a barber from 1321 until 1334 and thereafter (until his death in 1349) a surgeon.[66] Or it can be seen in the tag, "barberius et cirurgicus," claimed by Ferrer Alexandri of Barcelona in 1344 and

---

[62] "Scientificus opifex et probatissimus practicus in arte huiusmodi apothecarie, que tanquam membrum capiti arti medicine convertitur"; the image is that of Pere III, writing in late 1348 about the apothecary Pere Janer (C 887/95v). Pere is expressing gratitude specifically for Janer's service in the plague, but the apothecary had had a long relationship with the royal household (see above, chapter 3, n. 115).

[63] A case in point is Ramon de Podio of Gerona, whose father Pere had been an apothecary there 1323–35, as had his grandfather before that. Ramon identified himself as an apothecary 1332–40 (agreeing to train an apprentice in that trade in 1339), but by 1341 he had begun to term himself "fisicus," and by 1348 his medical patients ranged from the bishop to Jews of Gerona.

[64] In one case where a barber tried to enter the apothecaries' trade he seems to have failed: Bernat de Pla, "barberius qui consuevi esse apothecarius et barberius Barchinone," confessed his indebtedness to another apothecary "pro precio plurimum diversarum specierum seu rerum de dicto officio apothecarie quas diversis temporibus multis et diversis vicibus a vobis emi habui et recepi": ACB, manual de Bernat de Vilarrúbia Feb. 1334/5–April 1334/5, ff. 64v–65v (21 Feb. 1335).

[65] As *barbitonsor*, ARV, Just. Val. 29/75, 11 May 1322; as surgeon, ARV, Just. Civil 46, [17] kls. Jun. 1335.

[66] He is *barberius* in AHPG, Notari 8–1, 6 non. July 1321, and Notari 4–7, 2 kls. Sept. 1334; but he is *cirurgicus* in Notari 6–8, 2 kls. July 1334, and in his will of 1349 (Notari 5–58/95r–v).

by Guillem Bolurri of Puigcerdà in 1347.[67] In 1338 two men calling themselves barbers, one of Gerona and one of La Bisbal, thirty-five kilometers away, set up an association to practice together *ratione officii barberie et cirurgie*.[68]

We can study the process of transition closely in Santa Coloma de Queralt, where in March 1338 two *barbitonsores* – Berenguer Fontanet and Francesc Metge – created a *societas*, a joint practice that would split equally their collective income from barbering, bloodletting, cupping, or "serurgia." Berenguer was the senior man, the established figure, and had been a barber in Santa Coloma since 1325, but now he was declaring himself a surgeon; and, as a surgeon, he was permitted to give forensic testimony before a court two years later.[69] Francesc, far less experienced, had just moved to town from Cardona, and was trying to develop a new career. In that same summer of 1338 he contracted to serve the surgeon Pere Ritxart on condition that "instruatis me in dicto officio vestro serurgie," so that he could consolidate his position.[70]

In the 1330s, too, we begin to get details about concrete cases of barbers' practice. In the spring of 1336 Guillelma, the wife of Domènech de Montnegre of Gerona, was attacked and gravely wounded in the face and limbs. A friend brought her to a local *barberius*, Arnau de Prato, who treated her wounds and came regularly to her bedside for three weeks while she was recovering.[71] When a cleric of Besalú fell and broke his right arm in 1337, his friends asked the Besalú *barberius* Bernat Jordà to cure him; Bernat put the dislocated limb back into place and set the bone, healing him in a little less than a month.[72] Both these cases suggest that surgical competence was now expected in barbers, since in each case a particular practitioner was sought out by his client. On the other hand, there is also some reason to think that the professional situation of barbers was still a little ambiguous. Arnau de Prato was paid twenty *sous* by Guillelma's husband for his treatment, but Bernat Jordà had been paid nothing and was suing for his expenses and fees; his erstwhile patient gave as his reason for refusing to pay the fact that "[Bernat] now claims in his suit that he is a healer, a qualified surgeon, yet then he only called himself a barber."[73] (The court seems eventually to have found for Bernat.)

---

[67] For Ferrer: RP 321/111v, paying him for service in Roussillon from 29 Sept. 1343 to 24 Jan. 1344 at two *sous* per day. For Guillem: AHCP, Joan Montaner Liber firmitatis 1347–8 (13 April 1347).

[68] AHPG, Notari 5–34/22v–23v. The barbers are Francesc Conill of Gerona (recorded 1328–43, always as a barber) and Joan Marie of La Bisbal.

[69] The *societas* is recorded in AHPT 3855/256v (24 March 1338); he had first referred to himself as a barber, in AHPT 3835/96 (30 July 1325). In his testimony to the court as *cirurgicus* he swore "prout humana fragilitas et cursus cirurgie nosse sinit": AHPT 3854/181v (18 Feb. 1340).

[70] AHPT 3857/148v (2 Sept. 1338).

[71] ADG, Sèrie C (procesos), 161 (new numeration); Arnau gave his testimony 6 July 1336.

[72] ADG, Sèrie C, 191 (new numeration); case of 25 Feb. 1338.

[73] "Ipse [Bernardus] conetur dicere in sua petitione quod sit medicus et bonus cisurgicus et tamen se al. barberium apellavit": ibid.

Such evidence of an expanding medical or surgical role for barbers makes understandable the introduction of controls on their specifically health-oriented activities, which similarly first become evident in the 1330s. At the turn of the century their practice had been supervised by king or municipality no more than by the *fueros*. Jaume I might have licensed a town barber in the environs of Montpellier (at Lattes, in 1274),[74] where a general policy of medical control was already well established, but no such policy existed in his peninsular realms, not even by the time of his grandson Jaume II. Easy entrance into the occupations of apothecary and barber perhaps explains their early coalescence into loose brotherhoods (*confratrias*), which in turn could lead to a voice for them in municipal government, as in Barcelona.[75] In Valencia the barbers were the most numerous health practitioners, and were already organized as one of fifteen civic *confratrias* by 1283; the barbers' brotherhood was suppressed early in the reign of Jaume II, along with most of the others, but it was given a new charter in 1311 and allowed to meet at the city's Augustinian priory.[76]

Confratrias like the barbers' had originally had pious rather than professional aims, and the 1311 charter specified several such goals of the brotherhood – relief for the poor, services for the dead; in Valencia and elsewhere, regulation of the craft's activities was not internal but came from outside authority. Barbers tended to disregard holidays and to seize any opportunity to practice, so that towns repeatedly enacted ordinances meant to compel their observance of Sundays and other feasts or fasts as days of rest. Lerida had laid this down for Jewish and Muslim barbers as well as for Christians by 1257;[77] Valls compelled its four barbers to agree to a similar rule in 1299.[78] Individuals, however, continued to evade such regulations. In Calatayud (Aragon), where the town had prohibited shaving or cutting hair at night or by candlelight, the *barbitonsores* appealed collectively to the king to ensure that everyone be made to obey.[79] By 1327 the barbers of Huesca evidently had some power of self-regulation – "inter se ordinarunt seu statutum fecerunt" – but they too had to appeal to the king to enforce upon all Christian and Jewish barbers of the town their prohibition of Sunday hair-cutting and shaving, practices which, they protested, brought "opprobrium sive etiam detrimentum" upon their Christian clientele.[80] The same

[74] Letter of 7 June 1274 (C 19/130v).

[75] The *speciayres* seem to have had representatives on the *Consell de Cent* as early as 1257: Comenge, *Medicina en Cataluña*, p. 83.

[76] García Ballester and McVaugh, "Nota," pp. 76–7, 87–8, where the document is mistakenly dated 1310 (21 Feb. 1310 is actually 1311, since in Valencia as in most parts of the Crown of Aragon the new year was dated from the Annunciation = 25 March).

[77] Pleyan de Porta, *Apuntes*, pp. 480–1, citing C 5/37.

[78] Carreras y Candi, "Ordinacions," p. 202.

[79] C 432/24v (23 April 1328).

[80] 7 Aug. 1327 (C 191/33v). Conversely, in Tortosa the Muslim *barbitonsores* complained that Christians were trying to enforce Christian feast days upon them and were promised redress (C 358/159v; 28 Jan. 1319).

concern that the Sabbath be observed by barbers and indeed by all tradesmen can be seen in legislation for Catalonia and Valencia in the previous century. Such controls, however imposed, bore only upon the religious implications of the barbers' activity, not upon its medical aspects.

By the 1330s, however, barbers had generally been brought under more narrowly medical supervision. The Valencian *furs* of 1329 insisted for the first time that "no barber shall practice medicine or surgery if he has not been examined by the examiners of practitioners and found competent."[81] Behind this provision would seem to lie a concern, not for the barbers' routine practice of bloodletting, but for the extension of their services into the sphere of medicine, brought on by the absence in many parts of the kingdom of an adequate supply of qualified physicians and surgeons. A command from Alfons III three years later reveals that now bloodletting itself was being scrutinized more carefully. Reacting to complaints that "several individuals, daring to act as *barbitonsores* and to exercise that office even though unskilled in the art, fail to observe the proper times for carrying out phlebotomy and bloodletting, on account of which some incur danger of death and others of illness," the king moved to subordinate barbers to the standards of academic medicine. His strikingly detailed language must certainly indicate consultation with medical advisors:

> no *barbitonsor* . . . may dare or presume to bleed or phlebotomize anyone in the city of Valencia or its suburbs in the first thirty canicular days or in those days called "Egyptian" or during the full moon, or . . . at a conjunction of the moon, unless evident necessity requires it or physicians advise it.[82]

In Barcelona, where barbers were less numerous than in Valencia and represented a much smaller proportion of the health providers of the city, their medical character was acknowledged even sooner. The city's ordinances of 1323 added a new element to previous restrictions on their practice: besides being forbidden to shave or trim hair (*raure ne adobar*) on Saturday night or Sunday, or on any feast when ovens didn't bake, or to leave blood outside their houses or shops, they were prohibited from bleeding anyone on certain special days, except on instructions from a physician.[83] This last provision shows that in Barcelona as in Valencia the medical side of a barber's trade was increasingly becoming a municipal concern. In 1342 the city became even more medically

---

[81] García-Ballester, McVaugh, and Rubio-Vela, *Medical Licensing*, p. 61.

[82] Published by García Ballester and McVaugh, "Nota," p. 88. Lists of the "Egyptian days," two days in each month considered unlucky or dangerous – for starting a journey or an undertaking, or being bled – can be found in Western manuscripts from the ninth century on (Thorndike, *History of Magic*, I:685–6; Steele, "Dies Aegyptiaci"). Arnau de Vilanova agreed that "prohibet medicus flebotomiam fieri tempore excellenter calido sicut hora meridiei et in diebus canicularibus": *De consideracionibus*, pp. 189–90.

[83] AHCB, Llibres de consell, I–8/11r–v. The first provision is already laid down in I–1/6v (December 1301); the first and second appear together in I–1/81 (January 1303).

precise in specifying that no barber should bleed a client at the moon's four quarters.[84]

Furthermore, by the late 1330s Barcelona had recognized that its barbers were becoming medical practitioners who were offering services that required a surgeon's expertise, and in the new regulatory climate of that decade (above, pp. 98–101) the city had begun to require confirmation of their skills before allowing them to practice their craft. The certification of competence granted the "barberius cirurgicus" Bernat Ferrer in October 1338 gives the details of the procedure: the city *consell* chose three practitioners and two citizens, municipal representatives, who subjected the candidate to a long examination and formally pronounced him "capable of treating and curing any wound, simple or compound, and all other conditions pertaining to his art."[85] The three practitioner-examiners were, like the candidate, addressed as "barber-surgeons," but they had been practicing simply as "barbers" for over twenty years.[86] Eight years later it was the same tribunal, virtually to a man, to which Romeu de Lirana – "*cirurgicus* civitatis Barchinone" – was directed when he sought permission to practice surgery in the city.[87] Whatever distinction had once existed between barbers and surgeons had now largely disappeared, just like the corresponding frontier between surgeons and physicians. In the Crown of Aragon, the medical world of 1340 presented a spectrum of roles, with one shading off into another.

The continuum of practice

In trying to understand the nature of the broad community of practitioners that we have been describing, it will be useful to set it against the wider context of the development of occupational communities (guilds) generally in Catalonia

---

[84] "Negun barber ne son missatge no gos sagnar neguna persona a dia de senyal ne en ple de luna ne en quint ne in girat de luna." AHCB, Llibres de consell, I–16/41r–v.

[85] "Sufficiens quantum ad medicandum et curandum omnia vulnera, tam simplicia quam composita, et alia ad ipsam artem pertinenciam": C 869/158r–v. The certificate, dated 22 Oct. 1338, has been recopied into its subsequent confirmation by the king (8 July 1340). No doubt Barcelona's size made it natural that the examination of barbers should have been seen there before anywhere else in Catalonia, but it was not alone in its concern. In September 1346 Pere III responded to a complaint from Vilafranca del Penedès about "barbers and others" who, ignorant of the theory and practice of surgery, were presuming to treat patients – to their great harm. Pere agreed that such barbers would first have to be examined in the art "iuxta constituciones Cathalonie" before practicing surgery (C 643/158v).

[86] The three are Pere Sinola, Bernat Guerau, and Bernat de Pla; the two municipal representatives are Berenguer Basset and Bernat Vives. Pere Sinola can be found in documents of 1316–42 and Bernat Guerau of 1334–44, both always identified as barbers. Bernat de Pla appears as barber 1327–46, but calls himself "cirurgicus" in two documents of 1340 (this is the same man who attempted to set up as an apothecary before 1335; see above, n. 64).

[87] Italics added for emphasis. C 882/141v–142 (2 Jan. 1347). The examining board was described as "Berengario Basseti, Bernardo Vives, Bernardo de Plano, Petro Sinola, et aliis examinatoribus civitatis pretacte ad hoc deputatis."

and neighboring Languedoc during the later Middle Ages.[88] Their formation originated in or was at least encouraged by the tendency of members of the same craft to live – and practice their art – in the same street. In the early fourteenth century the occupations first began to find a formal identity by organizing a *confratria* of their members, an entity that could act in law and could receive and hold monies: the contributions of the members paid for the annual celebration of their patron saint's feast, and also helped to provide in the case of the poverty, illness, or death of one of their number.

The occupations themselves were still loose and unorganized at this time, with few difficulties placed in the way of newcomers – apprentices or immigrants – who might want to enter them. They did not yet have the character of a society sworn to its own regulations. Regulation of the individual crafts did not originate in monopolistic self-interest but in the concern of town governments (or monarchs) to control the quality of goods and services and to prevent fraud and inconvenience or danger to their citizens. Typically, town councils laid down regulations which became the crafts' earliest statutes (sometimes at the crafts' request), and in swearing to them artisans were really swearing not to go against the laws of the town. Such external control over the affairs of a craft – exercised through municipal agents, sometimes through craft-representatives – went virtually uncontested by its members.

Consistent with this lack of internal regulation was a looseness of occupational hierarchy within the crafts. In neighboring Languedoc, at least, thirteenth-century artisans fell into two broad categories: masters (*magistri*), who owned their own shops, and apprentices (*discipuli*), who had contracted with a master to learn his art. Aged anywhere from fourteen to twenty-five, an apprentice would typically pay a small sum to the master and promise one to four years of service in return for training and the necessities of life, after which time he could practice the craft independently upon payment of a small fee; but apprenticeship was not yet a necessary precondition for practice. At the beginning of the fourteenth century a new category of artisan began to appear, the assistant (*operator*, *discipulus collocatus*). Sometimes – but not always – this man had previously trained as an apprentice. He was an independent craftsman who did not own his own shop, but served a master for a salary (or rarely for a share of the profits) for a specified period of time; when the agreed-upon time

---

[88] Freitag, "Die katalanischen Handwerkerorganisationen," attempts a unified treatment but recognizes that for developments before the 1330s any reconstruction is speculative; the real focus of his study is the second half of the century. Bonnassie, *Organización*, has little to say about the period before 1400; Tintó i Sala, *Gremis*, is only a sketch. I have found particularly suggestive the work of Gouron, *Réglementation*, which begins its close examination of the crafts in the twelfth century and carries it down to the sixteenth: Gouron's Languedoc stretches from Toulouse to Montpellier, and the picture he presents accords so well with the little that has been written about Catalonia to the south that I have depended heavily upon it in the summary that follows.

was up, the assistant could do what he wanted – contract again to serve the same master or another, or set up in business for himself. This occupational fluidity meant that it was not unheard-of for individuals to abandon one craft and take up another.

From the second half of the fourteenth century on, however, we find the occupational associations of Languedoc and Catalonia closing and hardening. The charitable *confratria* becomes only one side of a different legal entity, the guild, which is assuming a certain independence or autonomy from municipal interference and is controlling its own affairs, most obviously perhaps by strictly limiting admission. Apprenticeship followed by an examination or the creation of a master-work comes to be a requirement for anyone who would enter the guild, and it is correspondingly virtually impossible to move from one craft to another. It is much more difficult for newcomers to town or for assistants or apprentices to cross the threshold into the craft association; the distinction between the latter two categories erodes, as both are increasingly exploited by and dependent on their masters. By the middle of the fifteenth century the new form of the guild is established in the south.[89]

This model of development fits very well the features of the early fourteenth-century health trades that we have had occasion to touch on – their lack of corporate status, their supervision by royal and municipal authorities, the indefinite and permeable boundaries between them, and the absence of formal criteria for identifying a master in a trade. It is borne out when we focus our attention on individual trades, like barbers, already discussed above, or apothecaries. The density of apothecaries was nowhere greater than in Barcelona, and already by 1302 they were grouped with grocers and chandlers in sending representatives to the city council there, yet like the barbers or the physicians they still had no corporate identity. Tales of privileges conferred on them as a collectivity in 1319 and 1337 cannot be substantiated, and the myth that the apothecaries were named a *collegium* by Pere III seems to have arisen out of confusion over the royal ordinance of 1351 that set up a three-man panel (a merchant, a physician, and an apothecary) to supervise their practice but did not recognize them as a body capable of self-governance.[90]

Our model explains, further, the observable continuum of practice across the occupations, as apothecaries and physicians, surgeons and barbers, moved into new fields. And it suggests too that we ought to be able to observe a continuum

---

[89] Wolff, "Recherches," pp. 129–33, 139–42, gives particular attention to the fifteenth-century consolidation of the barbers' guild in Toulouse, which apparently came into being shortly before 1400.

[90] Sorni and Suñé, "Farmacia desde Alfons," pp. 68–70. Such earlier municipal regulation of the trade as existed in Barcelona is outlined in Sorni and Suñé, "Farmacia desde Jaume." Much of the evidence concerning the eventual emergence of the apothecaries' guild has been drawn together by González y Sugrañes, *Contribució*, pp. 31–136.

of independence *within* each occupation, a spectrum of practitioners ranging from the fully independent, self-proclaimed master, down through assistants, students, and servants of gradually diminishing expertise and ambition. If so, at any one time there would have existed many more people involved with the occupation than actually claimed a title, people who were functioning as at least auxiliary practitioners.

We will begin to see these auxiliaries if we look more closely at the practitioners themselves, who normally appear in the documentation not as isolated, self-sufficient individuals, traveling and working alone, but rather as the centers of small companies of people, typically accompanied by as many as three assistants.[91] These assistants fill a variety of roles, but they are all extensions of the practitioner-master and as such are bound to assimilate their master's science and represent it to the public. By defining their activities we can study a portion of the medical spectrum that is normally invisible.

Artificially, one might distinguish two ranks, two types of assistant in a practitioner's entourage that are distinguished by more or less consistent verbal usage as the *scutifer* and the *nuncius*. The former, also occasionally referred to as a *famulus*, was evidently a simple servant, a drudge-of-all-work with little independent activity; he contracted with his master for service in exchange for simple subsistence and scarcely anything more.[92] Jacme Oriol, a cleric from Orís, agreed in 1317 to serve master Joan, *physicus* of Vic, for a year "pro scutifero necnon servitore vestro"; he was to receive food and clothing but no money, and in return would serve faithfully without stealing his master's money; he would go where he was sent and obey all licit commands.[93] One typical duty for a servant was protecting his master against the likelihood of attacks in the streets – the king routinely granted many practitioners who had to visit their patients' homes by night as well as by day special permission to arm themselves and a *famulus* ("ensem et alia arma prohibita portare"), a practice normally forbidden by the city.[94]

---

[91] For example, Guillaume de Carcassonne, called from Lerida to Montblanc to attend Alfons, came attended by a *scutifer* and two "footmen"; the king paid the expenses of all four: RP 303/33 (July 1333). Quite exceptional was Bernat de Figuerola of Manresa, who hired *five* men "pro mancipiis" to defend his person and do his bidding (AHCM 184, 2 id. Dec. 1343).

[92] Though Amphosius, a physician of Castelló d'Empúries, agreed to pay a *scutifer* 100 *sous* for a year's service; but this is unusual (AHPG/CE 35/60r–v; 7 Feb. 1319).

[93] ACFV 69, 8 id. Nov. 1317. Housing for the servant is never specified and must have been taken for granted – see Martí de Soler, whose servant stayed "secum" (ACFV 220, 2 non. Sept. 1332).

[94] Such a privilege, for example, was granted to the apothecaries Antoni Pautrer of Valencia, 25 July 1329 (C 479/94r–v), and Ramon de Podio of Gerona, 13 April 1338 (C 863/206), each with one *famulus*. Bonanat Metge, surgeon of Barcelona, had the privilege conferred on him and a *discipulus* by Jaume II in 1324, confirmed by Alfons III in 1331, and reconfirmed by Pere III in 1336 (C 859/204v). Because they had to travel in the day to collect herbs or at night to tend to patients, the Barcelona apothecaries Joan de la Geltrú and Felip Jutge were given permission in 1325 for themselves and their *nuncii* to go armed; two years later the privilege was extended to

The term *scutifer* in documents evidently often conceals an apprentice (the term *discipulus* sometimes does so as well). Apprentices' contracts committed them to virtually the same utter subordination to their master as a servant's, in largely identical language. But in addition to their food, clothing, and shoes, they could expect their master to teach them his trade "as best you can given your knowledge and my abilities," as the standard contract guardedly puts it;[95] they might also receive a small sum or their tools if they completed their apprenticeship.[96] In addition, what frequently sets apprentices apart from mere servants is their youth – they are usually committed by a parent – and the much longer term of service to which they are committed, usually somewhere from three to seven years.

The subtler details of apprenticeship varied, however, depending on the master's own needs – for apprentices were not there just to learn. Occasionally a practitioner was given a cash payment for accepting an apprentice, for to a family with a son's future to ensure it was often worth a financial sacrifice to buy him the chance at a career: Guillem de Ecclesia, a Barcelonan miller, promised six pounds in support of his son Simon's living expenses when he apprenticed him to the surgeon Bononat de Villa.[97] But even without a cash incentive, practitioners took on apprentices because they could thus guarantee themselves submissive and inexpensive labor for several years to come. Guillem Moraria, a Valencian apothecary in need of help, went so far as to hire an agent in Morvedre (present-day Sagunt), thirty kilometers away, "to get and bring back ... a boy who will stay with me to learn my occupation" – not, probably, out of an unselfish wish to sponsor a child.[98] Not even a university-trained physician, like Pere Gavet, disdained the opportunity to take on an apprentice.

A few practitioners' careers are known in such full detail as to make

cover Joan's brother Gaubert as well, plus two "discipulis negociatoribus seu gestoribus" for *each* of the three apothecaries (C 230/43). Mutgé Vives, *Ciudad de Barcelona*, p. 185, describes the city's unhappiness with such royal privileges.

95 "Prout melius poteris secundum scienciam vestram et meam subtilitatem": AHPT 8599/45v (27 Sept. 1335).

96 An apprentice to the Gerona apothecary Ramon de Ulmo was to receive 30 *sous* in the last of his five years' apprenticeship (AHPG, Notari 4–4, kls. July 1340); an apprentice to the Zaragoza apothecary García Perez d'Olivan was to receive 50 *sous* in his seventh year. Many apprentices did not stay the course.

97 ACB, manual de Guillem Borrell Oct. 1332–Dec. 1332, document of 2 kls. Nov. 1332: this reports that five of the six pounds promised on 22 May that year have already been paid over to the surgeon. Ramon de Ulmis of Olot was paid 200 *sous* from someone wishing to learn his art of surgery in five years' service (AHCO, B–29, cuaderno 60, 5 kls. Jan. 1342).

98 "Ad recipiendum sive conducendum . . . unum puerum qui maneat mecum pro adiscendo predictum officium meum apothecarie": ARV protocolos 2830, 21 Oct. 1318. But in general it is barbers who can be found paying for an apprentice, perhaps because the occupation was relatively unattractive: Jaume Graner of Vic paid an apprentice 30 *sous* to stay with him for two years (ACFV 47, 5 non. Oct. 1307); Bernat de Ecclesia of Castelló d'Empúries, 20 *sous* for one year (AHPG/CE 73 bis/46); Berenguer Fontanet of Santa Coloma, 30 *sous* for one year (AHPT 3848, loose leaves).

startlingly clear how normal an apprentice's presence in an entourage might be. Pere Ritxart was practicing surgery in Santa Coloma de Queralt as early as 1329 and was still in practice there when the plague broke out: in those twenty years he treated patients from a very wide catchment area, from Serrateix in the north to Santes Creus in the south and as far east as Sant Cugat Sesgarrigues,[99] and was apparently never without an apprentice at hand. In July 1330 Arnau des Torrent of Balaguer contracted with him for five years; in September 1335, for the same period, Pere Porta of Tarragona; in September 1339 Paschasio Pereç of Aguiló for three years, and in November Ramon Germà of Prades, likewise for three years; in October 1343 Guillem de Netya of Castanyera for three years; in September 1345 Nicolau Romei for five years; and in January 1348 Bernat ça Torre from Santa Coloma. Pere Ritxart's reputation must have been considerable, given so wide a practice; no doubt at least some of these apprentices (a few of whom came from even farther away than his patients) sought him out – the apprentice from his home town of Santa Coloma paid him 100 *sous* for the privilege. Nevertheless, it is impossible not to believe that Pere found it to his own advantage always to have a servant at hand who was more or less trained help. In certain respects an apprentice was more valuable than a simple *scutifer*. An ordinary servant (especially an adult with some education, like the *clericus* Jacme Oriol) could no doubt pick up a smattering of his master's craft in a year, enough perhaps to help out if it were a simple one like barbering. However, an apprentice could be trained in five years to practice some independent medicine or surgery, lightening the practitioner's work load while keeping up his income; that this in fact might happen is shown by Pere Ritxart's contracts with his apprentices, which anticipate that they may receive fees from patients for their services and swear them to turn such fees over to their master without holding anything back for themselves.[100]

On the very same day in 1339 that Paschasio Pereç agreed with Pere Ritxart "ad discendum officium vestrum serurgie," Francesc Metge signed a rather different contract with Pere; Paschasio's first responsibility was to witness the document. During the next year Francesc would, like an apprentice, be given his food, drink, shoes, and clothing, "et instruatis me in dicto officio vestro serurgie prout melius poteritis" – but if he received any fees, he would retain one-third, and in turn his master would give him one-tenth of anything *he* was paid. We have already been introduced to Francesc: he was a barber of Cardona who had

---

[99] These towns are, respectively, 60, 25, and 40 kilometers from Santa Coloma. Pere also had patients from Sant Martí de Maldà (30 km. away), Sant Martí de Sesgueioles (20 km.), Cervera (18 km.), Vilagrasseta (12 km.), Rocafort de Queralt (10 km.), Rourich (2 km.), and several other small villages in the same wide area; his cases included a wide variety of problems – wounds of the head, eyes, throat, feet; kicks from animals – and he ended his career calling himself "sirurgicus et fisicus."

[100] AHPT 3890/156v (31 Oct. 1343); AHPT 3865/142r–v (3 Sept. 1345).

moved to Santa Coloma and was attempting to move into the practice of surgery. Like an apprentice, Francesc was in training, but at a graduate level, and it would be wrong to think of him as merely an apprentice. The value of his services is shown by Pere's willingness not only to let him keep some of his own fees, but to turn over to him a portion of his own; there is still an association of master and assistant, teacher and disciple, but there is obviously an element of collegiality and shared responsibility as well.

Commonly, better-prepared assistants like Francesc were known as *nuncii* (or sometimes *discipuli*). Because they already had some – often considerable – acquaintance with the craft, they could be trusted to act independently, within limits, and to be a surrogate for their master: as one surgeon's assistant promised, "faciam servicium que vos facere debetis in dicto officio."[101] And their experience made them valuable enough that, if they did not negotiate for a share of the profits, like Francesc, they could insist on a reasonable salary.[102] Like apprentices, they might be given a variety of duties, but these would generally be responsible ones calling for some initiative – transporting merchandise,[103] caring for a sick mule,[104] collecting debts and fees owed their master for goods or medical services.[105] And characteristically they would be given charge of the shop (*operatorium*) in their employer's absence (or of a branch in another city),[106] rendering formal accounts of fees taken in on his return.[107] For a *nuncius*, the natural next step in a career was setting up on his own account, and sometimes the temptation to take that step to independent status brought him into conflict with his master: when the apothecary Guillem de Mari joined the infante Alfons on the expedition to Sardinia in 1323, he left his *nuncius* Pere Ferrer to run his shop in Iglesias – but when Guillem returned, Pere refused to turn over the shop, its supplies, or its receipts.[108]

For some, like Francesc Metge, serving an employer as *nuncius* was no doubt a means of gaining additional training in their craft, but for most it was

---

[101] ACFV 61–I, id. Nov. 1313: Bernard Alexandri, surgeon of Perpignan, agreed to serve Guillem Viaderii of Vic for a year, evidently by subcontracting from Guillem to act as town surgeon. Guillem had been promised 200 *sous* yearly by the town if he would practice there (ACFV 53, 9 kls. Dec. 1311), but was now moving to Sanahuia, where he was living as late as 1316. Bernard – to whom Guillem paid half his Vic salary, 100 *sous* – was still in Vic in 1319.

[102] Two years for 160 *sous*, AHPT 3855/217 (10 Feb. 1338); two years for 300 *sous*, AHPT/Valls 28b/22 (5 kls. Mar. [1340?]); two years for 480 *sous*, AHPT 3890/90v (11 Sept. 1343), though here the assistant is not called "nuncius."

[103] The *nuncius* of Guillem Galaubi of Vic was robbed of fifteen pounds' worth of cloth that he was carrying for his master: ACFV 80/53 (30 June 1321).

[104] Letter of 13 May 1334 (C 502/240).

[105] AHCM 187, 16 kls. Oct. 1343; ACFV 57–II, 4 kls. Sept. 1313.

[106] Thus Guillem de Restany, apothecary of Valencia (recorded 1298–1325), also had an *operatorium* tended by two *nuncii* in Castelló de la Plana, which he visited only occasionally: C 205/159 (29 April 1308), 149/103 (27 April 1312), 150/5v (11 June 1312).

[107] Document of 11 Mar 1344 (AHPT 8603/3v–4).

[108] Letter of 21 March 1325 (C 373/114).

primarily a way to acquire enough capital to set up in business independently. Berenguer de Rixach was a struggling apothecary in Puigcerdà 1330–2; then he moved on to Cervera and eventually, in 1338, to Santa Coloma. Here he agreed to assist a local apothecary, Ramon Roqueta, for two years "pro ypothecario seu nuncio ypothecarii . . . regendo operatorium vestrum," in exchange for food, clothing, and 160 *sous*.[109] Two years later Ramon acknowledged that his *nuncius* had rendered a satisfactory accounting for the shop, and the contract was dissolved; then Ramon and Berenguer entered jointly into a *societas*, with Ramon investing his stock and money and Berenguer a much smaller sum.[110] The profits were to be divided 3:1 in Ramon's favor, but even so this was all the commercial foothold Berenguer needed, and he now prospered as he had not been able to in Cervera or Puigcerdà – buying, selling, investing, taking on an apprentice of his own, before disappearing in the plague.[111] We can follow others along the same road who gained experience as well as money – Antoni Pautrer, for example, as he serves the apothecary Joan de la Geltrú as *nuncius* in Barcelona in 1319, becomes acquainted with the wider medical world, including the court physicians whom Joan supplied, meets and marries the niece of one of them (Martí de Calça Roja), and finally establishes himself as a successful apothecary in Valencia.[112]

Thus a reasonable career path for someone who was formed by apprenticeship would have been to spend five years or so training under one master, and then perhaps – if he stuck out the term of his apprenticeship – a few more years working for pay for a second master, before finally striking out on his own and passing into the visible portion of the medical spectrum. For a practitioner formed within a family tradition, the route could be shorter and more direct: some basic knowledge would presumably have been assimilated while growing up, and the first years of drudgery as an apprentice could be reduced or eliminated, while the need for capital in order to set up independently would not be so pronounced. The de Soler family of Vic produced half a dozen practitioners, physicians and surgeons, in the first half of the fourteenth century. The founder of the tradition, the surgeon Guillem de Soler, first appears in the city records in 1313, when his son Guillem is simultaneously identified as a skinner

[109] AHCP Mateu d'Alb Liber debitorum, id. Oct. 1330; AHCP Bernat Blanch Liber firmitatis 15 kls. July 1332; AHPT 3855/217 (10 Feb. 1338). In the last of these documents he names as his *fideiussor* an established apothecary of Cervera, Berenguer Solsona, who may have employed him there.

[110] AHPT 3860/25v (24 April 1340); AHPT 3926/21 (29 April [1340 or 1341]).

[111] AHPT 3865/36v (10 May 1345); the apprentice had himself become an apothecary in Santa Coloma by 1377. Berenguer thus followed a somewhat different career route to success from his employer Ramon (above, at n. 58).

[112] Antoni appears as *nuncius* to Joan, tending to King Jaume in an illness, 8 Oct. 1319 (C 259/259); fifteen years later he is prospering in Valencia, furnishing electuaries, confections, syrups, and other medicines to the royal household (C 503/86r–v). His relation to Martí is established in the latter's will of 11 March 1337 (ARV, Just. Civil 64/4v–6v). He was still alive in 1349.

(*pelliparius*). The younger Guillem remained in that trade until at least 1318 and probably 1320,[113] but by 1322 he had abandoned it and, called "sirurgicus," was associated in practice with his father. In October 1324 he first contracted independently to provide surgical treatment, though his father (who witnessed the document) seems to have been hovering prudently in the background.[114] His father died the next summer,[115] and Guillem began a successful independent practice that lasted until the 1340s and led to service with King Pere III.[116] Here the transition from apprentice to independent practitioner took no more than eight and perhaps as few as three years – though of course Guillem entered the craft as a mature individual rather than as a child.

All these cases confirm that there was as yet no abrupt gulf separating health practitioners from their assistants, any more than there were sharp lines separating one health occupation from another; rather, there was considerable continuity of experience within a broad and rather amorphous community. The criteria that distinguished a surgeon from his *nuncius*, on the one hand, or from a physician, on the other, were still fluid, dependent if anything on economic rather than independent professional factors. Such circumstances favored the communication of knowledge and skills, and ensured that some degree of understanding of the new medical and surgical learning was bound to spread throughout this community of practitioners.

---

[113] The year "1318" is documented by ACFV 69, 15 kls. Aug. 1318 (the volume is erroneously labeled "1317"). In 1320 Guillem entered a profit-making *societas*, though with no trade-label attached (ACFV 201, 3 id. Oct. 1320).

[114] ACFV 205, 15 kls. Nov. 1324: the younger Guillem here contracts to cure a case of hernia ("trenquedura del cifach del ventre"), while his father is present to witness the document. Note the use of the term "cifach": it derives from Arabo-Latin anatomical writings and refers to the peritoneum; see Avicenna's *Canon*, III.13.i.i, or, in the more recent surgical literature of the West, Henri de Mondeville's *Chirurgia*, I.8. Does the use of the term imply a degree of participation in a learned surgery by these practitioners?

[115] The will, giving his son all rights "racione officii mei et ipsius sirurgie," is ACFV 3507/6 (13 Sept. 1325).

[116] The de Soler family went on to become a surgical dynasty whose activities spanned the century; Carreras Valls, "Bernat Serra," pp. 26–7, gives a few references, but has little to say about their origins – they were not, as he believed, of noble stock. After his father's death, the younger Guillem was successful in independent practice, first in Vic and then by 1338 in the service of Jaume III of Mallorca, where he stayed until at least 1341 (C 1054/239, C 1304/64–5). In 1343, however, on the eve of the invasion of Mallorca, he had come into Pere III's service and was sent to treat the Emperor Ludwig IV (C 874/89, 1059/33v). He then accompanied Pere on the Roussillon invasion in 1344 (RP 322/113, 179v), dying before 1349.

Guillem II had two sons who also became surgeons. Bernat was practicing in Vic with his father 1338–40, but by 1347 he had moved to Barcelona, where he worried lest the municipal examiners make difficulties about accepting his credentials (C 644/94). Another son, Pere, accompanied his father on the trip to Emperor Ludwig and then returned to Vic to practice. It was apparently he who, in 1346, asked permission to practice the art of *medicine* in Barcelona (below, p. 239), but it was as a surgeon that he billed a citizen of Vic for having successfully cured him of three plague buboes (*busanyes*) in July 1348 (ACFV 320, 5 id. Aug. 1348). In January 1349 he was given a pension of 500 *sous* for services to the king (C 887/128). A full study of this family, which continued to practice surgery for at least half a century more, would be of great interest.

5

The response to illness and the maintenance of health

Diagnosis and prognosis

In December 1314 a Barcelona merchant named Bertomeu de Deu began to suffer from an abscess or aposteme (*apostema*) in his jaw, which gradually became so severe as to affect his throat; his mouth and neck became so swollen that he could not eat, could only slowly sip broth with a spoon. He was cared for at the beginning by the surgeon Pere del Hospital, whose treatment did no good and who almost immediately abandoned his worsening patient; then Jaume Servià, another surgeon, took over the case, looking after him assiduously but with no more success.[1] Four days after the onset of his illness, which Servià diagnosed as "squerentia," Bertomeu passed into unconsciousness. Broth was still given him, and medicines of the surgeon's prescription, but he lay thus for two more days without improvement. On the eve of St. Lucy's, 12 December, Servià administered two clysters to his patient, together with some mulberry syrup; one of the clysters caused an efflux of matter, but the other had no further effect, whereupon the surgeon announced that Bertomeu was approaching the crisis and could be expected to die that night. Leaving his patient's house, Servià told Bertomeu's friends and family assembled there to get him out of bed, to support him and carry him about, and to slap his face and pound on brazen vessels in an attempt to awaken him; but Servià can have had little faith in these measures, since he sent his assistant back to the house several times during the night to listen at the door for the tell-tale lament for the dead. Bertomeu's friends eventually tired of carrying him around, banging fruitlessly on pots; the signs of death began to appear on his face, and his brother-in-law Ramon de Pujol said that it was shameful to torment a dead man so, but Pere Fluvià

---

[1] Pere del Hospital is known from another case where he joined physician Bernat ça Llimona and surgeon Bernat de Pertegaç in treating wounds (letter of 2 Aug. 1315; C 156/156r–v). He may originally have come from Gerona, where he held property in the early 1330s; he was still alive in 1333 (ACB, manual de Guillem Borrell April–June 1333, 3 kls. April 1333). Jaume Servià is otherwise unknown.

retorted that if they stopped carrying him about the surgeon could say his death was their fault, and besides he still had a pulse. However, Bertomeu's immediate relatives were sent out of the house, according to custom, to await the announcement of his death, and his friends arranged for the usual candles for his bier.

We know so much about the details of this episode, which plunges us directly into the experience by ordinary people of illness and medical care, because of its remarkable outcome. While Ramon de Pujol was sitting down, exhausted, on the bed, Bertomeu's mother and sisters were praying at the Dominican convent in Barcelona and invoking the help of Ramon de Penyafort, the famous member of that order who had died in 1275. At that very moment Bertomeu came back to his memory and senses – hearing, seeing, and responding to those around him, and reporting a vision of Brother Ramon protecting him from a demon who wanted to kill him. Within four days Bertomeu was up and around, healed. His cure was the first of the miracles claimed for Ramon de Penyafort at his canonization proceedings in 1318: Bertomeu, his wife, father, mother, and sister, Ramon de Pujol and Pere Fluvià, with others, were all examined closely on the events of three years before, and their accounts agree well enough to yield a fully circumstantial narrative of a serious illness in medieval Barcelona.[2]

One lesson to be taken from Bertomeu's story is that medical miracles formed part of the public's realm of possibilities. Within five years of the death of Ramon de Penyafort, a notary had already collected dozens of tales of miraculous cures through his intercession, from as far away as Ripoll and Lerida, and even Zaragoza in Aragon: cures of fevers, tumors, epilepsy, dysentery, and scabies, cures of the crippled, deaf, blind, and dumb.[3] With such stories circulating so widely, people could easily imagine that the saints might intervene in healing – not only laymen, like Bertomeu's family, but physicians, too. Another miracle attributed to Brother Ramon that was closely examined in 1318 was the cure of Margaret, the three-year-old daughter of a Barcelona physician, Joan. Master Joan testified personally that, twenty-five years or so before, his daughter had been sick

> so that she suffered from a fever for a long time, and then had a flux of the belly, or dysentery; and one day a little after noon she appeared to be dying and *in extremis* . . . and [he] recognized that the signs of death were appearing, for she lost

[2] My description of events is based on the documentation in Rius Serra, *San Raimundo de Penyafort*, pp. 209–23; the diagnosis of "squerentia" comes from the testimony of Bertomeu's brother-in-law (p. 213), probably in error for "squinancia," quinsy. (I have not been able to consult Piquer, "Metges i malalties.") By the early fourteenth century, canonization proceedings had developed reasonably sophisticated methods for collecting, testing, and corroborating testimony: see Finucane, *Miracles and Pilgrims*, pp. 36–7, 52–4, 173–81, describing the evidence-collecting techniques employed in 1307 for the canonization of Saint Thomas Cantilupe.

[3] Rius Serra, *San Raimundo de Penyafort*, pp. 286–327; see below, p. 142.

her sight and her teeth darkened, her nose grew sharp, and she took on the color of death, so that [he] and the others there knew that she must be dead, since there were no signs of life.

She lay apparently lifeless from the ninth hour until sunset, while her mother Romia prayed at the grave of Brother Ramon, and then she began to breathe, to see, and to talk; her fever and dysentery came to an end, and she lived for another fourteen years. Asked if these marvels (to which four neighbors also testified) could have been due to the art, practice, advice, or medical learning of physicians, master Joan said no, "for [he himself] was then teaching and practicing medicine, and he saw the said Margaret dead . . . and then come back to life, which must have taken place supernaturally, by God's power."[4] Obviously we need not believe in the miraculous character of these cures to acknowledge that fourteenth-century doctors as well as patients recognized the possibility of other routes to health besides the assistance of the medical community.[5]

But an equally important lesson to keep in mind is that many patients looked first to practitioners when ill, not to God and the saints.[6] We must not underestimate their conviction of the efficaciousness of the medical care available to them. Hope of heavenly intervention to cure serious illness was a last resort, not only for laymen but for clerics. Regular clergy normally could expect routine care from their chapter's *infirmarius*, or from a lay practitioner contracted by the chapter; regular and secular clergy alike might in grave cases be seen by local physicians, or might be given dispensation to travel to seek medical care elsewhere, "on account of your illness and your body's needs."[7] Physicians were more dependable than prayer.

It is not unreasonable to ask – and it often *is* asked – why medieval society felt this confidence in its medical practitioners; what could a fourteenth-century physician or surgeon possibly offer to his patients? We can start to answer this question by seeing what they sometimes contracted to provide. In the agreements drawn up between the town of Castelló d'Empúries and a series of town physicians in the first quarter of the fourteenth century, the physician promised "that he would well and properly, as far as he was able, examine and judge all

---

[4] Joan's testimony is presented in ibid., pp. 247–9; the whole of the testimony on his daughter's illness covers pp. 247–52.

[5] Palmer, "Church, Leprosy and Plague," emphasizes the coexistence of religious and secular healing, but principally in response to epidemic disease and plague from the late fourteenth century through the sixteenth.

[6] See Park, *Doctors*, p. 51, who makes the same point about the society she is studying; and Finucane, *Miracles and Pilgrims*, p. 67.

[7] ADB, Collationes 3/23v (20 May 1327). Again, ADB, Collationes 4/22 (22 May 1331) and ADG, Sèrie U (Regesta litterarum), 10/5v (30 March 1346): rectors in the dioceses of Barcelona and Gerona, in ill health, are allowed to live outside their parish so as to remain under the constant supervision of physicians in larger cities.

the urines that were brought to him by the inhabitants of the said town; would give them advice on bloodletting as well as on diets; would generally provide regimens and *consilia*; and would visit twice any sick inhabitant of the town who asked for him."[8] Contracts like this one show us that the ordinary responsibilities of the physician were prophylactic and preventive: the public asked first of all to be maintained in health, to have their health monitored by uroscopy and regulated as necessary by diet and phlebotomy. The aim was to avoid crises like Bertomeu de Deu's quinsy.

Uroscopy was probably the physician's most frequent activity – it is not for nothing that so many medieval illuminations portray him squinting into a urinal. By the 1340s (and no doubt before) the king's physicians were expected to inspect the royal urine every morning.[9] It was a procedure well adapted to the interests of a professionalizing corps attempting to demonstrate the importance of specialized learning, for it had a considerable body of technical writing to support it: the uroscopic tracts of Theophilus, Isaac Judeus, and Gilles de Corbeil were three of the thirteenth century's most widely circulated books. Moreover, uroscopy possessed its own distinctive apparatus (including colorimetric charts) and terminology. The *De cautelis medicorum* ascribed to Arnau de Vilanova advises the reader who finds himself unable to interpret a urine specimen satisfactorily to fall back on the diagnosis of *opilationem in epate* ("obstruction in the liver") – "and particularly use the word, *opilatio*, because they do not understand what it means, and it helps greatly that a term is not understood by the people."[10]

By appraising the color, sediment (or other content), and consistency of a urine sample, the physician could infer his patient's state of health, since urine was the filtrate of the body's constituent humors and an index to their balance or disproportion. The analysis could be carried to great lengths and made the basis for a pathology rich in diagnostic detail, as in Walter Agilon's successful *Summa*

---

[8] "Quod bene et legaliter pro posse suo videbit et iudicabit omnes urinas que sibi apportabuntur per omnes habitatores dicte ville et quod dabit eis consilia tam super flebotomiis quam etiam dietis et generaliter regimina et consilia et quod visitabit bis illos infirmos habitatores dicte ville de quibus fuerit requisitus": AHPG/CE 92, 3 non. Aug. 1317.

[9] "Et cascun dia de mati la urina nostra esguarden per tal que la disposicio de nostre cors regonegen e si hauran vist en nostre cors alcun piyorament decontinent curen de remey salutari proveyr": Pere III, "Ordenacions," p. 76.

[10] "Et specialiter utere hoc nomine opilatio quia non intelligunt quod significat et multum expedit ut non intelligatur locutio ab eis": Arnau de Vilanova, *De cautelis*, f. 217ra; translated by Sigerist, "Bedside Manners," p. 135. The authenticity of *De cautelis* is still debated. Sigerist followed Henschel in distinguishing four sections in it, of which the third is an abstract of a Salernitan treatise. The first section, paraphrased here, seemed so cynical that Henschel was unwilling to believe it could be Arnau's, though Sigerist was able to entertain the possibility. The second section now proves to be virtually identical with the last lines of Arnau's commentary on Hippocrates' first aphorism (Arnau de Vilanova, *Repetitio*, f. 281rb), so perhaps the attribution of the first section to Arnau can tentatively be accepted as well.

medicinalis,[11] but it also permitted fairly simple discriminations and could be used by empirics, some of whom were beginning to absorb the rudiments of academic medical science. Gueraula de Codines, the woman of Subirats near Barcelona arraigned by the bishop in 1304 for irregular medical practice, was asked if she knew anything of the art of medicine:

> she said no, except that she could diagnose a patient's illness from his urine.
> Asked by what signs, she said that citrine urine indicates a continued fever, *vermeyla* a tercian fever, *rubia* the first stages of a quartan fever, though later this indication disappears; and that white spumous urine indicates an aposteme.

Such language evidently impressed her rural clientele. Three years later, she was brought back before the bishop, to whom she swore that she limited herself "to interpreting urines and feeling the pulse and giving advice to those suffering with all kinds of illness . . . ; asked if many patients were coming to her, she said yes, especially to have their urine interpreted."[12]

Why did the public, in turn, find this procedure so satisfactory? What sort of pressures made it necessary for Jaume II to exempt the physician Vidal Rouen from orders closing his street in the Jewish quarter of Barcelona, on the grounds that "many people have to show him the urines of sick people and to ask him for advice for them"?[13] Partly, no doubt, because it seemed inherently plausible to people that the urine should be an index to the condition of the body from which it came. But the procedure had the further practical advantage that by bringing the urine to the physician, the patient or his family had the opportunity to test the supposedly expert knowledge of the practitioner. Arnau's *De cautelis* makes it plain that clients expected to be able to hear the physician infer age and sex as well as state of health from a urinal, and it suggests that they might substitute another person's urine (or an animal's, or wine, or stewed figs) for the patient's in order to see if the physician would recognize the trick.[14] The practitioner's expertise still needed to be proved – but once proved, of course, it tended to

[11] A measure of the *Summa*'s circulation is perhaps Arnau de Vilanova's attack upon it in the 1290s: he vehemently criticized students who steeped themselves, not in the works of Hippocrates and Galen, "ymmo pocius in cartapellis et summis que potissime magni voluminis sunt, sicut in historiis Gilleberti et fabulis Poncii et Galteri": *De consideracionibus*, p. 133. The two writers associated with Walter Agilon in this passage are Gilbertus Anglicus and Ponce de Saint-Gilles. Note that Gilbertus is found in two and Walter in one of the Catalan libraries mentioned above, chapter 3.

[12] Asked where she had obtained her knowledge of medicine, Gueraula replied, "a quodam medico extraneo, qui venit per mare ad Villam Francham, nomine En Bofim, bene sunt xxx anni." The documents concerning Gueraula's practice are published and discussed by Perarnau, "Activitats," pp. 58–64, 67–73. The bishop's investigation of Na Serra Bona of Madrona, who rumor said "utitur officio medici et iudicat urinas" (ADB, Visitationes 1 bis/58v; 24 March 1306), shows that Gueraula was not the only woman to employ the technique.

[13] "Plures gentes habeant ei hostendere hurinas infirmorum et requirere ab eo consilium pro eisdem": C 211/337v (16 June 1315).

[14] Sigerist, "Bedside Manners," pp. 134–7.

ensure the patient's trust and confidence.[15] Only when the public had become convinced that learned physicians' training gave them an unquestionable expertise did this sort of testing become unnecessary.

But prognostic judgments were not based just on immediate examinations and tests like uroscopic evaluation. The physician needed to be aware of his patient's normal complexion, the qualitative balance proper to him when healthy. His complexion or temperament was reflected in his aspect and manner, and could be estimated on first examination,[16] but it was preferable to have built up such a knowledge by observations over many years – the citizens of Gerona who wanted permission for Vidal Cabrit to return to their city emphasized that he had studied their complexions for a long time.[17] Acquaintance with a patient early in life also conferred a familiarity with his basic temperament. When the infant king Alfonso XI of Castile fell ill in the autumn of 1315, his grandmother María de Molina wrote to Jaume II asking for the services of Heinrich of Germany, a physician who had settled in Tarragona – "for you" (wrote King Jaume to Heinrich) "were present at his birth and know his complexion, for the better maintenance of his health."[18]

It was also important to know a patient's occupation and manner of life, for the connection between what one did for a living and one's health was well established. Arnau de Vilanova pointed out that not only are smiths, glaziers, sweepers, gilders, and other artisans often made ill by their trade, but some other apparently harmless occupations can also be risky: notaries, who may sit in poor light reading or writing documents all day, risk the progressive loss of their sight, while at the same time they often come to suffer from kidney and bladder problems since the press of business forces them to go for long periods without relieving themselves.[19] The first of these problems, at least, could sometimes be helped – by means of magnifying crystals, in use as

---

[15] O'Boyle (*Medieval Prognosis*, pp. 1–2) begins his general account of prognostic technique at the end of the thirteenth century by making this point; Edelstein (*Ancient Medicine*, pp. 69–70, 80–2) has argued convincingly that prognostic skills served a similar purpose for the Hippocratic physician (and patient).

[16] See Arnau de Vilanova, *Speculum medicine*, ff. 33v–35 (cap. 99). Complexion could even be evaluated by letter, as in Arnau's *Consilium sive cure febris ethice*.

[17] "Qui eorum complexiones diucius novit": AHAG, Correspondencia, Lligall 1, f. 33 (3 Oct. 1330). Cardoner Planas, "Linaje," p. 358, finds Vidal Cabrit a Gerona surgeon in 1326; Vidal subsequently appears as physician and surgeon to the infante Jaume d'Urgell in 1344 (AHPT 3864/242v), and he was still practicing in both capacities in Barcelona in 1347 (C 649/147).

[18] Above, chapter 1, n. 44. Again, when the infante Joan was ill in 1321, and his physician asked Joan's father for instructions, the king turned for help to Martí de Calça Roja, "qui complexionem ipsius . . . plene novit" (C 246/276; 28 Sept. 1321).

[19] Arnau de Vilanova, *Speculum medicine*, f. 26va (cap. 84). Arnau may here have been bringing into a contemporary setting Galen's recognition of illnesses that arise from retention of urine "propter opus quodlibet aut propter bonorum hominum verecundiam aut quia maneret ante regem vel in loco iudicis aut in convivio": *De interioribus*, in *Opera Galeni* (Venice, 1490), vol. II, f. 137ra.

aids to sight in Catalonia since at least the first decade of the fourteenth century.[20]

Uroscopy could confirm that a patient was generally healthy, then, or, together with other tests – assessing the quality of the pulse, studying the patient's aspect, and so forth – could lead the physician to a diagnosis of illness and a prognosis. Then as now it was important to the patient to have a name given to his condition, although in the late thirteenth century most patients showed little awareness of specific disease labels. The 134 healing miracles attributed to Ramon de Penyafort and taken down in 1279–80 by the Barcelona notary Jaume de Portu suggest the index of morbidity as perceived by the public:

tumors, abscesses, ulcers	21
fevers	21
localized pain	17
unspecified illness	16
problems with sight	13
pain in jaws or teeth	9
localized paralysis	6
pregnancy/childbirth	6
epilepsy	5
problems with hearing	3
accidents	3
others	14

Included among these last were isolated cases of particular complaints: of dropsy, serpigo, vertigo, hernia, lupus. People also sometimes spoke of their fevers with a certain precision: seven had suffered with quartan, two with double tertian fevers.[21] But the vast majority of health problems that worried Catalans in 1280 did not fit into neat nosological categories.[22]

The diffusion of medical learning in the early fourteenth century seems to have increased the precision with which conditions might be named or explained. For the unsophisticated, an imaginary *opilatio in epate* or a misunderstood *squerentia* might still suffice, but more attentive patients got the jargon right – like the weaver who reported himself miraculously cured of the ulcer (*morbum corrosionis*) in his left leg "that they call *fistula*."[23] Simply

---

[20] Simon de Guilleuma, "De l'ús de les ulleres"; see also Rosen, "Invention." Note that "tres uyerias abtas ad studendum" are included in the surgeon Bernat Serra's inventory (Carreras Valls, "Bernat Serra," p. 17).

[21] The regularity of the malarial fevers not only allowed sufferers to define their illness carefully, it also encouraged them to invest with meaning the number of times the fever recurred in any particular bout: see MF, II:98, doc. 142.

[22] Rius Serra, *San Raimundo de Penyafort*, pp. 286–327.

[23] Ibid., p. 321.

giving a physiological interpretation to a client's symptoms made them seem less frightening, of course,[24] but refinement of diagnosis gave a better chance of intelligent treatment, too, as Jaume II appreciated. When his daughter Isabel told him of her eye disease "that the physicians call *cateracta*," he replied asking for more details. "We have called to us a number of practitioners [*medici*] of our realm," he wrote, "so get an opinion quickly from some expert practitioners there as to what this illness is, and what its nature is, and what they think its cause is, so that you can explain it clearly to us in your letters" – and, as he later told her husband Friedrich, so that he could see whether any Spanish practitioners were skilled in treating that particular condition.[25]

For of course diagnosis and the accompanying prognosis had practical as well as psychological import, and were expected to be confirmed by the course of a patient's illness. In formally promising Pere de Serret that his son would recover from the horse's kick he had received forty days before, the surgeon Pere Ritxart was staking his reputation on the outcome.[26] Unfulfilled expectations could destroy that reputation. When Bernat de Toncadella was wounded in the left arm, the surgeons agreed that his only hope for a cure lay in amputation, and his death following the operation was attributed to their negligence or lack of skill.[27] Some physicians were therefore more cautious about prognostic promises than others. Mosse Avinardut had claimed, sight unseen, that he could cure Ruggiero II di Loria, but his son Alazar, more prudently, asked to see the patient first – "he wants to see the said Ruggiero," wrote the king in June 1323, "so that once he has seen and thought about his illness he can decide whether it seems to him to be curable." Apparently Alazar decided not to commit himself to the case, and wisely, for Ruggiero died the next year.[28]

Indeed, it was particularly important for practitioners to be able to identify the signs of imminent death in a patient, and not merely so that the patient might be given the opportunity for a final confession; it enabled them to dissociate

---

[24] "El lunes primero passado en la manyana nos sentiemos alguna poca de calentura e de agreviamento en nuestra persona e havemos assi passado con viandas de dieta que conviene entro a huey dia sabado, que no avemos sentido tanta callor, e segun dizen los phisigos est accident es de la qualidat de la sangre, por que entienden que periglo nenguno no avemos": the infante Pere is reporting on his health to Alfons III, 23 April 1334 (Girona i Llagostera, "Itinerari," 19:203–4).

[25] "Rogamus ut confestim congregatis aliquibus expertis medicis et electis discerni faciatis que sit infirmitas et natura eiusdem et quid estiment causam dedisse eidem, et de hiis . . . nos clare et liquide per vestras litteras velitis reddere cerciores": Jaume to Isabel, 11 Dec. 1326 (C 318/30v–31); Jaume to Frederic, 7 Oct. 1327 (C 318/31). These documents are published by Zeissberg, "Register," pp. 87–9.

[26] Document of 6 Aug. 1332 (AHPT 3845/83).

[27] Document of 7 July 1331 (C 446/27r–v).

[28] "Videre vellet dictum nobilem Rogeronum ut visa et cognita eius infirmitate deliberaret si sibi infirmitas curabilis videretur": letter of 5 June 1323 (C 177/299v). For more detail on the illness, see above, chapter 4 n. 12.

themselves more or less honorably from the case.[29] Miquel de Sala reported to
the Penyafort commission that in July 1306 he had come down with a quotidian
fever which after a week culminated in coma; for eight to ten days he lay
unconscious in his home, unable even to take medicine. During that time his
physicians – Bernat ça Llimona and Esteve, *physici multum prudentes, de
melioribus medicis Barchinone*[30] – determined that since he was dying
(*incurabili et quasi pro mortuo*) he no longer needed treatment, and they
resigned his case, just as first Pere del Hospital and then Jaume Servià would
give up on a dying Bertomeu de Deu ten years later. Miquel's physicians based
their prognosis upon the facts that, as his daughter reported, "he twitched
[*faciebat tractus*] as the dying do, and the signs of death appeared on his face."[31]
The "signs" are those we have already found identified by master Joan in the face
of his dying daughter, going back to Hippocrates' *Prognostics* – "the nose
sharp, the eyes sunken, the temples fallen in, the ears cold and drawn in and their
lobes distorted, the skin of the face hard, stretched and dry, and the colour of the
face pale or dusky."[32]

Preventive medicine

Besides diagnosis and prognosis, what did a physician have to offer to those
who might consult him? The town contract we have already cited went on to
speak of providing advice, *regimina* and *consilia*. These duties remind us that
the physician had been charged with preserving health as well as curing illness,
and that the public was no less concerned with preventive medicine than it is
today. A typical collection of advice on maintaining one's health is available in
the *Regimen sanitatis* drawn up about 1305 by Arnau de Vilanova for Jaume II.[33]
The first part of the text describes how those things "que necessario approximant
corpori humano" – air and baths, activity or exercise, sleep, food and drink,
evacuations, and the emotions – can be regulated to keep a person healthy. These
six items were routinely brought together as the "six non-naturals" in elementary

---

[29] There are Hippocratic roots for this precaution: cf. *Prognostics*, 1, in *Hippocratic Writings*,
p. 170. Amundsen and Ferngren, "Evolution," pp. 34–40, suggest that this attitude changes only
in the fifteenth century.

[30] On Bernat ça Llimona, see above, chapter 2, n. 28. Esteve ("Stephanus") is perhaps to be
identified with the *magister* Stephanus of Barcelona whose wife testified before the diocesan
court on 24 July 1326 (ADB, Not. Com. 4/43v–44).

[31] "Faciebat tractus quod faciunt obeuntes et in eius facie apparebant signa mortis"; "tractus"
recalls Hippocrates' *Prognostics*, 4. For Miquel, see the documentation published by Rius Serra,
San Raimundo de Penyafort, pp. 242–7.

[32] *Prognostics*, 2, in *Hippocratic Writings*, p. 171. For one surgeon's prognostic criteria for death,
see below, chapter 7, p. 212.

[33] A Latin edition of the *Regimen sanitatis ad regem Aragonum* is being prepared by Ana Trías
Teixidor. A useful account of the work and of its diffusion and influence is given by Paniagua
Arellano, *Maravilloso regimiento*.

medical theory, but their treatment in the *Regimen* has nothing of the scholastic about it: Arnau seems deliberately to have adopted homely, non-technical language for the king. Perhaps, too, he anticipated the still wider audience that the *Regimen* in fact almost immediately enjoyed. More manuscripts of the *Regimen* survive than of any of Arnau's other Latin works, and it was early translated into vernacular languages. Jaume's queen, Blanca, asked the Geronan surgeon Berenguer ça Riera to render the work into Catalan "so that this regimen can be helpful to those who don't read Latin," and his translation was completed by 1310.[34] Even a Hebrew translation of the work (made in Avignon in 1327) was available in the king's lifetime – reminding us again that the Jewish and Christian medical worlds were not really distinct.[35]

Because the non-naturals govern health, it follows that they can corrupt or restore it as well as preserve it, and thus each of the six could be a matter of concern in daily life, as the royal correspondence reveals. Air, for example, had widely differing merit, depending on geography and the time of year. Thus in summer the mountain air of Prades in the Pyrenean foothills was acknowledged as superior to the climate of the Catalan coast, even though ordinarily its cold air might be cause for worry.[36] Other mountain cities presented special dangers: at Seu d'Urgell, sunk deep into the Pyrenees, the trapped air was particularly unhealthy, so stagnant that bedding had to be hung out to ventilate lest it rot.[37] Other cities had bad reputations for different reasons. The autumn fogs that, then as now, beset the town of Lerida, on the Segre, disturbed many; even though Lerida was ventilated by an east wind, it was "diffamada de moltes malauties." Leridan physicians defended their city by explaining, not that its air was corrupt, but that it was too fertile a locale: as a general rule, they argued, having fruit and viands in plenty "is a powerful factor tending to spawn disease and to keep you from growing old." Its trees, too, had been blamed for corrupting the atmosphere, until the poplars along the river were finally cut down.[38] In general, it was the "mirabilis aeris temperancia" of Valencia that the king's doctors prescribed for him.[39] Of course, your own birthplace, whose climate matched your complexion, could always be counted on to return you to health, and this

---

[34] "Per ço que aquest *Regiment* . . . pusca tenir o fer profit a aquels qui non entenen latí": Arnau de Vilanova, *Obres Catalanes*, II:100.

[35] The translation was made by Israel ben Joseph Caslari, whose introduction to the work is edited and translated by García-Ballester, Ferre, and Feliu, "Jewish Appreciation," pp. 102–5.

[36] "Cum nos apud montanas de Pratis proponamus de presenti dirigere iter nostrum et ibidem per aliquod spacium estivalis temporis residere": letter of 23 June 1302 (C 269/72v). Jaume was very conscious of the "temporis estivalis periculum" – see the letter of 13 July 1322 (C 247/110); or MF, II:325, doc. 448 – as well as of winter cold (letter of 30 Sept. 1314 [C 299/145v], where for fear of the effects of the winter on the infantes Joan and especially Ramon Berenguer, "cui frigora contraria existunt," they are to be brought from Montblanc to Barcelona).

[37] Jaume d'Agramunt, *Regiment*, p. 63.

[38] "És una rahó molt forts d'engenrar malauties e de no venir a veyllesa": ibid., 63–4.

[39] MF, I:59.

was the motive that sent Urraca de Entença back to Alcoletge when she fell ill in 1336.[40]

Like air, baths – particularly thermal springs – had the potential to affect health, and were an especially important resource of the physician. The Italian baths of Pozzuoli, outside Naples, had long been famous, and Arnau de Vilanova recommended their use to Charles II of Naples when the monarch was diagnosed with scabies in 1308,[41] but the Crown of Aragon had its own spas. The hot waters of Caldes de Montbui, in use since Roman times, lie only thirty kilometers from Barcelona, and were resorted to frequently by members of the royal household.[42] The kings themselves, however, seem to have preferred the spa of Estarach (now Caldetes); Jaume II provided 100 *sous* to repair its facilities in 1317. Five years later, in a vain attempt to cure the dying queen Maria, he had its water brought especially to Barcelona, and baths built in the palace in which to reheat it.[43] Alfons III visited it, too, in the last year of his life, on the advice of his physicians.[44]

Exercise was of medical concern because in arousing the natural heat it enhanced digestion and the expulsion of waste; the more one eats, the more exercise one needs (and vice versa).[45] But many modern patterns of exercise would probably have struck medieval physicians as unhealthily extreme. People who follow a normal regimen and require only moderate activity should stop their exercise as soon as it becomes painful or tiring. Furthermore, they should try to exercise the upper and lower body equally – hunting on horseback, Arnau de Vilanova assured Jaume II, is excellent in this respect. The king could evidently have indulged the royal passion for hawking in the confidence that he was ensuring his own health.[46]

The emotions – *accidentia anime* – belong among the non-naturals, Arnau explained in his *Speculum medicine*, because of their fundamentally somatic

---

40 "In quo nutrita extitit et cuius aeri eius complexio se confirmat": letter of 27 June 1336 (C 1053/150v–151). Medical experts urged Jaume II to bring his daughter Constança from Castile to Valencia – "in qua nata fuerat et nutrita" – for the same reasons: letter of 9 Jan. 1315 (C 242/74v–75). Cf. the king's letter to Don Juan Manuel, published in MF, II:115, doc. 170.

41 AA, III:176–7, which does not identify the sources. Charles' first letter to Jaume II, on 8 Feb. 1308, specified that "multa scabie affligamur"; it is now ACA pergaminos Jaume II extra-inventario 76. His follow-up letter, published by Finke and dated 18 Feb. (17 Feb. by Finke), is now ACA pergaminos Jaume II extra-inventario 41.

42 MF, I:38, on Yolanda, and letters of 7 March and 27 April 1318 (C 279/134v, 181r–v).

43 MF, I:263. The construction is announced in a letter of 8 Dec. 1317 (C 259/27).

44 Above, chapter 1, at n. 137.

45 Arnau de Vilanova, *Regimen sanitatis*, f. 82r–v (cap. 2); *Speculum medicine*, ff. 5v–6 (cap. 15).

46 Vincke, "Sobre la caça," is based primarily on secondary sources and can give only a hint of the extraordinary attention the king gave to hawking. For instance, between 1300 and 1314 he sent for falcons and gerfalcons from Montpellier, Mallorca, Flanders, England, France, and Provence (C 115/379v; C 235/215v; C 238/221; C 239/242; RP 277/32). It ought to be made clear, however, that there is no evidence that Jaume went hawking because he thought it would be good for him; nor does the *Libro de la caza* of his son-in-law Don Juan Manuel allude to its healthful character.

character.[47] All originate in a judgment by the brain's cognitive faculty that some object is desirable or harmful, a judgment that causes a corresponding physical reaction in the heart. For example, something terrible that cannot be avoided or withstood evokes sadness, which is a constriction of the heart that leads to a diminution of blood and spirits diffused to the internal and external members, thereby chilling and drying the whole body; it can no longer digest food, and so wastes away. Joy, anger, shame, distress – every emotion corresponds to a particular physiological process; but because of the tight connection between psychology and physiology the link goes both ways, so that wasting away of the body in turn produces sadness. It is only the moral philosopher, however, who is concerned with the production and expression of psychological states; the physician's task is to study the emotions insofar as they lead to physiological ones, sensible changes pertaining to the health of the body that may conceivably result in illness. And in fact Arnau's *Regimen* for Jaume II (written at almost the same time as the *Speculum*) takes precisely this tack, advising the monarch to avoid anger because it overheats the body, sadness because it chills and dries.[48]

Foods have such varied properties that it is not always easy to distinguish them from medicines. Some foods merely nourish the body, while others act on it medicinally as well. Likewise with drinks: all help to prepare food for better digestion, but while some (like water) only lubricate, others (like wine) also nourish, and still others (vinegar) behave like medicines.[49] Consequently there are many general rules that one must keep in mind to remain healthy. Eat only when hungry, and not to excess; chew thoroughly, and do not consume a variety of dishes at one meal, for otherwise digestion will be impeded; make sure that your foods are not only easily digestible, but also appropriate to your constitution. The character of particular foodstuffs is examined at length in the second part of Arnau's *Regimen* for King Jaume. Bread, legumes, fruits, vegetables, meat, fish – each category includes certain things to be avoided as far as possible. Legumes are unsuitable for the healthy body, though round white peas are not as bad as the rest. Vegetables should be eaten cooked, not raw. Fruit should be consumed not for pleasure or even for nourishment but as medicine, to maintain one's health[50] – though it seems clear from the royal correspondence that the monarchs ate what they enjoyed. They were fortunate that the Valencian *horta* could supply so much of the produce they wanted.[51]

---

[47] Arnau de Vilanova, *Speculum medicine*, ff. 23v–25v (cap. 80); see also Salvador de les Borges, *Arnau de Vilanova moralista*, pp. 39-42; and, more generally on the psychological/physiological relationship, Paniagua, "Psicoterapia."

[48] Arnau de Vilanova, *Regimen sanitatis*, f. 83 (cap. 6).

[49] Arnau de Vilanova, *Speculum medicine*, f. 6r–v (cap. 17).

[50] Arnau de Vilanova, *Regimen sanitatis*, ff. 83v–85r (capp. 8–15).

[51] Thus, for example, in the summer of 1337 Pere III asked his Valencian bailiff to send him a load of melons, another of peaches, grapes, squash, and eggplant, and two of Greek wine (C 1054/102v). As Pere wrote, "Jacsia que menjar de fruytes no sia per meges molt approbat,

There are similar recommendations for wine. Drink wine only when truly thirsty, and only light wines, especially white or rosé; it is better to mix a weak wine with a little water than a strong wine with much water.[52] Wine, indeed, might almost be considered a medicine, conferring as it does so much good on the body: it strengthens the natural heat, clarifies the blood, opens the body's inner passages, and relieves the mind. It benefits all ages, at all times and in all places.[53] But wines that are specifically medicinal can also be made, by steeping herbs or fruits – rosemary, eyebright, wormwood, pomegranates – in them. Such wines can be prepared in a hurry, by heating the herb in white wine, but the best are made by placing the herb in the must of wine and allowing them to ferment together.[54] Because such wines required special preparation, they were not always readily available; Jaume II had to order one from Valencia when he was unwell in Tarazona (Aragon) in 1304.[55]

Such recommendations gave precision to what the public already understood as constituting a healthy diet. At one level, popular tradition recognized certain foods as soothing or strengthening to the weak or sickly: chicken soup, for example, and gruel.[56] But popular attitudes were also molded by the gradual dissemination of medical theory. In his novel *Blanquerna*, finished in 1283, Ramon Llull described his hero's upbringing and included rules for health that appealed to basic physiological principles for their rationale. Children in their first year should have only milk, from a healthy wet-nurse of good moral

---

elles, però, per gràcia dels hòmens són perduytes a tast humanal naturalment ordonades: per què en les regions en les quals se fan de bona costuma e en dinar e en sopar comunament són ministrades": quoted by Conde y Delgado de Molina, "Fonts," p. 29; this collection of essays has much information on what Catalans actually ate in the fourteenth century. Bertran i Roigé, "Menjador de l'almoina," shows what sort of diet was provided to the poor: mutton for meat, beans and onions for vegetables.

[52] Arnau de Vilanova, *Regimen sanitatis*, ff. 82v–83r (cap. 5).

[53] One of the cures worked by Ramon de Penyafort benefited a boy named Bendit who detested wine, and who, because he didn't drink it, "fluxum et dissenteriam ac debilitatem corporis tam gravem incurrerat, quod de eo mortis periculum visibiliter timebatur"; his loving mother prayed for him to Brother Ramon, whereupon the boy immediately demanded wine, drank it down, and was returned to health (Rius Serra, *San Raimundo Penyafort*, p. 295).

[54] These views are paraphrased from the *De vinis* ascribed, with some plausibility, to Arnau de Vilanova. If authentic, it would seem to have been written in the period 1309–11, and dedicated to King Robert of Naples. It was an unusually popular work in the later Middle Ages, and was translated into several vernaculars. Part of it was translated into German in the fifteenth century, combined with accretions from another source, and it was this composite version that was in turn translated into English by Henry Sigerist as Arnald of Villanova, *The Earliest Printed Book on Wine*. This translation preserves only twenty-six of the forty-one medicinal wines described in the Latin edition, and omits entirely the introduction to the work, which explains the general rationale for and preparation of these wines.

[55] Letter of 13 Aug. 1304 (C 258/150v).

[56] The *Libre de Sent Sovi*, a Catalan cookbook that in its original form dates back perhaps to the 1320s, offers recipes for "brou amellat a hom deliquat," "brou de gualenes per confortar," and "farines ha hom levat de malaltia." See Grewe, *Libre de Sent Sovi*, pp. 191–4, 223, or Faraudo de Saint-Germain, "'Libre de Sent Sovi'," pp. 21–2, 26, for the texts.

character, "for, lacking a strong digestion, infants in their first year can digest no other foods that parents may give them, such as bread sopped in milk or oil, or other similar things that they are made to eat; and this is why children have weak kidneys, have pustules, tumors, or boils, and their humors begin to ascend and damage their brain and their sight, and to bring about many other illnesses in them."[57] As an older child, Blanquerna was given only bread in the morning (so that he would not lose his appetite for dinner). At mealtimes he was made to eat something of every dish, so that his nature would not grow accustomed to just one thing; "he was forbidden to drink either strong wine or heavily watered wine, or [to use] strong sauces that destroy the natural heat."[58] Llull himself had a broad if informal and idiosyncratic knowledge of medical thought, but his account here is meant for a lay vernacular audience and shows that that audience had a general understanding of the same system of physiology and pathology that its physicians had mastered in detail.[59]

Diet was one of the subjects on which the physician of Castelló contracted specifically to counsel the citizens; the other, bloodletting (phlebotomy), was, like diet, a routine means of maintaining a person in health. A gross imbalance of the humors was one important cause of illness, and a regular prophylactic bleeding (and purging) of the healthy ensured against humoral accumulation. From the frequency with which fleams appear in domestic inventories, it seems likely that the procedure was often carried out by the members of a household on one another.[60] It was still advisable to consult a physician, however, for a long line of technical treatises agreed that in many situations phlebotomy should not be carried out unless therapeutically imperative: in the case, for example, of persons of melancholy complexion, the very young or very old, pregnant women, the malnourished or those who have just dined; nor in winter, or on extremely hot days – the refinements were such that to be safe a physician's advice was crucial, in this as in other aspects of regimen. But by following a general program drawn up by a physician who was careful to take into account your natural complexion, you could feel some confidence in the prospect of a healthy future. Dying in November 1348, Bishop Arnau of Gerona added a

---

[57] "Car, per defalliment de fort digestió, los infants en lo primer any no poden coure ni digerir les viandes altres, com són sopes de pa mullat ab llet o oli, que hom los dóna, o altres semblandts viandes que hom los fa menjar per força; e per açò són los chichs ronyoses e ab buanyes, e han vèrtoles y vexigues, e accarreren-los les umors de pujar amunt, e destroheixen-los lo cervell e la vista, y no res menys los causen moltes altes malalties": Llull, *Blanquerna*, I.2 (ed. Salvador Galmés, I:30–1).

[58] "E fon-li vedat lo vi fort y lo massa amerat, e forts salses que destruexen la calor natural": ibid., I:32.

[59] Demaitre, "Idea of Childhood," makes it clear that medieval medical literature understood children and adults to require different hygienic, dietary, and therapeutic régimes.

[60] ACB, manual de Bernat de Vilarrúbia, 4/1327–7/1327, ff. 30v–34v; ACB, manual de Bernat de Vilarrúbia, 3 non. Aug. 1340–18 kls. Jan. 1340, ff. 12v–13 – each with "unam benam abtam fleubotomie."

codicil to his will, leaving thirty-five pounds to master Guerau de Sant Dionis "qui multo tempore nos tenuit in suo bono regimine et dieta."[61]

Therapy: regimen, purges, and phlebotomy

Health, as all medieval medical students learned, is only a relative state,[62] and thus only an indistinct line separated the preservation from the restoration of health. Regimen was still what a physician first thought of adjusting if his patient fell ill: according to every introductory medical text, the physician should prescribe diet, drugs, and surgery for his patients – in that order.[63] In principle, foods and drugs could be distinguished: foods were converted by the body to its nature, while drugs converted the body to theirs. In practice, however, the distinction was difficult to make, for many foods could, like drugs, act medicinally upon the body, although only when larger quantities than usual were administered.[64] Moreover, diet could be used in conjunction with other therapies when a patient was seriously ill. Abulcasis' *De cibariis infirmorum*, for example, dealt with the application of diet to a full range of systemic illnesses (quartan and quotidian fevers, leprosy, dropsy, etc.), as well as to afflictions of the stomach, liver, and other individual organs; Bernard Gordon, Arnau de Vilanova's slightly later contemporary at Montpellier, arranged for the treatise's Latin translation (via Catalan) by Berenguer Eymerich, a Valencian physician who maintained his professional activity in Valencia city down to the 1350s.[65]

Into the hazy area between foods and medicines fell sweetmeats, preserved and candied confections available from apothecaries and typically combining fruits or nuts or other flavored or scented material with sugar or honey.[66] Such preparations could be consumed in astonishingly large quantities. During the single year 1322, for example, one Barcelona apothecary, Joan de la Geltrú, sold to Jaume II 28½ pounds of *dragea* (a confection based commonly on almonds), 29 pounds of *batafalva* (based on anise), 13¾ pounds of *pinyonat* (based on pine nuts), 17 pounds of rose sugar, 12 pounds of *rosata novella* (roses, sugar, and

---

[61] ADG, Sèrie G (Lib. Notularum), 22/12v (13 Nov. 1348).

[62] Ottosson, *Scholastic Medicine*, pp. 162–6.

[63] "In ordinacione vero regiminis curativi debet ordinem servare quo ad particularia regimina quibus completur opus curacionis. Tres enim sunt, ut habetur a Galieno in prologo regimenti acutorum: scilicet regimen in dieta et regimen in administracione medicinarum et regimen in manuali operacione": Arnau de Vilanova, *Repetitio*, f. 279vb; MS Munich CLM 14245, ff. 32v–33. Cf. Johannitius, *Isagoge*, tr. 3, in *Articella* (Venice, 1523), I, f. 4va; Hali Rodoan, comm. Galen, *Tegni*, III, text 148, in idem, III, f. 143rb; Avicenna, *Canon* I.4.i.i (f. 67va).

[64] "Omnis medicine ratio est quod non sit nata converti in substantiam et fieri pars nostri corporis, et in hoc distat a cibo . . . Et etiam de ea non tolerat corpus tantam quantitatem ut cibi": Arnau de Vilanova, *De simplicibus*, f. 233vb. Arnau examined the distinction between the two more carefully in *De intentione medicorum*, II.ii, ff. 37rb–38ra.

[65] Above, chapter 2, n. 46.

[66] On this subject generally, see Pérez Vidal, *Medicina y dulcería*.

licorice, flavored by cinnamon, ginger, nutmeg, and some other materials), and smaller quantities of half a dozen other comfits.[67] These sweets were obviously eaten for pleasure – Alfons III ordered cases of them for his wedding guests[68] – yet their medicinal powers were pronounced enough to warrant their inclusion in the apothecaries' pharmacopoeia: the standard *Antidotarium Nicolai* describes *rosata novella* as beneficial for an upset stomach, general weakness, and thirst.[69] *Diacitron*, one of Jaume II's favorite confections, is recommended in Arnau de Vilanova's *Antidotarium*: lemon peel soaked in water is cooked in sugar syrup and rose water until the mixture thickens, and spices are added for flavor. It is good, says Arnau, for hot passions of the stomach, cardiac passion, and choleric flux.[70] Sugar and sugared drinks (*iulep*) themselves were beneficial to the stomach and to digestion,[71] so that all these sweets could be complacently devoured in the happy knowledge that they conferred health as well as pleasure.

Digestive medicines were of such concern because humoral physiology asserted that the proper assimilation of food was a first requirement for living things, and regular or copious excretion was thus interpreted as a sign of health since it revealed the proper functioning of the natural faculties. Like foods, therefore, laxative preparations might be prescribed for the well or for the ill. Taken prophylactically, they strengthened the natural powers of the body; administered in illness, they gave visible assurance of the body's return to health. Aloes, rhubarb, and *cassia fistula* seem to have been the purges most commonly used in the Crown of Aragon; the last of these was considered mild and safe, and Jaume II took it with increasing frequency during the last ten years of his life.[72] Purges are not foods but medicines, of course, and their powerful physiological effect made it desirable that even prophylactic doses be overseen by physicians. Feeling a purge to be necessary to his well-being in March 1334, Alfons III

---

[67] RP 287/43v, 55, 77; RP 288/50, 103.

[68] Letter of 1 July 1329 (C 493/131).

[69] *Antidotarium Nicolai* (Venice, 1471), f. 29v; reprinted by Van den Berg, *Middelnederlandsche Vertalung*, p. 127. See Pérez Vidal, pp. 211–13, for more detail on the use and popularity of *rosata novella* in Spain.

[70] Arnau de Vilanova, *Antidotarium*, f. 248; this section may have been assembled not by Arnau but by his Aragonese disciple, Pedro Cellerer (above, chapter 3, p. 82). See also Pérez Vidal, *Medicina y dulcería*, pp. 157–62.

[71] Cf. above, chapter 1, p. 18.

[72] Aloes was used least often; the king sent "duas aloes" to Urgell to Teresa, the infante Alfons' wife, in 1318 (C 259/143–5). The others appear routinely in court expenses: e.g., rhubarb in C 300/125–6 (for May 1316), RP 284/89 (for May 1320), and RP 287/77 (for spring 1322); *cassia fistula*, in RP 281/120v (for June 1317). C 147/196–7, for June 1311, orders 6 ounces of rhubarb and 2 pounds of *cassia fistula*. *Cassia fistula* was considered a mild, general purge; aloes was thought to purge phlegm from the stomach and bile from the head. Over rhubarb there was more confusion, as Roger Bacon complained in the late thirteenth century. "Nam Aristoteles dicit quod purgat fleuma, et Greci. Nullus autem de auctoribus medicine exprimit in libris Latinorum quem humorem purgat. Sed opinio medicorum Latinorum est quod coleram": *De erroribus*, p. 164. The same point is made by Johannes de Sancto Amando, *Expositio*, f. 224va.

summoned Joan Amell to him urgently at Teruel; four days later, having had no response from his *phisicus maior*, he wrote more insistently to Amell (and, to be safe, to another physician as well) to come immediately to administer the drug.[73]

It was their evacuative powers that made purges such important medical tools in illness, for they helped the body rid itself of the unhealthy humors that were manifest, for example, in an aposteme. The infante Jaume suffered from an aposteme while traveling through the southern part of the Crown during the second half of 1318, and his physician, Bertomeu de Bonells, treated him with repeated doses of laxatives. In Teruel, Bertomeu prescribed syrup of violets, *cassia fistula* and other stronger purges, and sugar; in Sogorb, two further doses of *cassia fistula* and sugar, as well as other laxatives; in Borriana, *cassia fistula* once more; in Valencia, a laxative electuary with cordial fortifying medicines; then *cassia fistula* again in Castelló de la Plana – surely an exhausting course of treatment, in every sense of the word.[74]

Phlebotomy, like purgation, was something carried out in sickness as well as health, and for the same underlying principle of eliminating unwanted humors.[75] Specific purges existed to expel phlegm, choler, or melancholy, but if a disproportionate quantity of blood itself was the cause of illness, phlebotomy was called for.[76] Now the gravity of the patient's condition might make it necessary for the usual contra-indications of age or climate to be overridden, and here again the learning of the practitioner was needed to decide what risks could be accepted. Thus what seems technically to be a purely mechanical surgical procedure, an incision, proves from another perspective to be a medical one, a therapeutic evacuation like purgation. In his *De consideracionibus operis medicine*, indeed, Arnau de Vilanova used phlebotomy as the exemplar of all therapeutic activity in explaining what general approach should guide the physician in treating a patient, by whatever means.

This co-optation of phlebotomy by learned medicine, which apparently was influenced by the teachings of the *Canon*, was already having occupational consequences by the early fourteenth century, if Henri de Mondeville is to be believed: "there are only a few who consult surgeons about phlebotomy (unless they are being treated for a surgical problem), because the wealthy, nobles and clerics, usually follow the advice of physicians or even common barbers in such

---

[73] Letters of 19 March 1334 (to Joan Amell; C 529/8v) and of 23 March 1334 (to Joan Amell and Domenico de Crix; C 529/10r–v).

[74] Letter of 5 Dec. 1318 (C 362/118v–19).

[75] In one historically important instance, Pere III was bled for a morbid eruption close to his eye, an illness which frustrated an attempt by Jaume of Mallorca to kidnap him: Pere III, *Crònica*, III.18 (in Soldevila, *Cròniques*, p. 1044).

[76] For what follows, see Pedro Gil-Sotres' introduction in Arnau de Vilanova, *De consideracionibus*, pp. 9–120.

cases."[77] The poor or the tight-fisted still chose to think of blood-letting as an operation requiring little expertise, and went to a barber, whose fees were low.[78] But for Arnau, such *vulgares medici et barbitonsores* fail to understand what the *sapiens medicus* knows, that phlebotomy no more than any other therapeutic procedure is governed by absolute, hard-and-fast rules; such rules must always be adapted thoughtfully and knowledgeably to the circumstances of the individual patient.[79]

Therapy: drugs

Only after considering regimen, phlebotomy, and purging did the physician turn to drugs. Here in particular there was an immense technical literature available to him, but it is difficult to know whether the typical practitioner made much use of it. Part of this literature dealt with simple medicines (usually herbs) and with their medicinal properties, which were founded either upon their primary qualities – hot or cold, dry or moist (in any of four degrees of intensity) – or, as with purges, upon a further *proprietas* that was independent of the drug's elemental nature. The *De viribus herbarum* of Macer Floridus (a book in Bernat Serra's library) briefly describes about eighty such medicines; the *De simplicibus* attributed to Arnau de Vilanova analyzes much more systematically the properties of 600.[80] Yet there is very little indication that physicians actually prescribed simple medicines, least of all for their primary qualities. When they employed simples, they did so for some special effect revealed by experience or reported by a trustworthy authority.[81] Arnau gave an account of many such effects in his *Experimenta*: that millefolium taken for three or four mornings on an empty stomach cures hemorrhoids, for example, or that the water prepared by distilling scabiosa prevents summer apostemes.[82]

In general, medieval medicine valued compound medicines over simple ones – that is, medicines built around one or two drugs as a base but typically with others added to modify, reinforce, or channel their effects. Such compounds included, for example, the *triasandali* prescribed for the infante Jaume or the

---

[77] "Pauci quaerunt a cyrurgicis consilium de fleubotomia facienda, nisi qui morbum cyrurgicum patiuntur, quoniam divites, nobiles et prelati in hoc casu acquiescunt consilio medicorum, et vulgaris barberiis ut plurimum se committunt": quoted by Gil-Sotres in ibid., p. 14 n. 19.

[78] "Istam operationem cyrurgici usque ad barberios repulerunt propter duo: primum quia est operatio pauci lucri; secundo quoniam ibi est magisterium paucum et leve et casuale": ibid., p. 15 n. 22.

[79] Arnau de Vilanova, *De consideracionibus*, p. 202.

[80] Gil-Sotres has raised some questions about the atttribution of this work to Arnau; ibid., pp. 91–2.

[81] See Crisciani, "History, Novelty, and Progress," pp. 127–30.

[82] McVaugh, "*Experimenta*," pp. 114, 115.

diaborregenat ordered for the infante Joan.[83] Recipes for these were available in the *Antidotarium Nicolai*, but many physicians preferred their own formulations. "I have had the best apothecary in Montpellier make up the perfect *diazinzibereos* to strengthen your stomach," wrote Guillaume de Béziers to Jaume II, "which you can take as much of as you want to help your digestion."[84]

Many apothecaries must have kept a record of their prescriptions, and one such *receptari* survives from fourteenth-century Catalonia. It was assembled in Lent 1348 by the apothecary Bernat des Pujol of Manresa, seventy kilometers northwest of Barcelona, and lists 230 recipes. Bernat made almost no mention of the conditions for which these medicines were prescribed, but he did usually record the patient's name and sometimes those of the prescribing physicians, "mestres e betxeleres e daltres nobles e bons pratichs e cirurgians":

> RX: of root of butcher's broom, asparagus, and grass, each 1½ handsful; of cinquefoil, a handful; of the four cold seeds, greater and lesser, each three drams; of anise, fennel, and caraway, each ½ ounce; of rose licorice, 1 ounce; of white pepper, just enough; of flowers of violets and borage, each 1 ounce; twenty plump damson plums; just enough raisins; half an ounce each of white vinegar and pomegranate wine; of loaf sugar, one-half pound; of rose honey, one quart. Make up a pound of syrup. For a man of Sallent, prescribed by master Jacme Traver.[85]

At least two other physicians besides master Jacme ordered drugs from Bernat, for a diversity of patients – lay and clerical, men and women, rich and poor. The recipes typically incorporate a dozen or so ingredients; the majority are vegetable simples, but some standard compound drugs – *diarodon abbatis*, *yera*

---

[83] "Electuario confortativo de triasandalis" (5 Sept. 1317; C 362/75r–v); "sex librarum de diaborregenat et quinque libr. de sucaro rosato ad opus infantis Johannis" (9 Nov. 1308; C 297/3v–4). The first would have incorporated three varieties of sandalwood, mixed perhaps with rose sugar; the second, borage mixed with honey. Cf. Johannes de Sancto Amando, *Expositio*, f. 205ra.

[84] "Domine per confortacione stomachi vestri feci fieri meliori apothecario montispessulani optimum diazinzibereos quo audacter poteris uti ad confortacionem digestionis": CRD Jaume II, Apéndice general 94. Johannes de Sancto Amando, *Expositio*, f. 203rb, offers a recipe of honey and ginger in a ratio of 20:1, plus a few other spices. Jaume routinely consumed ginger-based comfits for his digestion: "aliquibus confectis zinziberatis" (1 July 1303; C 294/127v); "una zinziberata" (5 March 1309; C 297/78v–79); "una magna zinziberata" (21 Nov. 1310; C 147/85r–v).

[85] "Recipe radicis brusci sparagi graminis ana M 1 et s; quinque foliorum ana M 1; quatuor seminum frigidorum maiorum et minorum ana ʒ. 3; anisi, maratri, carui ana ʒ. s; liquiritie rose ʒ. 1; seminis piperis albi q. s.; florum viol. boraginis ana ʒ. 1; prunorum damascenorum bone pinguidinis viginti; vuarum pasarum mundatarum q. s; aceti albi, vini malorum, ana ʒ. s; panis zuquare libra s; mellis rosacei q. 1; fiat sirupus usque ad libram 1. per un hom de Salent, per ma de mestre Jacme traver": Comenge, *Receptari*; the document is reproduced on p. 19, rendered into Catalan on p. 17 (my transcription differs slightly from Comenge's). My English equivalents for the Latin names of herbs are inevitably only informed guesses.

pigri Galeni – are included too. All told, there are over 250 ingredients employed among the 230 recipes; the number might seem high to have been available in a small town relatively remote from the great Catalan capital, yet at just this time in Santa Coloma de Queralt, an even more remote town about one-third the size of Manresa, an apothecary's actual inventory included a comparable number of different drugs.[86] That Bernat often gives instructions for topical administration – "fiat clister," "fiat sacculus super frontem," "fiat emplastus extensus super alutam ad formam scuti," "fiat epithima super tota parte anteriore capitis" – suggests that most of the patients were being treated for localized disorders rather than qualitative imbalance.

As a matter of fact, it was in theory possible to create a compound medicine of any given degree from simples of known degree, so that if physicians had diagnosed such qualitative imbalances in their patients they could have prescribed compounds as well as simples to treat them. Fusing earlier theories of the Arabic writers Alkindi and Averroes, Arnau de Vilanova wrote an entire treatise on the mathematics of calculating what quantities to mix of two simple medicines, opposite in quality, in order to produce a compound drug of whatever intermediate degree was desired; his system had some adherents in the Crown of Aragon, but it cannot have been widely used.[87] Illnesses of pure qualitative distemperancy, while part of a theoretical nosology, do not seem to have been commonly diagnosed.

Not all prescriptions were drawn up to restore ill health, except in the broadest sense of the word "health"; people went to their physicians for cosmetic preparations, too. The *De ornatu mulierum* attributed to Arnau de Vilanova is a rather miscellaneous assemblage of recipes, ranging from the cosmetic to the gynecological, for men as well as women: against stinking breath, falling hair, or spots on the skin; to ensure an erection, give pleasure in coitus, evoke (or restrain) the menses.[88] A scrap of paper reused by a Zaragoza notary in 1337 had two such cosmetic prescriptions carefully written out on it, one for discolored teeth and the other perhaps for bad breath. Presumably this was the sufferer's own copy, given him by a physician or written down by him, perhaps out of the *De ornatu* itself, for one of these prescriptions corresponds exactly to one of

---

[86] AHPT 3869/225v–27.

[87] Arnau de Vilanova, *Aphorismi de gradibus*. Vernacular notes in MS Gerona, Arx. Cap. 75, show that Arnau's system was understood in fourteenth-century Catalonia; so does the use made of it by masters in the medical faculty at Lerida in the second half of the century (Dureau-Lapeyssonie, "L'œuvre"). On the question of its application, see McVaugh, "Quantified Medical Theory."

[88] The content of this work (and that of a similar one, *De decoratione*) has left many scholars uneasy about accepting Arnau's authorship (see Paniagua, *Arnau de Vilanova*, pp. 78–9); but whoever its author, *De ornatu mulierum* certainly circulated in conjunction with other works of fourteenth-century Montpellier, as shown by its presence in MSS Vat. Palat. 1331 and Leipzig KMU 1161.

Arnau's.[89] It is one of our very few direct evidences as to how a learned medicine moved from the book to the patient.

The Manresan *receptari* has attracted particular attention because included among its many recipes for local townspeople is a leaf listing five recipes prepared for the infante Jaume d'Urgell, third son of Alfons III; it has been suggested that they were prescribed when he passed through Manresa in late 1347 on his way to his brother Pere III's wedding. The infante died suddenly in Barcelona that November, and his sudden death, coming immediately after his leadership of the rebellion against his brother known as the *Unió*, gave rise to rumors that he had been poisoned by Pere – the latter's *Crònica* says tersely (and perhaps a little coolly) that Jaume died "fort mal aparellat de malaltia."[90] However, the rumors were probably unfounded, for archival evidence makes it plain that Jaume had had a long history of poor health. When he was only ten and in the care of his elder brother Pere at Daroca, he was attacked by a frightening *discrasia*; twelve-year-old Pere wrote imperiously to three Zaragozan physicians – masters Junta, Azarias Abeniacob, and Juceffus Baron – commanding their immediate presence to treat his brother's *languor* before it worsened.[91] And by the beginning of 1346 Jaume's health had begun an accelerating decline, forcing him in February of that year to give up many administrative responsibilities.[92] In April, at Jaume's request, the bishop of Gerona allowed his personal physician, Guerau de Sant Dionis, to travel to the infante, collecting medicines from Barcelona on the way; the bishop had not expected his physician to leave his side for long, and was much put out that a month later Guerau was still attending to Jaume.[93]

---

[89] The paper containing the recipes was reused by a notary who on its other side drafted a document that he then recopied into his manual on 10 June 1337, at which point he loosely inserted the scrap with the recipes (ANZ, manual de Pedro Sanchez de Monzón, 1337, f. 36r–v). The second of the two recipes, for "dentes discalceatos," is virtually identical with a recipe in *De ornatu mulierum* (f. 270rb) "contra cancerem gingivas corrosas et discoriatas." I have not found a source for the first recipe.

[90] Bisson, *Medieval Crown*, pp. 107–8; Pere III, *Crònica*, 4.34 (in Soldevila, *Cròniques*, p. 1101; tr. Hillgarth and Hillgarth, p. 420 n. 44).

[91] Letter of 23 Sept. 1331 (C 577/201v–202); by the 26th Jaume was better. For Junta, see above, chapter 1, n. 120; Pere called him back to treat a *discrasia* in his own person 23 June 1333 (C 578/141v), of which he was cured in two weeks. Juceffus Baron had cared for the boys before, in 1326 (CRD Alfons III judíos 202); I have found no trace of him after 1331. Rabi Azarias had been a physician in Zaragoza since at least 1311 (C 148/229v); at the request of the Dominicans there, he was given charge of the synagogue de Benvenist, though the congregation complained that his medical responsibilities took him away too much (9 June 1317; C 162/296v). He went to Sardinia with Alfons in 1323, and treated Alfons' wife Teresa the next year. Thereafter he became an important agent for the king in royal dealings with the Aragonese Jews, but he maintained his medical practice; after his visit to Pere and Jaume in 1331, he was called to Molina de Aragón in 1337 to treat their brother, Joan (RP 310/64v). He is last encountered in 1339. See also Rius Serra, "Aportaciones," pp. 340, 349–50.

[92] Letter of 13 Feb. 1346; C 1060/152v–53.

[93] For more detail, see below, chapter 6.

The illness attested by the *receptari* of Manresa may be this very episode from spring 1346 rather than one from 1347, as previously supposed, for Guerau is one of the six physicians from all over Catalonia named in the *receptari* as prescribing drugs for Jaume d'Urgell:[94] the medicines included an aperient syrup, a plaster, a clyster, a philtre, and two pounds of a julep. It has been argued that their particular ingredients imply that the infante was suffering with a malignant quartan fever, but this inference does not really seem secure.[95] It is worth pointing out, however, that the medicines prepared for him are no different in content or complexity from what other, humbler, patients were taking; this *receptari*, at least, does not present evidence that rich and poor received different drug therapy.[96]

Even if mistaken, the suspicion that Jaume had been poisoned shows what people felt possible: poisons were understood to be in common use, and physicians were expected to respond to the threat they represented, since poisons were generically akin to medicines. One favored remedy against them was theriac, which was indeed a nearly universal medical panacea.[97] Its quality, however, could be highly variable.[98] Jaume II could find none that was satisfactory in Tortosa in September 1304 and wrote urgently to the bailiff of Barcelona, the master of the Templars, and the lord of Empúries, all three, begging each to send him "the best and finest theriac that can be found."[99] Jaume may not have feared poison in this instance, but it was a continuing preoccupation of the great; the following year Armengaud Blaise translated

---

[94] The physicians were "mestre Guerau [de Sant-Dionis] de Gerona mestre en medicina [1318–49], lo prior de Solsone, mestre R. de Berga, mestre Martí de Vich [Martí de Soler, 1334–47], mestre P. de Pau de Tarrega [1328–47], mestre Cresques jueu metge del seyor Rey darago [1341–8, probably from Figueres]." Comenge, *Receptari*, p. 49, reproduces the document; a portion is also reproduced in his "Historia de la medicina en Cataluña," p. 183.

[95] Comenge, "Historia de la medicina en Cataluña," pp. 181–9; Miró i Borràs, *Receptari de Manresa*, esp. pp. 18–20.

[96] Apothecaries' prices seem to have held more or less constant through much of Jaume II's reign: he paid 6½, 5, and 5 *sous* per pound, respectively, for *rosata novella*, *diacitron*, and *batafalva* in 1308 (RP 271/87r–v), and 6, 6, and 4 *sous* respectively for the same in 1326 (RP 293/49); his son Alfons III paid 5 for *diacitron* and 4 for *batafalva* in 1335 (C 581/67–9). Apothecaries must have made very little profit from medicines.

[97] See my introduction to Arnau de Vilanova, *De dosi tyriacalium*, pp. 57–65.

[98] Some men proclaimed themselves specialists in its manufacture, accusing their competitors of selling a false or misleading product; after one such accusation, "Johannes magister in arte conficiendi triagam" had his product certified by the justices of Valencia in 1329, confirmed by the king in 1333. The confirmation is published by Rius, "Més documents," pp. 139–40, doc. 1; Jordi, "Curioso documento," discusses the document (seeming not to know of Rius) and cites similar supervision of the preparation of theriac at Paris in the 1370s.

[99] Letter of 20 Sept. 1304 (C 258/164). Theriac was best taken six hours after eating, after which it was necessary to fast for another six; see the letter of master Juan d'Ordas to the *primogenitus* Joan in 1370 (C 1230/82r–v), of 20 Nov.; quoted in part by Comenge, *Medicina en el reino de Aragón*, p. 63, and in full by Roca, *Medicina catalana*, p. 155, who however systematically misread ".vi." as ".iii."). Juan d'Ordas was from Huesca, and had been practicing medicine since at least 1343 (ACA, Cancillería, Procesos de infanzonia, legajo 21, no. 1).

Maimonides' *De venenis* for Pope Clement V.[100] And only a year before Jaume of Urgell's death an attempt had been made to kill his uncle, Jaume II's son Ramon Berenguer, by putting poisons (*metzines*) in jugs and pitchers of wine and water.[101]

Nor was it just the powerful who feared poison: the preoccupation was alive at all levels of society. When a royal judge died in the summer of 1314, the Zaragozan apothecary who had prepared a draught for his illness was immediately suspected.[102] Jews and Muslims, already objects of suspicion, were particularly easy targets for the accusation of preparing *metzines* under the cover of medical care.[103] But behind all the rumors there was a certain element of truth: poisons were indeed in use at court, in the monastery, and in the home – to procure abortions if nothing more.[104] "The fourteenth century," one Catalan historian has written, "could well be called the century of poisons."[105]

Therapy: surgery

A patient's last resort was surgery, in the Middle Ages as in Hippocrates' time. A standard, rather ominous definition of the surgeon's role was "the joining together of broken parts, the separation of parts unnaturally joined, and the removal of whatever is superfluous";[106] in desperate cases, calling in a surgeon automatically evoked fears of pain and danger from knife or cautery. Consequently its practitioners sometimes made a point of insisting that their methods were not necessarily invasive: Jaume II hired the surgeon Guillem de Valls to treat the face of the infante Ramon Berenguer (perhaps for a skin condition) only

---

[100] Wickersheimer, *Dictionnaire*, [I] p. 41, lists manuscripts of the translation and reports the date 1305; James, *Descriptive Catalogue*, p. 118, reports the date "Barcelona, 1307," in his transcription of the translation's *explicit* in MS Peterhouse 101, but the archival evidence suggests strongly that Armengaud had left Barcelona the year before.

[101] C 1164/39v, 99v.

[102] Documents of 4 and 14 Sept. 1314 (C 241/231, 236v).

[103] For Muslims, see RL, II:67–8; for Jews, C 1304/196r–v (20 April 1342). Particularly vivid is the accusation made against Juceffus Barlanga of Calatayud in 1327; the relatives of his Christian patient, who had died, were convinced that the patient's enemies had suborned Juceffus and had engaged him to poison the medicines he administered: CRD Jaume II judíos 140.

[104] If any one poison was feared, it was realgar (arsenic sulfide), which the Barcelona *consell* was already attempting to control strictly in 1312: Jewish apothecaries could neither buy nor sell it, while Christian apothecaries could sell it only to physicians – and then the physician had to swear he would use it only medicinally and could not resell it (AHCB, Llibres de consell I–2/35). Forty years later two monks of Sant Miquel de Cruilles conspired to poison their prior, and asked the woman tending the apothecary shop for realgar. She replied that "non erat ibi vir suus et sine ipso non auderet vendere realgar," so they attacked the prior (unsuccessfully) with a sword instead: ADG, Sèrie C (procesos), old C 12 no. 7 (7 Nov. 1353).

[105] Miret y Sans, *Sempre han tingut*, II:48. Miret made his remark after discussing two poisoning cases of the 1370s. Cf. Cardoner, *Història*, p. 105.

[106] "Intentio operationis cirurgorum est circa tria, scilicet circa coniunctionem solutorum, circa separationem coniunctorum praeter naturam, et circa extirpationem superflui": Teodorico, *Chirurgia*, capitulum proemiale; f. 134vb.

after Guillem assured the king that he could bring about a cure "without cutting or burning."[107]

In fact, surgeons did much more than cut and sear, as we can see from the *Chirurgia* of Teodorico Borgognoni, the text that provides the most appropriate introduction to surgical practice in the Crown of Aragon. The *Chirurgia* starts by repeating the traditional characterization of surgery as an invasive procedure, but the contents of the work reveal a very different reality. The first two books discuss the cause and treatment of wounds and ulcers, fractures and dislocations – conditions which today too we consider as surgical. Book three, however, covers not only the surgical treatment of tumors and abscesses and hemorrhoids, but also the cure of what we would probably think of as dermatological problems: burns and blisters, scabies and scrofula, lupus, freckles, and even diseases like leprosy; for "infections which take hold upon the human body in plain view," as Teodorico put it, fell to the surgeon to treat.[108] We thus encounter again the surgeon's overlapping competence with the physician, who likewise might treat such conditions as hemorrhoids and leprosy, and in the fourth (final) book of the *Chirurgia* the overlap is even more pronounced: here Teodorico describes the purely medical treatment (with drugs or occasionally bloodletting) of headache, ophthalmia, gout, paralysis, and epilepsy.

Hence it is instructive to compare the responses of a physician and a surgeon to a complaint, like hemorrhoids, that both might treat. The final chapter of Arnau's *Regimen sanitatis* is a chapter *de lapsibus emorroydarum* that was drafted expressly for Jaume II, who had suffered from this condition for at least a decade.[109] It gives us the opportunity to see a doctor prescribe for a painful chronic (but not rapidly progressive) illness, and to recognize the authority of the scholastic paradigm in the sphere of medical practice. In most cases, writes Arnau, the pain of hemorrhoids can be controlled by maintaining a normal healthful diet, in particular avoiding sharp, salty, or too-sweet foods; but "often we fall away from the proper regimen," leading the hemorrhoids to flare up, and therefore the patient should know how to treat them. If they bleed copiously, styptic foods and syrups can be ingested, or styptic medicines applied externally; if they swell but do not bleed, and cause severe pain, they can be lanced, drained with leeches (*sanguisugis*), or relieved with medicines – or the engorging blood can be removed from the body by phlebotomy of foot or hand. It is dangerous, however, to try to remove them by cautery or surgery; caustic ointments are preferable, since they are less likely to obstruct the affected veins and cause them to swell anew.[110] Arnau's advice here is less elaborate than that available in a

---

107 Letter of 16 April 1315; C 242/128v. See above, chapter 1.
108 "Infectionibus que in manifesto corporis humani contingit": Teodorico, *Chirurgia*, f. 135ra.
109 See above, chapter 1.
110 *Regimen sanitatis*, ff. 85v–86r (cap. 18). Cf. the even milder remedy set out in his *Experimenta*, above, n. 82.

scholastic compendium like Avicenna's *Canon*, but it is not essentially different in its approach to treatment and diagnostic detail.[111] Teodorico's chapter on hemorrhoids, on the other hand, while suggesting a dozen remedies to open them and dry them up, considers their surgical removal as well. In this instance, therefore, the surgeon was prepared to offer everything that the physician could – and more, too, if the patient really wished it.

The picture presented by Teodorico's surgery is confirmed from archival records of actual surgical cases in the Crown of Aragon. Not all the allusions to a surgeon's practice name the condition he was called upon to treat, to be sure, and the bulk of those which do so refer merely to wounds, of head, trunk, or limb. The frequency with which assaults occurred is a startling feature of life in communities of all sizes, large and small, and together with infrequent detail as to their savagery – eighteen pieces of bone had to be removed from Juan del Frago's skull – reveals how violent a society it was.[112] (Juan lived to accuse his attacker, which at least speaks well for the skill of one particular surgeon.) However, the records also identify a number of specific complaints for which a surgeon was consulted: some of these we would still think of as surgical (bladder stone, hernia, breast cancer), but others reveal the same "medical" side to medieval surgery that is indicated by Teodorico's text. If the surgeon of Zaragoza who contracted to cure a case of "inpetigo o serpige" on the face (1346) had consulted the *Chirurgia* for advice, he would have discovered the same sort of non-invasive pharmaceutical therapy set out there that a physician would have found in the *Canon*.[113] Indeed, some surgeons were perfectly willing to accept cases far more "medical" than anything included in Teodorico's handbook: Guillem Arnau of Santa Coloma agreed to try to cure Pere Comill of "the illness called stupidity or madness" for a fee of 200 *sous* – to be paid if he had success within the year.[114]

All this is general surgery, for there seems to have been virtually no specialization in the Crown of Aragon.[115] Jaume II had difficulties in locating a surgeon

---

[111] Avicenna, *Canon*, III.17, capp. 1–10 (ff. 333–5).

[112] Letter of 1 Sept. 1330 (C 523/109). An equally vivid reminder of everyday violence is the case of one Berenguer, "positus in articulo mortis eo quia sum letaliter uno vulnere cum petra in capita vulneratus nescio per quem et ipsam vulnus sit mihi factum in villa Tarrege de nocte casu fortuitu": ACA pergaminos Jaume II 4120 (26 April 1325). Given, *Society and Homicide*, has helped me think about violence and social response in medieval society.

[113] ANZ, manual de Pedro Serra 1343, f. 117 (June 1346). Teodorico, *Chirurgia*, III.50 (ff. 175v–76); Avicenna, *Canon* IV.7.3.3–4 (ff. 494v–495). The *Canon* chapter treats only *impetigo*, but Teodorico links *impetigo* and *serpigo*, like the Zaragoza surgeon.

[114] "Quem promisistis curare de infirmitate stulticie seu d'oradura quam patitur": letter of 21 Feb. 1334 (AHPT 3847/242, 242v).

[115] Cardoner Planas, "Ejemplos," pp. 201–3, shows that a specialization in the treatment of hernias ("trencadures") was not uncommon in early fifteenth-century Catalonia, but he finds no instance of it earlier than 1393. García-Ballester, McVaugh, and Rubio-Vela give two instances from

in his realms who could treat his daughter's cataracts, and there is no sign that the man he finally settled on was particularly well known for his treatment of eye problems.[116] In 1342, when King Pere sought an eye-specialist to treat Roger de Sant Vicenç, the only one he could identify in his realms was a Muslim slave in Vilafranca del Penedès (it may not be a coincidence that the prevalence of trachoma in the Middle East had created a specialized ophthalmology there).[117] Four years later, domestic resources having failed, Roger was given permission to travel to Montpellier for his eyes; there, at least, "an abundance of physicians and surgeons expert in such problems is to be found."[118]

The earliest exception to such general practice may have been dentistry. Dentistry had traditionally been the undifferentiated province of barbers and surgeons alike, but there is some reason to think that in the 1340s foreigners specializing in oral surgery felt that the Crown of Aragon might provide a profitable new market for their skills.[119] Simon Virgilii arrived in Valencia from Florence in 1346, announcing his expertise "in the science of surgery, particularly in ailments of the mouth, teeth, glands, tumor of the throat, and scrophula," and, after an examination by the city's medical establishment, was licensed to treat these illnesses.[120] Two years later Pere III gave permission to a surgeon from Cagliari in Sardinia to treat "morbis dentium" anywhere in his

Valencia in the 1380s (*Medical Licensing*, pp. 90–3, 96–7; note that both specialists are immigrants from Italy). In the first half of the fourteenth century, however, it is always general surgeons who are found treating hernias (cf. above, chapter 4 n. 114).

[116] This man (Jaime de Rocha) is only once called "metge de mal de uylls" in the curial documentation, after his abortive trip to cure Isabel (Nov. 1330; RP 298/95); at all other times he is simply "cirurgicus." Note that Henri de Mondeville was concerned that many "de curis cyrurgicis periculosis sine scientia intromittunt et maxime de curis aegritudinum oculorum, quarum curae sunt periculosae, difficiles et fallaces, ita quod in ipsis curandis cyrurgicus sufficiens et expertus rarissime reperitur": Pagel, *Chirurgie*, 40:661. A useful survey of the speciality in the West is still Pansier, "Pratique de l'ophthalmologie," who says, "nous voyons Arnauld de Villeneuve constater que s'il a vu souvent des spécialistes abattre la cataracte, rarement il a pu constater que cette opération ait donné des résultats heureux" (p. 14).

[117] Rius, "Més documents," pp. 162–4, docs. 57–9. See further Meyerhof, "History of Trachoma Treatment."

[118] "Fisicorum et cirurgicorum expertorum in talibus poterit copia reperiri": letter of 7 July 1346 (C 881/21).

[119] For early references to dental practice by barbers and surgeons, see above, chapters 1 (barber's tools) and 3 (Jaume d'Avinyó and young Isabel). Surgical specialization already existed in southern Italy by 1300 and was explicitly recognized in licenses to practice: those published by Calvanico, *Fonti*, identify skills ranging from "medendis ungulis et carnositatibus crescentibus supra oculos" (doc. 1546) to "cura egritudinum lapidis vexice et crepaturarum" (doc. 669).

[120] "In sciencia cirurgie et specialiter ac signanter in infirmitatibus oris, dencium, glandularum, tumoris gule, ac scrophularum": letter of 17 May 1346 (C 881/3v). Documents relating to Simon's later career as dentist to Pere III and his family in the second half of the century are discussed by Rahola i Sastre, "Odontòlegs." Simon died in 1375.

realms.[121] Of native practitioners of the specialty, however, there is virtually no trace.[122]

Other therapies

It is easy to understand why the activity of those who claimed the titles of "surgeon" and "physician" should be best documented. Their world's recognition of those titles is mirrored in the letters, contracts, wills, and the like that take formal notice of their practice. On the other hand, we know very little about the practice of the local healer, the village empiric whose cures were perhaps only a minor part of his (or her) role in the community, even though such practitioners were still undoubtedly providing health care to much of the population. The scraps of information that we have, however, reveal a multitude of folk practices ostensibly far removed from the new, rational, learned medicine. They tended to be carried out by people who by religion or gender were excluded from the emerging profession: Muslims, like Ali de Lucera of Daroca, whom we find treating headaches with talismans in 1311;[123] or women, like Benvinguda of Mallnovell, who claimed to have cured twenty sufferers from heart palpitations (*pantex de cor*) with incantations and natural magic.[124] As the case of Gueraula de Codines has already shown us, however, these healers were likely to have assimilated something of the new medicine to their own traditional practice. A line between "scientific medicine" and "superstitious magic" would be impossible to draw.[125]

And in their turn academics did not automatically disdain such things as amulets or incantations, not even an Arnau de Vilanova. In May 1301 Arnau had arrived at Anagni (near Rome) to defend himself before Pope Boniface VIII against the attacks made on his writings by the Paris theologians in the previous fall. He used his medical skill to ingratiate himself with the pontiff, who was suffering from kidney stone. During the month of July Arnau secluded himself in the pope's castle at Sgurgola and drew up a *regimen sanitatis* addressed to Boniface's complaint, probably the work now known as *Contra calculum*; he also prepared a golden sigil for the pope as well as a belt (*bracale*) to wear it on, with both of which Boniface was delighted: "I am wearing them and

---

[121] Document of 26 Dec. 1347 (C 885/133), repeating a privilege granted nine days before (C 885/108).

[122] Rahola i Sastre has called attention ("Odontòlegs," pp. 298–9) to a document of 1344 identifying "mestre Barthomeu Peres caxaler" ("queixaler" = dentist) in the king's service; Bertomeu was apparently still alive and active in 1380.

[123] Above, chapter 2, p. 52.

[124] Perarnau i Espelt, "Activitats," pp. 55–7. Benvinguda also claimed to be able to treat headache, St. Anthony's fire, and inflammations of the throat (*mal de cap, foc salvatge i gotornons*).

[125] This point is emphasized in regard to the healing arts by Kieckhefer, *Magic*, p. 64.

they are keeping me free from the pain of the stone as well as from my other pains – they are letting me live."[126] Charms and talismans are not in fact included among the remedies prescribed in *Contra calculum*, but not necessarily because Arnau felt it somehow "unscientific" or unprofessional to subscribe to them publicly;[127] subsequently, in his ambitious *Speculum medicine*, he made no secret of his conviction that "the lion seal passed on by Hermes when applied to the loins straightway eases the pain of those suffering from stone."[128]

We can learn how Boniface's golden lion seal must have been manufactured from the treatise *De sigillis*, also printed among Arnau's works. This short text gives meticulous instructions for the preparation of twelve talismans of gold or silver, each bearing a different zodiacal sign and begun as the sun entered that sign. The instructions for producing the lion seal are typical:

> The sixth seal is for Leo, 22 July. Take gold and make a seal with it as described above; carve the form of a lion in it according to the conditions set out above for the first seal, of Aries, and while it is being hammered say as follows: *Stir up thyself*, lion of the tribe of Juda, *and awake to my judgment, even unto my cause, my God and my Lord* [Ps. 34:23], *and plead my cause* [Ps. 42:1] . . . On the side with the lion, around the circumference of the lion seal: Choel, Saint James; and around the other side: *The Lion of the tribe of Juda, the Root of David, hath prevailed* [Rev. 5:5], alleluia; and in the middle: Heloy, sadoy. The properties of this seal are, generally, that it is good against all passions of the stomach, sides, back, kidneys, and excessive menses, and against the heat of the sun and acute, intense fevers, and against all apostemes, and many other things. It is worn over the kidneys.[129]

---

126 Finke, *Aus den Tagen*, pp. 200–9, discusses Arnau's professional relation to the pope; the sigil and belt, and the pope's reaction, are described in the text published on pp. xxvi–xxxvii. Lerner, "Pope and the Doctor," is a splendidly evocative picture set in a broad context.

127 Unlike the cardinals at the papal court, who "valde mirati fuerunt . . . de magistro, qui se talibus immiscebat" (Finke, *Aus den Tagen*, p. xxx).

128 "Sigillum leonis ab hermete traditum si lumbis applicetur protinus mitigat dolores in calculosis": Arnau de Vilanova, *Speculum medicine*, f. 7ra (cap. 18). Arnau repeated in *De parte operativa* (f. 127ra) that "presentia sigilli leonis lumbis appositi non permittit sensum percipere lesionem calculi."

129 "Sextum sigillum est leoni, 11 kls. Augusti. Accipe aurum et fac inde sigillum ut supra et sculpatur in eo forma leonis observatis conditionibus que supradicte sunt in primo sigillo Arietis et dum malleo ferietur dic: *Exurge* leo de tribu iuda *et intende iudicio meo Deus meus et Dominus meus in causam meam et discerne causam meam*. [Psalmus, *Iudica me Deus et discerne causam meam* etc.] Et ex parte leonis in circumferentia sigilli leonis, Choel, sanctus Iacobus, et ex alia parte in circumferentia: *Vicit leo de tribu Iuda radix David*, alleluia, et in medio: Heloy, sadoy. Proprietates huius sigilli in generali sunt he, valet ad omnes passiones stomachi, laterum et dorsi et renum et menstruis multis et contra ardorem solis et febres acutas et peracutas et contra omnia apostemata et multa alia. Portetur in renibus": Arnau de Vilanova, *De sigillis*, f. 302ra, which gives "Deus" in place of "Dominus" in the quotation from Psalm 34. The words bracketed in the quotation may well be an intruded marginal gloss.

De sigillis may well be genuinely Arnaldian;[130] in any case it certainly reflects the debates over the therapeutic use of talismans taking place among Latin and Jewish scholars in Montpellier *c.* 1300, aroused by the appearance of a version of the Latin *Picatrix* (an Arabic text on astral magic translated fifty years before at the Castilian court of Alfonso el Sabio).[131] These debates – whose echoes persist for at least a century – turned on whether it might not be superstition and idolatry to believe in the efficacy of such medals; but many physicians seem to have decided that their use was perfectly legitimate.[132] It is not easy to draw a sharp distinction between the physicians' ritual prescriptions, their charms, and those employed by a rural empiric like Gueraula de Codines – except perhaps that theirs had been legitimated by incorporation into written and quasi-learned tradition.[133]

On the other hand, it is difficult not to conclude that a more technical astrology (and the "occult sciences") played very little part in medical practice during the first half of the fourteenth century. We find only occasional indications that celestial influences were being considered by physicians, and then only influences of the most general kind, as in the Valencian prohibition of phlebotomy on canicular and other unlucky days (above, p. 126). There is certainly no sign that contemporary doctors – or their patients – believed it was important to correlate planetary positions with the course of a disease. Undoubtedly Arnau de Vilanova was well acquainted with the literature on medical astrology, and he actually wrote one book on the subject, a *De iudiciis astronomie*; this gives the reader a qualitative description of the heavenly motions, agreeing that they affect our health or the efficacy of the drugs that our physicians prescribe, but it concludes by saying that many of these relationships are too obscure or too complicated to be useful, and that the most a physician really needs to keep in mind as he treats a patient is the current zodiacal sign of the moon.[134] Significantly, obsessed though he was about his family's health, Jaume II seemingly paid no attention to possible astrological considerations

---

[130] Paniagua, *Arnau de Vilanova*, pp. 71–2, drew together evidence indicating that Arnau knew well and often used the lion seal but not the other eleven in the *De sigillis*. For this reason, and because he felt that the use of sacred texts as magical formulas was foreign to Arnau's thought, Paniagua rejected its authenticity. Since then, however, Montpellier's fascination with medical magic has been well documented, and the case for the work's genuineness remains open. Arnau's interest in magic and astrology was first studied seriously by Diepgen, "Arnalds Stellung."

[131] Pingree, "Diffusion," esp. pp. 90–3; Demaitre, *Bernard de Gordon*, pp. 97–9.

[132] Delmas, "Médailles astrologiques."

[133] So too Kieckhefer declares (*Magic*, p. 57) that "much of the magic in medieval Europe . . . was not regularly limited to any specific group," and he goes on to demonstrate the use of magical practices by barbers, surgeons, and even academic physicians in their work.

[134] Paniagua, *Arnau de Vilanova*, pp. 73–4, accepts the *De iudiciis astronomie* as genuinely Arnaldian, and points out that its emphasis upon the importance of lunar position recurs in Arnau's *Medicationis parabole* (pp. 59–63). Arnau owned the *Centiloquium* (Chabás, "Inventario," #319) and at least one other astrological work (ibid., #33; Carreras Artau's identifications ["Llibreria," p. 72] seem to me somewhat overconfident).

(a youthful enthusiasm for geomancy seems to have been abandoned),[135] and this lack of interest contrasts sharply with the fascination with astrology and astronomy that his descendants Pere III and Joan I would display.[136] It may be that the mid-century epidemics encouraged physicians to explore new and perhaps – as they may have thought – more effective medical technologies.

In what has been discussed above it has not seemed necessary to ask about the "actual" effectiveness of medieval therapy. Our own conceptions of sickness and health have changed so much in seven centuries that it is not truly possible for us to assess the skills of fourteenth-century practitioners, and if we try to do so we may unknowingly apply irrelevant standards of judgment. Can we really appreciate medieval estimates of the success of a prognosis or treatment? Consider, for example, the Montpellier master Jordan de Turre, who enjoyed a wide reputation in his day as a successful physician – an unusually large number of references to his recipes and *regimina* have been preserved. In the fall of 1318 Jordan was summoned to Barcelona to join other physicians in treating Jaume II, who had been desperately ill for two months with a fever. All we know of the physicians' course of treatment is that in mid-November they prescribed an electuary containing powdered gold and pearls, and that the king almost immediately thereafter began to regain his health. Our judgment today of the effectiveness of that electuary is likely to be different from the recovering king's, and we will be less ready than the court to believe in master Jordan's skill; but it is the belief of the fourteenth century that matters historically. Jordan's share in Jaume's recovery could only have confirmed his reputation and strengthened his patients' confidence in him, and this presumably helps explain why, when Jaume's son Alfons III became seriously ill in 1335, Jordan was recalled to Barcelona for consultation. This time, however, Jordan seems to have abandoned the case as hopeless and returned home, and the king vindicated his prognosis by dying in January 1336 – a further confirmation, of course, of master Jordan's expertise.[137] It is ultimately the public response to medical practitioners that is our best evidence as to their effectiveness.

---

[135] *AA*, II:920.

[136] See Rubió i Lluch, "Cultura catalana," pp. 231–2, and "Joan I Humanista"; and Roca, "Johan I y les supersticions" and *Johan I d'Aragó*, pp. 363–415.

[137] McVaugh, "Two Faces." Fifty years after Jaume's illness, his grandson's wife, Elionor of Sicily, became ill in Barcelona, and for her too was prescribed an electuary rich in gems – emeralds, sapphires, and others (Roca, "Notes medicals historiques: Medicaments reyals"). Was this perhaps a further recollection of the old king's recovery?

6

Patient-practitioner relationships

The physician's authority

In the last forty years the "doctor-patient relationship" has become a focus of attention for students – and for critics – of modern medical practice. It is now generally understood that doctors and their patients alike may contribute to a greater or lesser extent to the interchange between them. Critics have found it disturbing that medical training encourages physicians automatically to assume a controlling, dominant role and to expect acquiescence or compliance from their clients, and consequently the recent trend of medical ethics has been to insist that patients should be furnished full information about their condition so that they can participate in treatment by giving it their "informed consent." This contemporary fascination with the interrelationship is misleading. The relationship between healer and patient is one of the elements that in any age help to determine how treatment proceeds and whether it succeeds, and it is beginning to pique the interest of some medical historians, but they must be on guard against the temptation to read modern norms into the past, as though "informed consent" were a universal in all medical care. It might properly be argued that different forms of the doctor-patient relationship are appropriate at different moments, or in different societies.

In today's society, which has set a standard for medical qualification, the act of consulting a physician already implies a certain concession of expertise and authority by the patient. In the early fourteenth century, however, as indeed ever since classical antiquity, no such standard existed. A university degree would eventually provide it, but it did not do so in 1300, when academically trained physicians were still rare in the Crown of Aragon; only in the second quarter of the century have we found signs that their training was coming to be thought of as a standard to be required of all practitioners, and even then the older habits of individual negotiation with a practitioner must have persisted for some time among their clients. In the first decades of the century, therefore, every physician would at the outset have had to convince his patients that he knew something they did not – what was wrong with them, and how it could be cured – and that they should concede him authority and power over them in treatment. He could not have felt at ease until he was sure that his patients fully believed in him and accepted his authority: as Galen put it in his commentary on Hippocrates' first aphorism, in treating a patient "it is not just necessary that *you* do all the right things, the patient has to obey you and never go against your commands."[1]

Indeed, medical students of the time had just this lesson reinforced by their teachers. They encountered the Hippocratic *Aphorisms* early in their training; Arnau de Vilanova used the opportunity to explain to those beginning their education at Montpellier *c.* 1300 why it would be important to them to keep control over their patients from the outset of every case, and he suggested techniques for doing so. Degree or no, they would still have to prove themselves to their clients, as physicians had always done: Arnau did not foresee a time when academic credentials would automatically produce unquestioning trust. The techniques he taught his students to adopt, his practical advice for them, had been distilled from collective craft experience and were certainly not peculiar to him, but were and had been passed on by example in whatever manner practitioners were being trained. His instructions may have been given to university students, but they applied to all practitioners.

Arnau explained to his students what their role should be by likening the *officium medici* to the *officium naute*: a physician, like a sailor, has been given charge of something which he rules or directs by selecting and manipulating certain variables.[2] The sailor alters the sails in conformity with changing winds; the physician modifies his course of treatment in conformity with changing circumstances, according to the knowledge of the medical art that he has built up with study and experience. This role is not merely an ideal; it determines how the physician must behave towards his patient, for he must always be in control of his patient's actions. For example, because no course of treatment is totally predictable – the physician is always altering his choice of regimen or of medicines as the state of the disease or the condition of the patient happens to evolve – patients are likely to prove skeptical of a doctor who appears unable to select a correct treatment and stick to it. Therefore, Arnau counseled his listeners, a physician must "preserve his authority and guard against his patients' (or their friends') becoming mistrustful when he changes what he does, as change he must."[3]

---

[1] "Non solum oportet facienda ex parte tui fieri, sed etiam tibi infirmum obedire, neque in aliquo decet eum obviare tibi": Galen, commentary on Hippocrates, *Aphorisms* [tr. Constantinus Africanus], I.i, in *Articella* (Venice, 1523), (II) f. 3r.

[2] The analogy goes back to antiquity: cf. Galen, *On Examinations*, pp. 49, 147; or Hippocrates, *Tradition in Medicine* 9, in *Hippocratic Writings*, p. 75.

[3] Arnau de Vilanova, *Repetitio*, ff. 279vb–280ra; MS Munich CLM 14245, f. 33r.

The need to maintain control of the relationship, a control that Arnau saw as ultimately in the patient's own interests, is most critical at the onset of the illness, when the patient is seeking assurance that a name can be given to his condition and when the physician has to prove his own expertise.[4] Arnau took special pains to guide his students step by step along the path they should follow in arriving at an initial diagnosis in any particular case. When a physician is first summoned to attend someone, he should extract from the messengers sent him all the information he can about his patient's condition, and review this in the light of medical science. Then, arrived at the bedside, he should examine the patient. He should not begin by taking the pulse, for if (as is likely) the patient has been waiting anxiously for him, the pulse will be abnormal. Instead, he must first ask the patient to describe his state and then make (as far as decency permits) a physical examination: on this basis he should try to identify the illness and assign its cause, and, if he succeeds, he can proceed to prescribe a therapeutic regimen. If however he cannot come to a decision without further study, he must prescribe *something*, so as not to lose the patient's confidence (*ne patiens remaneat desolatus aut forte diffidat*), and he can recommend foods that will maintain the body's strength. In this latter case, since the patient's friends may ask him for his opinion, he must choose his words carefully, taking pains not to lie[5] – say that he needs to study the patient a little further before drawing a conclusion, or say that the symptoms are unclear rather than that he doesn't understand them. Then, in private, he must go over the symptoms again in the light of reason; Arnau recommended drawing up a tabular presentation of the symptoms of all illnesses that can be consulted privately, which should lead the physician eventually to an unequivocal diagnosis.[6]

Nevertheless he may still be unable to decide at this point what the symptoms mean, and in this case he should consult with a colleague, or, if there is none nearby, he should encourage the patient to call in a second opinion. Meanwhile he should continue to study the case, assuring the patient's friends that he wants simply to eliminate all possible doubts before revealing his diagnosis and prescribing drugs. This should strengthen his patient's belief in his expertise, but if it fails to satisfy, and if the physician encounters the beginnings of mistrust, he may prescribe a placebo "to keep the friends from muttering, and the patient from suffering any nervousness or anxiety." At this point he should be especially careful in what he says:

⁴ The relationship between these two things and their importance for the success of treatment are emphasized in Hippocrates' *Prognostics*, I.ii, and repeated in Galen's commentary thereupon: *Articella*, (II) f. 141ra–b.

⁵ This scrupulousness would seem to be inconsistent with the deliberate use of jargon to confuse the patient that is recommended in *De cautelis medicorum* (above, chapter 5); if the latter work is indeed authentic, perhaps the ideal was one thing and practice another.

⁶ Arnau de Vilanova, *Repetitio*, ff. 178vb–179ra; MS Munich CLM 14245, f. 30r–v.

for when he doesn't know how long the illness will last or when it might return, he should never promise that any particular treatment is going to be the last, because when the treatment is complete the patient will lose hope if he hasn't gotten better, and the physician will be accused of falsehoods. Thus the prudent physician will always tell the patient and his friends that he is using this drug or that in order to bring about a preliminary state, so that the patient can look forward to a further important treatment and will not give up hope; and meanwhile, if health returns, the physician will win praise for his preliminary treatment as having reinforced the powers of nature.[7]

Then the patient will maintain a belief in his physician's knowledge of the art, and if he begins to improve will praise his skill.

To his patients, Arnau presented a slightly different image from that to which he trained his students; while not denying physicians' need to maintain power over their patients, he emphasized that they were bound to exercise it responsibly:

The doctor should be trustworthy in his treatments, taking pains not to wound through his carelessness or to injure through his lack of skill, nor to kill by using unwise artful tricks. He must take responsibility for his lack of skill, and if he employs lethal potions for unlawful ends he will be held guilty of the blood, and a murderer. He must behave honestly in the bedroom, suppressing the flame of desire lest he be burnt by a touch or smitten by a glance. He should keep silent where necessary so as not to reveal what should not be known, keeping such things sealed in his heart. He should not hurry to use drugs or desperate remedies, but should always follow the more cautious counsel, nor should he use the knife to treat wounds that may be healed with mild applications. The trustworthy doctor will not look for new remedies, for novelties can be dangerous.[8]

---

[7] "Cum enim ignoret quantum debeat morbus durare vel quod etiam in futuro poterit apparere, nunquam promittere vel asserere debet ab aliquo particulari opere quod exercet quod sit opus finale secundum suam intentionem . . . quia terminato isto opere . . . nisi sanitas sequeretur, haberet infirmus desperandi vel tristandi occasionem, et medicus notaretur de mendacio vel falsitate. Et ideo medicus prudens semper dicit infirmo et aliis quod ordinet usum talis aut talis antidoti ad talem vel ad talem preparationem introducendam in egro, ad hoc ut ipsum egrum et alios retineat semper in spe ulterioris et necessarii operis, ut animo non fatigentur aut perturbentur; et interim si apparuerit effectus sanationis, commendabitur medicus de recta administratione preparatoria corporis et adiutrice nature": Arnau de Vilanova, *Repetitio*, f. 279va; MS Munich CLM 14245, f. 32r.
[8] "Sit medicus in sua curatione fidelis ut caveat ne per imperitiam sauciet, per negligentiam vulneret, vel dolosis fraudibus imprudenter occidat. Tenetur enim medicus ex imperitia obligari in cura, et si potiones letiferas machinationibus dolosis ingesserit reus ipse sanguinis horrendus et ipsius homicida. Sit honestus in thalamis; delitescat in eo flamma libidinis ne tactu ardeat nec aspectu mordescat. Sit in silendo cautus ut taceat que revelare non expedit et futurus cognitor futurorum secretorum. Occultaque colliget in scrinio cordis pectoris sub sigillo claudat. Ad farmacias non sit immaturus, et ad finalia remedia non declinet festinus, sed semper ad curatiora consilia; nec sunt ferro curanda vulnera que fomentorum possunt blandiciis recipere sanitatem. Novis experimentis fidelis medicus non studeat, quia solent novitates pericula inducere." Arnau de Vilanova, *Contra calculum*, cap. 3, f. 305vb.

There are obvious echoes of Hippocratic ethics in this passage, yet there are new features too: the implied acceptance of professional incompetence as criminal, and the insistence that medical treatment must be conservative not only in favoring mild remedies but in avoiding therapeutic innovation as too risky.[9] It does not matter that there may be a deliberately apologetic element here (Arnau was explaining his role to a powerful client – Pope Boniface VIII – at a delicate moment), for the ideal that he sets out shows us what patients wanted to hear.

Surgeons had perhaps to be even more conscious than physicians of the need to maintain control, because their patients' behavior could be especially trying. Henri de Mondeville complained that patients often felt capable of understanding and independently improving on his apparently simple procedures – over-tightening his bandages, or leaving strong unguents on a sore longer than desirable on the principle of getting more of a good thing, and generally carrying his prescriptions to unhealthy extremes. Not many shared the sophistication of professional colleagues, who automatically accepted the importance of unquestioning obedience to a doctor's orders once they had decided to place themselves in his hands. Henri wrote approvingly:

> A certain famous doctor suffering from an aposteme put himself under the care of master Jean Pitard while I was assisting him, and when we wanted to explain our prescriptions to him, he told us, "Didn't I pick you out to treat me because I thought you were qualified and trustworthy? Go ahead and treat me as though I were a stupid rustic – if I knew what your prescriptions were made from I might trust them less and so gain less advantage from your treatment."[10]

Less understanding and more mistrustful patients had to be won over with threats of what would happen if they disobeyed instructions, promises of rapid relief if they did as they were told, and assurances of their doctor's competence and experience in similar cases. Only when a patient has fully accepted the surgeon's authority can the latter in his turn feel confident about his ability to be of help.[11]

The patient's trust is important for a further reason: his emotional state helps determine whether his health will improve or decline. Hippocrates and Galen both taught the importance of maintaining a patient's spirits, and Arnau and Henri agreed – Henri, indeed, would evidently have been prepared to lie to keep

---

[9] For more on the tension between stability and innovation in the medicine of this time, see Crisciani, "History," esp. pp. 134–8.

[10] "Ita enim se commisit magistro Joh. Pitard me discipulo suo praesente quidam maximus medicus et famosus, qui habuit apostema, et cum sibi vellemus receptas nostrorum localium eidem revelare, ipse dixit: Nonne Vos elegi prae aliis pro me ipso tamquam legitimos et fideles? Operemini ergo in me consideratis considerandis sicut in rustico penitus ignorante! Si forte scirem, ex quibus Vestra localia sunt confecta, inde minus confiderem et per consequens minus deberet proficere opus Vestrum!" Pagel, "Chirurgie," 40:710; French translation in Nicaise, *Chirurgie*, p. 171.

[11] Pagel, "Chirurgie," 40:692–4; Nicaise, *Chirurgie*, pp. 144–8.

his patient thinking positively about his prospects. This concern for their patients' mental outlook left practitioners uncomfortable with the church's insistence (dating from Lateran IV, 1215) that they admonish the sick to confess their sins to a priest before they begin to treat them. The church argued that some illnesses sprang from sin, and that confession and absolution might therefore bring about a cure, but physicians were well aware that warning their patients to confess could easily lead them to imagine a mortal illness and to lose all hope of recovery.[12] To judge from the regularity with which bishops and local councils insisted that practitioners obey the requirement, doctors felt more concern about their patients' physical than their spiritual health.[13]

Fees and trust

Formed both at Montpellier, Henri and Arnau shared an academic ideology of the *ars medicine* that assumed that the learned practitioner possesses a special ability to identify the cause and so the cure of illness; and from this follows the need, as Arnau expressed it, for "the patient's obedience, which subjects his body to the commands of the physician [*artificis*] inasmuch as the latter's labor and study is directed towards the former's good."[14] Such an attitude was and is consonant with the universal human tendency to want, when ill, to invest

[12] The original injunction, canon 22 of Lateran IV, was collected in *Decretalium* V.38, cap. 13 (*Corpus Juris Canonici*, II, ed. Friedberg, col. 888). The decretal itself acknowledges the concerns felt by physicians, but insists that "anima sit multo preciosior corpore." It and its treatment by later canonists are discussed by Diepgen, *Theologie*, pp. 48–56.

[13] Amundsen ("Medieval Catholic Tradition," pp. 88–90) suggests that medieval physicians followed the injunction faithfully, but given its frequent reiteration in the fourteenth century it is difficult to feel confident of this. In the Crown of Aragon it can be found repeated by the diocese of Valencia in a document of 1300 (ACV, perg. 2399; Olmos y Canalda, *Pergaminos*, doc. 913), quoting a previous reenactment by a provincial council of Tarragona (probably of 1246; see above, chapter 2 n. 86); by another Tarragonan council of 1308–12 (Pons Guri, "Constitucions conciliars," pp. 301–2); by the bishop of Lerida in 1325 (Sainz de Baranda, *España Sagrada*, p. 183); and by the bishop of Gerona, who told the priests of his diocese to remind physicians of this for four consecutive Sundays in June 1346 and found it necessary to repeat the publicity in May 1347 (ADG, Sèrie U [Regesta litterarum], 10/54 and 11/19v–20).

Among contemporary practitioners, Henri de Mondeville paid at least lip-service to the church's requirement, making that his one exception to the need to keep up a patient's spirits ("nec sit [patiens] sollicitus de aliquibus negotiis nisi de spiritualibus solum, ut de confessione et testamento et consimilibus ordinandis, quaecunque ordinari debent secundum fidei catholicae documenta": Pagel, "Chirurgie," 40:692; Nicaise, *Chirurgie*, p. 145). Amundsen attributes similar views to Arnau de Vilanova on the basis of a passage from part III of *De cautelis*, but, as Sigerist pointed out ("Bedside Manners," p. 133), part III is actually a twelfth-century text here masquerading under Arnau's name. Perhaps significantly, when in his *Repetitio* Arnau took his students step-by-step through their first encounter with a patient, he nowhere mentioned the need to induce a confession.

[14] "Infirmi obediencia, qua corpus situm debet subicere vel exponere preceptis artificis, cum ipsius labor et studium ordinetur ad bonum eius": Arnau de Vilanova, *Repetitio*, MS Munich CLM 14245, f. 27 (the passage is omitted in the printed editions).

responsibility and authority in someone else; most patients are likely to have been happy to turn their worries over to someone else, once he had convinced them of his special competence. But how could the doctor be truly confident that any particular patient had accepted his authority and would follow his advice compliantly and unquestioningly?

The assurance was supplied by the doctor's fee, which was of symbolic as well as economic importance to both parties. The two aspects of the fee are mingled confusedly in the *notabilia* that are so distinctive a feature of Henri de Mondeville's *Chirurgia*; because of their obvious preoccupation with fees and payments, these *notabilia* have given Mondeville – and the medieval surgeon generally – a reputation for cynicism and avarice.[15] But it is not so much how high a fee the patient will pay, as *that* he pay, that is Henri's major concern. Once the patient has invested something in his physician, he will be reluctant to disobey him or to abandon him for another; once he has been paid, the physician can feel sure of his patient. To Henri, it is the act of payment that affirms the bond between the two, a tangible sign of commitment given and received: "munera sumpta ligant."[16]

Yet Henri acknowledges too that patients vary enormously in their appreciation and understanding of medicine, and it is their expectations that determine if and when they will ever thus commit themselves definitively to a particular doctor. Many, perhaps most, do not do so. Some patients think that God is the author of all illnesses and therefore shun all medicine, turning only to surgeons in the case of accidents and wounds: "God gave me my illness," they say, "and He and only He can cure me, if He chooses."[17] Of those who believe in medicine, only a very few recognize that, in surgery as in natural philosophy, "frustra fit per plura quod potest fieri per pauciora"; few understand that training and expertise matter, and therefore consult only one or perhaps two surgeons of established merit. Most patients, instead, go all the way to the other extreme, and even in minor illnesses call in all the doctors they can find, on the principle that ten masons can build a wall ten times as fast as one; they are likely to consult anyone who labels himself a "cyrurgicus," whether he is learned or illiterate – the assertion of skill and the display of technical jargon are enough.[18] Such patients never commit themselves to anyone, and if they recover they typically feel no obligation to pay any of their surgeons a fee: "a patient's one thought is

[15] For a variety of perspectives on Mondeville's advice, see Welborn, "Long Tradition"; Hammond, "Incomes," esp. pp. 155–6; Talbot, *Medicine*, pp. 102–4, 138, 141; Amundsen, "Medical Ethics," pp. 941–2; Rawcliffe, "Profits of Practice," p. 62.

[16] Pagel, "Chirurgie," 40:694; Nicaise, *Chirurgie*, p. 147.

[17] Pagel, "Chirurgie," 40:663–4, 718; Nicaise, *Chirurgie*, pp. 101–2, 182–3.

[18] "Vulgus credit, quod sermones eorum, quos non intelligunt, sunt efficaciores sermonibus intellectis": Pagel, "Chirurgie," 40:665; Nicaise, *Chirurgie*, p. 103.

that he be cured; once he is cured he stops worrying about it and forgets to pay, but until he is cured he can think of nothing else."[19] If he treats such patients, a surgeon's only course is somehow to convince them that his own particular skills, his own personal efforts, were decisive in bringing about their cure, and hence he often drags out the treatment and prescribes unnecessary medicines so that their resistance and skepticism can eventually be broken down.

This reasoning underlies Henri's famous advice about preventive medicine – a therapy that, he says, is ordinarily not in the surgeon's interest to practice, though it is best for patients. Preventive treatment should be offered to only five kinds of patients: (1) the truly poor; (2) your friends; (3) those whom you can trust to pay you when they recover; (4) the powerful, whom you have to treat, and who you know can never be made to pay you; (5) those who pay you in advance and in full. These groups include all those of your clients who have singled you out and placed an unreserved trust in you. Unfortunately, the majority of patients have to be convinced to pay by the treatment itself; "they pay once they are cured according to how difficult it seemed – a little if treatment was quick, generously if it lasted a long time" – and they would never appreciate preventive treatment at its true value.[20]

To depict Henri's attitude to his clients as shaped by "flagrant materialism," as some have done, distorts his values. No doubt he preferred wealth to poverty, but his more general goal was to give the surgeon control over treatment, making it practicable for him to do what he knows is best for the patient by convincing the patient that the surgeon's opinions (on illness, cure, and fee) can be trusted. Henri was by no means out to extort all the money he could from the sick, and he clearly felt somewhat defensive about the need to insist on the importance of money. When a patient places himself in your hands and raises the question of your fee, he explains, you should first decide privately what the treatment is really worth (given your status, the patient's circumstances, and the seriousness of his condition); then you should open the bargaining by asking twice that sum, being prepared to work your way back down to your original estimate.[21] Tactics like these were needed to adapt a new kind of learned skill to a market used to other crafts; they did not necessarily mark their practitioner as venal or mercenary, or even as particularly unscrupulous.

---

[19] "Patientis tota et principalis est intentio, quod curetur, et eo curato in ipso cessat hujusmodi appetitus et de solutione nihil et non curato animus ejus non quiescit": Pagel, "Chirurgie," 40:671; Nicaise, *Chirurgie*, pp. 110–11.

[20] "Solvunt post curam factam secundum quantitatem laboris et si curantur brevi tempore, modice, si longo tempore, abundanter": Pagel, "Chirurgie," 40:671; Nicaise, *Chirurgie*, p. 110. For a similar assessment, see Pagel, 40:722; Nicaise, p. 188.

[21] Pagel, "Chirurgie," 40:730; Nicaise, *Chirurgie*, pp. 200–1.

Contractual commitments

These writings on the doctor-patient relationship admittedly express an academic ideal; how far was that ideal realized in practice? Whether they had studied at Montpellier or not, few surgeons or physicians would have disagreed with Henri de Mondeville that a client who valued your skills and paid for them in advance was the best patient to have. One kind of such client was found among the great and powerful. From the beginning of the fourteenth century we can observe the count-kings paying a lifetime retainer (*violarium*) to as many as three or four physicians and surgeons (not to mention barbers and apothecaries) who were permanently subject to summons, although royal physicians like Joan Amell or Martí de Calça Roja had enough independence that one or even both at the same time could leave court on their own affairs. These practitioners were given occasional gifts, and their expenses were paid when they were in attendance on the king, but their retainer was due them whether or not they actually provided medical care – though it might often be far in arrears, and they might have to sue their patient's estate to collect.[22]

Another rewarding patron for the ambitious practitioner was the church. Some physicians were retained by a bishop and cathedral chapter just as others might be by a lay lord, and under similar conditions – except that while the latter might be required to come when summoned or to accompany the lord on his travels, the former were likely to be expected to reside permanently in the diocese. In 1296 the bishop and chapter of Gerona appointed a *medicum specialem* (the surgeon Ramon de Cornellà) at an annual salary of 100 *sous*.[23] Nine years later they worked out a much tighter contract with a physician, master Albert, for a canon's portion and a fee six times as large as Ramon's: Albert promised to live within the city walls and not to leave Gerona if a member of the chapter were ill, and to attend and treat the canons without charge, wherever they were, as long as they were within the diocese.[24]

Despite occasional difficulties over payment, the retainer system undoubtedly provided a comfortable financial cushion for a few practitioners, helped to establish their reputation by expressing trust in their skill, and still left them considerable freedom of activity.[25] It established a relationship in which they were the privileged party, for they can not infrequently be found ignoring summonses from their patron, apparently with no fear of being dismissed. The

[22] Comenge, "Formas de munificencia," pp. 8–10; cf. Rawcliffe, "Profits of Practice," pp. 67–72, though looking at a later period.

[23] ADG, Sèrie G (Notularum), 1/26r (April 1296).

[24] ADG, Sèrie G, 2/21v (23 April 1305). The Lerida chapter seems to have hired Guillem de Castellvell as its *fisicus* before 1297 (C108/84v).

[25] Rawcliffe, "Profits of Practice," p. 65, is less confident that doctors preferred the annuity over the fee-for-service approach to great clients, but she concedes nevertheless that the annuity had its advantages (p. 77).

history of the association between the bishop of Gerona and Guerau de Sant Dionis, who had university training and was the leading physician in the city from the 1320s until his death in 1349, shows how much autonomy a trusted practitioner might assume, a contract notwithstanding. Guerau was *phisicus sedis Gerunde* by 1318 at the latest,[26] but the relationship did not prevent him from routinely treating lay patients in Gerona and in nearby towns like Sant Feliu de Guixols.[27] In 1346, as the king's brother Jaume voyaged to Barcelona from his county of Urgell, suffering from the complaint that would kill him the next year,[28] Bishop Arnau of Gerona learned of Jaume's illness and sent master Guerau to the young count to administer appropriate medicines, on the understanding that Guerau would be away only a few days. In early April the bishop wrote urgently to Count Jaume and to Guerau: the physician had overstayed his leave and was to return immediately, for many were sick and some had died in chapter. The letters had to be repeated in even stronger and more pitiful terms in May – *every*one was sick or dying in the chapter – before Guerau eventually returned to Gerona. As Guerau must have known very well, the bishop was committed psychologically to his physician, and there was little danger that he would discharge Guerau and put himself under the care of someone untried – nor did he. A codicil to Bishop Arnau's will, two years later, left 700 *sous* to Guerau, gratefully acknowledging his faithfulness.[29]

Members of the general public could not afford to keep a physician on retainer, but some had enough faith in a particular practitioner to make a not dissimilar commitment, and to provide against future illness or injury by arranging with him for what was in effect inexpensive pre-paid health insurance. Physicians – who might or might not already have contracted with town authorities to advise their citizens on health matters (see below, chapter 7) – are sometimes found contracting with individuals to treat them for any health problem whatsoever in return for a flat fee paid in advance. Bernat de Berriac made such an arrangement in Castelló d'Empúries, for example, supplementing an annual salary from the town of 300 *sous* with a payment of between 5 and 20 *sous* from each of several dozen men, whom he promised to treat (together with their wives, children, and households) "for every illness that requires the art of medicine."[30] Such a system was probably not to the physician's financial advantage, for his fee to treat a single episode of illness would normally have been greater than these small sums. Fragmentary evidence suggests that it was young physicians starting out in practice and anxious to build up a clientele who

---

26 ADG, Sèrie D (Beneficial), 3/115, where "magister Geraldus phisicus sede Gerunde" witnessed the will of Bishop Guillem (26 Sept. 1318).
27 ADG, Sèrie C (Marmessories), sign. ant. T 147, ff. 18–19.
28 Above, chapter 5, pp. 156–7.
29 Above, chapter 5, pp. 149–50.
30 McVaugh, "Bernat de Berriacho," pp. 241–2, 252–4.

accepted this sort of arrangement; once established, they then adopted the more usual fee-for-service system.[31]

A second form of pre-payment for health care had already existed in the Crown of Aragon for some time. Since at least the late thirteenth century, individual soldiers in the royal army had contracted with the physicians and surgeons accompanying the host; themselves paid a certain daily sum by the king, they promised one day's wages to a practitioner (to be paid directly to him by the monarch) and in return were apparently guaranteed whatever medical care would prove necessary.[32] The noble Dalmau de Castellnou contracted with Joan Amell to serve his entire company on the Almería campaign of 1309 for its daily wage, 800 *sous*.[33] Very considerable sums could be earned in this way, at least on paper: the surgeon Bernat de Pertegaç was promised more than 9,000 *sous* from such clients during his service in Sardinia in 1323–4.[34]

Henri de Mondeville did not comment specifically on arrangements with the prudent and healthy like these just discussed, though he would presumably have endorsed them. The ideal client he seems to have had in mind in his *Chirurgia* is the one who, upon falling ill, has enough confidence in a particular practitioner to commit himself unquestioningly to his care, settling his fee at the outset. In practice, many patients did indeed begin by agreeing orally with the physician on his fee, though they could (or would) pay only a small part in advance. No doubt they were quicker to pay the whole if treatment was successful, but to

---

[31] Thus Maurat Vitalis, just opening his practice in Castelló d'Empúries in 1326, agreed to the same arrangement with a number of families (McVaugh, "Bernat de Berriacho," p. 245); perhaps significantly, the earliest documentation for Pere Gostemps' long practice in Manresa shows him *canceling* such contracts (AHCM 43, 10 kls. Jan. 1309). Rifat Selga, "Aspectos," pp. 97, 98, gives other examples of this arrangement from 1297 and 1342. Shatzmiller, *Médecine et justice*, p. 22, describes a similar arrangement in Manosque, which he interprets as insurance sought by the client.

[32] On this arrangement, see McVaugh, "Arnau de Vilanova's *Regimen Almarie*." Jaume's brother Pere had already utilized it in his raids into Castile in 1296: letter of 10 Oct. 1301 (C 268/208v).

[33] RP 623/78v, of 1 April 1310.

[34] Bernat was still owed much of this sum by the king in 1325, plus a further 2,784 *sous* 5 *deners* for his own participation in the campaign (C 421/16r–v, 17r–v). He seems to have been owed an additional 516 *sous* corresponding specifically to "lo sou de un dia de 62 cavalls armats e 5 alforrats" (C 559/100ff.) – the normal military wage was 4 *sous* per day for a knight who maintained a lightly equipped (*alforrat*) horse and 8 *sous* for one more fully armed (*armat*): see Dufourcq, "Prix," p. 507. Such figures may provide a hitherto unappreciated way of estimating the numbers of troops involved in a campaign (on the obscurity of which see Hillgarth, *Spanish Kingdoms*, I:241).

    Another form of contract in such circumstances can be seen from the arrangement made by Count Malgaulí of Empúries with the surgeon Pere Seguer of Castelló to accompany him on the expedition on which the count eventually died (1322): Pere (active 1316–47) was to receive 2 *sous*/day while the count was alive but 4 *sous*/day after his death, perhaps to support him after his patron's death while he made his way back home (AHPG/CE 2045/5r–v; 28 Jan. 1341). Yet another: when Manresa contracted with its surgeon Berenguer de Acuta in 1322, it stipulated that he would have to accompany military expeditions as part of his contract but could claim a salary for any treatments he gave to the army (AHCM, Llibres de Consell, 2, 13 kls. Mar. 1322).

judge from the frequency with which physicians presented bills to or collected fees from executors, payment was not always conditional on a cure.

Often, however, doctors in the Crown of Aragon were forced to give their patients a chance to assess their skill and knowledge. As Henri admitted, some patients want to judge your work before committing themselves to payment, want to know how quickly, with what difficulty, and above all *whether* you can cure them (the last question, understandably, was not something Henri stressed). In such cases, therefore, the two parties seem to have come to a broad agreement at the outset (or early in the treatment), involving a limited mutual commitment; usually their agreement was verbal, but occasionally formal contracts were drawn up, defining the obligations on both sides. Generally a practitioner would receive a certain sum for agreeing to undertake the treatment of a patient, with as much again, or more, to be paid him if the treatment proved successful. Or he might demand part or even all of the sum (or a pledge of comparable value) in advance, promising either to return a portion if the treatment were unsuccessful or, at his discretion, to continue the treatment indefinitely at no further charge.[35] Sometimes the contract was drawn up after treatment had already begun. Bernat Metge of Sant Celoni had treated young Astrugonel for an ulceration (?*naxensa*) of the leg for some time before he came to concrete terms with the boy's guardian (1333): they agreed that Bernat should be paid 100 *sous* immediately for the work he had performed to date, another 200 *sous* if he concluded at this point that the boy's condition was curable and undertook to continue the case, and a final 300 *sous* when the cure was complete.[36] Occasionally the practitioner even agreed to make the whole of his fee contingent upon a cure; the few instances of such a concession so far found all involve Jewish practitioners, who were in a relatively weak bargaining position *vis-à-vis* their Christian clientele.[37]

These conditional contracts suggest the problems that might arise when patients had not "submitted" fully to their doctor and were allowed to determine the success and value of their doctor's attentions. What does it mean to "cure," after all? Patients and practitioners could easily have different ideas on the subject. The question raised particular difficulties for academically grounded

---

[35] (1) AHPG/CE 177/126v (26 April 1346), where Mosse Cohen promised to return all 20 *sous* if he failed to cure fistula of the toes in a year. (2) ACFV 101, 5 kls. Dec. 1326, where a patient agreed with a physician on a fee of 100 *sous* and left a silver goblet in pledge (he died before the treatment began, and his executors reclaimed the pledge for 70 *sous*). (3) AHPT 3847/242v (21 Feb. 1334), where the practitioner could decide whether to continue to treat witlessness (*oradura*) or return 150 *sous* of 200 paid.

[36] AHCB XIII-3 (Manual 1333/4), ff. 4v–5 (15 Nov. 1333).

[37] Bonjuha was promised 15 *sous* once his patient had been cured (Nov. 1333; AHPT 3833/102v); on another occasion he was promised 10 *sous* under the same conditions (Sept. [1334?]; AHPT 8706/37). Jacobus de Tolosa, Jewish surgeon of Lerida, was promised 1,400 *sous* once a cure had taken place (Nov. 1326; ARV protocolos 10408/267) – in this case the size of the fee may help explain the patient's prudence.

physicians, who had been taught the impossibility of defining perfect "health," and perhaps this helps explain why conditional contracts are so much rarer for medical than for surgical assistance: surgeons were called on to address specific or localized conditions, where they and their patients could more easily agree on the goals of treatment.

One objective measure of therapeutic success that all parties could agree on was of course simply survival, and contracts with both physicians and surgeons sometimes merely equated the two, as in the case of the physician Guerau de Castro Viridi referred to above.[38] A similar surgical contract defines survival even more precisely: Guillem de Gradu of Manresa in 1334 paid a surgeon 100 *sous* to treat his wounds, with the promise of an equal sum if he should still be living three months after treatment (which he was not).[39] But surgeons, with more narrowly circumscribed tasks, could be given more specific objectives. When Creschas de Torre of Gerona dislocated his hip (*ancha*) in 1318 and was unable to walk, Guillem Guerau, a surgeon of Besalú, took on the case, and the two agreed that Guillem should receive his fee (1,000 *sous*!) as soon as Creschas found himself able to walk to the window with the aid of a cane.[40]

Yet as Henri's complaints have already warned us, there remained a real risk of discord over conditional contracts as long as the patient believed he was as capable as his doctor of evaluating the treatment he was receiving. This may have been a particular problem for Jewish practitioners, since apparently they often had to accept such contracts, but if it was brought to court it forced judges to seek a general and objective standard for health. In 1314 a Christian of Xàtiva refused to pay a Jewish surgeon, Mayr, his 200-*sou* fee because his wife's broken leg had not been healed as the surgeon had promised. Mayr complained to the king, and Jaume responded by instructing his officials to consult other surgeons as to whether Mayr deserved to be paid. In effect, the king was empowering an imagined community of surgeons to decide the success or failure of treatment, taking the judgment out of the hands of the parties directly involved.[41] The king's action is an early sign of a growing tendency for the public to give medicine and surgery a quasi-professional status, well before practitioners themselves had expressed any awareness of collective identity or occupational solidarity. The standard originally imposed by the king could become a natural precondition of the patient-practitioner relationship, as the

---

[38] If she lives, "conveniemus vobiscum de salario vestro iuxta laborem vestram" (8 Sept. 1345; AHPG/CE 220/13). See also AHPT 3842/79, 10 July 1330: Pere d'Odèn, *fisicus* of Cervera, received 50 *sous* to treat a patient and was promised 50 *sous* more if the patient survived.

[39] AHCM 144, id. Oct. 1334; the patient is mentioned as dead in a document of 12 kls. Mar. 1335 in the same volume.

[40] C 165/125v (12 Sept. 1318), and further C 369/102v–103 (16 Aug. 1321); and see below.

[41] Letter of 26 April 1314 (C 154/63).

public accepted the idea that neither the patient nor his doctor but a wider occupational community deserved to pass final judgment on the results of medical care.

The individual practitioner thus found his authority reinforced by a broader authority freely conceded to his craft. In 1330, the surgeon Arnau ça Riera, fresh from the medical school at Montpellier, contracted to treat a woman suffering with a large tumor in the right breast; her husband and son-in-law promised him 160 *sous* if he could cure her, and agreed that if in the end they did not believe treatment had led to a cure, the degree of "success" would be left to "the decision of two neutral [*non suspectorum*] surgeons or other practitioners."[42] In accepting this, the patient's relatives were yielding authority to surgery if not to Arnau personally, were conceding that surgical training did confer a special expertise superior to lay opinion as well as an objectivity that overrode craft loyalties. We can view such arbitration as an early public expression of an implicit professional status, if we like; explicitly, however, it is an open recognition of the surgeon's authority that should have left Henri de Mondeville well content.[43]

Indeed, a growing public confidence in medicine, and a submissiveness to medical authority generally, is not difficult to detect in cases from the early fourteenth century. In formal contracts for medical services the practitioner tends to dominate the relationship, and in extreme situations he may be given complete legal control over the patient's person. Berenguer Mestre, kicked in the head by an animal (1329), was formally committed by his wife, brother, cousin, and relatives to his doctor's "discretion and the medical skill given you by God, and placed in your power absolutely [*in posse vestro mitimus absolute*]";[44] Pere de Villario was legally absolved in advance for anything that might go wrong in cutting a boy for bladder stone, even for his death.[45] In more routine cases, where the relationship was defined by reciprocity of obligation, the physician still was ordinarily allowed the upper hand. Occasionally a contract specifies that though the patient can decide to withdraw from treatment, the physician's fees will still have to be paid.[46] The patient could guard against some excesses – e.g.,

---

[42] AHPG, Notari 1–7, 5 kls. May 1330.

[43] A different but related kind of occupational arbitration is, not of degree of success, but of level of fee: that is, was this service worth what the practitioner demanded? Shatzmiller, "Doctors' Fees," p. 205, presents arbitrations of 1305 and 1431 and from them infers that "this must have been quite a common procedure." I have so far found no instances of such arbitration in the Crown of Aragon.

[44] Letter of 13 Aug. 1329 (AHPT 3841/90v–91).

[45] AHCM 101, 6 id. May 1325. See also AHPT 3861/4 (May 1341), where the surgeon Guillem Arnau is "desospitat" if anything goes wrong; or AHPT 3862/10 (10 April 1343), where Guillem's uncle, the surgeon Pere Ritxart, can "scindere et coure [*sic*] et alias medicare et operare prout vobis et vestre sciencie videbitur." Shatzmiller, "Doctors' Fees," pp. 207–8, describes a similar provision (from Toulouse, 1431).

[46] As in the case of Arnau ça Riera and his patient with a breast tumor; above, n. 42.

unexpected costs, and fee-splitting with apothecaries – by insisting that the doctor's fee should cover all medicines that might turn out to be necessary, and he might sometimes stipulate a regular schedule of visits; on the other hand, the practitioner could always hold out for an additional sum for his expenses – cost of travel, food, and lodging for himself, his helpers, and their animals – on top of his charges for medical service.[47] The privilege occasionally accorded practitioners of deciding whether to refund an unearned fee or simply to go on treating the patient indefinitely is still another indication of how the advantage in the relationship rested with them.

Patients who put themselves unquestioningly into a practitioner's care and did not quarrel with his fees left no such formal contracts; their experience is more likely to be represented today in receipts or acknowledgments of indebtedness for treatment undertaken or completed – "invoices," as it were. Such documents, like the formal contracts but to an even more marked degree, tend to record treatment by *cirurgici* rather than by *fisici*: of twenty-eight such surviving from the town of Manresa in the period 1315–45, for example, twenty-six refer to surgical cases. It is not easy to understand the reason for this disproportion – it seems unlikely to be a direct index to the relative frequency of surgical intervention, and it may simply be that physicians more often received payment in advance (so that few acknowledgments of indebtedness survive), whereas surgeons were often forced to await the outcome of treatment before agreeing with their patients on a fee.

We have already recognized that a practitioner did not merely service a clientele limited to his place of residence or its immediate neighborhood, and it is from these "invoices" that we can judge how much territory a medical or surgical practice might cover. Reference has been made above to two surgeons, Pere Fontanet of Manresa and Pere Ritxart of Santa Coloma de Queralt, each of whom began his career in the 1320s and practiced for twenty years. In both cases, the homes of a number of their patients can be identified from such invoices, which make it plain that many sufferers were prepared to travel twenty-five kilometers or more for surgical care.[48] Manresa and Santa Coloma, as it happens, are less than fifty kilometers apart, at opposite ends of a skewed lozenge whose shorter axis, only thirty kilometers long, connects two other important Catalan towns, Cervera and Igualada. Surgeons in all four communities must in effect have been in competition with one another – or, looking at it from the patient's perspective, we might say that by the 1330s patients anywhere in this region who were willing to travel twenty-five kilometers for

---

[47] See AHCM 48, 13 kls. June 1315: Ferrer de Cogullons, surgeon of Castell d'Odèn, promises two visits a week to Pere Andreu for ten weeks, "vobis tamen satisfaciente mihi et cuidam iuveni sive nuncio meo in cibo et potu et animali quod ego ducam in cibaria sua."

[48] See above, chapter 2 at n. 33 and chapter 4 at n. 99, respectively.

attention could have selected the surgeon they wanted from among several possibilities.[49] Indeed, citizens of Cervera can be identified visiting Pere Ritxart for treatment in Santa Coloma, twenty kilometers away, just as inhabitants of Igualada can be found seeking out Pere Fontanet in Manresa. Even if a practitioner had a town to himself, he ran the danger of losing local clients to a distant colleague with a reputation for greater skill or lower fees.[50]

The invoices also allow us to generalize cautiously about the level of fees – at least about surgeons' fees, to which, as I have said, the bulk of this material pertains. Normally a surgeon seems to have asked 40 to 60 *sous* to take charge of a case (though in some instances, of course, a successful outcome would have increased his fee substantially), but in this cash-poor society he might sometimes agree to take part of his fee in kind – a pair of hens, for example – or in installments.[51] Physicians' fees do not seem to have been significantly different in scale, but so few of their bills have survived that we cannot be confident that they accurately represent the typical practitioner's charges. Indeed, even those few suggest how widely fees could vary, and that economic as well as medical factors could influence a patient's choice of doctor. Seven "invoices" survive from Santa Coloma de Queralt that specify the fee exacted by various physicians on taking charge of a case: their amounts are 130, 50, 50, 45, 10, 10, and zero *sous* (in the last case, a fee of 15 *sous* was to be paid only if the treatment were successful). Of these seven fees, the four lowest were charged by one man, the Jewish *phisicus* Bonjuha Astruc. This is perhaps yet another manifestation of the relatively weak position of Jewish physicians in relation to their Christian patients, which in this case forced them to offer cheaper treatment. In any event, it suggests the danger of generalizing indiscriminately about levels of fees from a tiny sample.[52]

---

[49] Unfortunately, neither Cervera nor Igualada today preserves much documentation from the first half of the fourteenth century, but they certainly had surgeons of their own: in Cervera, for example, we know of Oliver de Fuxio (1310–37?), Ramon de Riner (with a contract from the town, 1333–7), and Pere Agiló (1341).

[50] Scattered evidence seems to confirm that this was as true of physicians as it was of surgeons, though in the absence of physicians' "invoices" it is not easy to demonstrate. We know, for instance, that the physician Pere de Gostemps of Manresa was called to Calonge [de Segarra] in 1322 to treat its rector, although there was certainly a much closer physician in Cervera, Pere d'Odèn (active 1318–41); see Sarret i Arbos, *Historia de la industria*, p. 139.

[51] Mondeville told his readers that one should treat the truly poor for free; "a mediocriter tamen pauperibus licitum est recipere gallinas, anseres et capones" (Pagel, "Chirurgie," 40:670; Nicaise, *Chirurgie*, p. 110). AHCM 142, 14 kls. Mar. 1334, sets a fee of 100 *sous* and two hens; AHMA 336/35 (Aug. 1307), is for a fee to be paid 10 *sous* at Christmas, 15 more at the next Michaelmas, then 25 *sous* three weeks after that; ACFV 256, 2 id. Jan. 1331, provides that a patient will pay 50 *sous* to his surgeon or else serve him for two years, receiving food but no salary.

[52] Thus while it might be reasonable to suppose that fees were higher in Barcelona or Valencia than in the provinces, as Rawcliffe suggests for England ("Profits of Practice," p. 65), I have no good evidence to support this.

Patient dissatisfaction

As Henri de Mondeville complained, patients who had not paid for their treatment in advance often tried to avoid settling up once they were cured. Physicians and surgeons routinely pursued such defaulters through the courts, obtained royal injunctions for payment, or, when all else failed, waited patiently for their clients to die so that they could present a bill to the estate.[53] Apothecaries suffered in the same way. When the Countess of Empúries died in 1327, her apothecary Bernat Paytavin came forward with a bill (115 *sous* 9 *deners*) for a dozen prescriptions that he had never been paid for, one dating back to 1311![54] Bills for individual drugs were so small that it was often not worth an apothecary's while to go to court – exceptionally, Bernat de Sangueda of Vic sued a client for a mere 18 *sous* owed for seven prescriptions[55] – but when his bad debts were added up they could constitute a considerable sum: Periconus Roseyllo of Santa Coloma, who died in the plague, had 118 bills outstanding for which he was owed nearly 1,140 *sous*.[56] Apothecaries must have been happiest when they were paid for their drugs by the prescribing practitioner, who could then pass on the charge to the patient (though this must have been one of the practices that suggested collusion between the two to the public);[57] physicians presented larger bills to their clients anyway, and they thus found it more profitable to sue when the bills went unpaid.

When patients felt the need to justify their refusal to pay, they tended to allege, not that the treatment had been unsatisfactory, but that some technicality exempted them from the original bargain; in a curious way, therefore, their defenses are further evidence of public belief in the capabilities of medicine. In

---

[53] Some examples will illustrate the levels of response open to the practitioner: (1) a physician suing jointly with two surgeons for 470 *sous* promised by their patient but left unpaid "sine aliqua iusta causa" (2 Aug. 1315; C 156/156r–v); (2) Domènech de Gargila of Tortosa getting permission to distrain on the goods of an inhabitant of Morella for a 60-*sous* fee agreed on ahead of time but never paid (5 May 1335; C 574/20r–v). Domènech had practiced surgery in Zaragoza since at least 1314 before accepting a municipal contract from Tortosa in 1330 (C 352/86v, of 4 Aug. 1314; AMT, Clavaria 1330, f. 19); (3) the Zaragoza surgeon Sancho Oliverii (active 1319–37) getting a royal warrant commanding that his bills be paid "cum mercenario cuilibet dari debeat merces eius, et potissime medicis qui propter necessitatem honorandi existunt" (23 Sept. 1320; C 170/231, with an echo of *Ecclesiasticus* 38:1). Sometimes practitioners simply wrote off bad debts by selling or giving them to someone else who might find it easier to collect, as Bonjuha Astruc did with a bill that included 16 *sous* 2 *deners* for drugs, 45 *sous* salary, and 10 *sous* expenses (AHPT 8599, 5 kls. Sept. 1335).

[54] AHPG/CE, 12–F no. 7, ff. 6v–7.

[55] ACFV 202, 18 kls. July 1323.

[56] AHPT 3869/2, ff. 53–57v (inventory of 2 Sept. 1348).

[57] This was the way in which the physician Bernat de Bonells did business, whether with the infante Jaume (C 352/118v–119) or with his other, humbler, patients (letter of 1 Dec. 1316; C 355/88v). When the Valencian apothecary Francesc Sedacer tried to collect 81 *sous* 7 *deners* for prescriptions he had made up for the patients of Bernat de Girona, it was the physician he sued for payment, not the patients (ARV, Just. Val. 13, 3 id. Aug. 1312).

1338 a clerk of Besalú broke both bones in his arm while out in the country, and his servant went into town and brought back with him Bernat Jordà, *barberius*; Bernat set and bandaged the arm and watched over his patient for three weeks while the bones began to heal. Once cured, however, the clerk refused to pay either the 50-*sou* fee or Bernat's expenses of 10 *sous* on the grounds that it had been wrong for a barber to usurp a surgeon's role.[58] At the conclusion of another case mentioned earlier (p. 178), Creschas de Torre, though apparently cured of his leg injury by Guillem Guerau, claimed that Guillem had stopped coming to Gerona from Besalú to see how he was doing and so did not deserve to be paid; Guillem protested that his patient had dismissed him in order to escape the fee, and that he himself would have been happy to make the trip to Gerona "quandocumque requisitus esset."[59] Lawsuits of this sort let us understand why Henri de Mondeville urged that practitioners demand payment in advance from their patients, and yet they are certainly testimonies to patients' willing submission to medical care rather than the reverse.

And in fact concrete instances of patient dissatisfaction with health care are not easy to identify. Almost invariably the dissatisfaction expressed is with surgical rather than medical treatment; physicians are only rarely the targets of criticism, perhaps because in medicine the patient found it more difficult to judge for himself what was wrong with him and what his doctor should be doing about it. The surgeon's practice was much more exposed, as Mondeville had warned his readers: "the surgeon has to perform manual operations, and when he makes a mistake it is obvious to the sight or touch and can be blamed on no one but him, while the physician's mistakes aren't obvious to the senses and so can be put down to nature or to the patient's own forces; this is why surgeons have to work more slowly and cautiously."[60]

Even so, patients in the Crown of Aragon who felt that they had not been helped by their surgeon, and who sued for return of their fees, tended to complain they had been given, not poor, but insufficient treatment. The surgeon who agreed to treat Pere Ruiç of Valencia when the latter broke his left thigh was paid 80 *sous* on account; but the surgeon then left the city for three weeks, the leg did not improve (indeed, claimed Pere, it grew worse), and through his procurator Pere asked to recover his down-payment and 200 *sous* in expenses

---

[58] ADG, Sèrie C (procesos), new 191/old 54 num. 2, of 25 Feb. 1338. See also ADG, Sèrie C, new 16/old 53 num. 2, of Dec. 1308, for a similar instance.

[59] And see C 144/54 (2 June 1309), where a Christian who promised 500 *sous* to Abraham [Alzalay], *fisicus* of Calatayud, to cure his kinsman in Daroca protests that Abraham left the kinsman once he began to recover, even though it was agreed verbally that the physician wouldn't leave the town.

[60] "Habet cyrurgicus manualiter operari, et quia error hujus operis oculo et digito apparet nec potest alteri quam cyrurgico imponi, et error medici operantis sensui non apparet et potest imponi naturae et virtuti corporis regitivae, ideo necesse est cyrurgicum cum majore deliberatione et cautius operari": Pagel, "Chirurgie," 40:671; Nicaise, *Chirurgie*, p. 112.

besides.[61] Another Valencian surgeon, traveling in Castile, met a man in Valladolid suffering in his right eye, and promised to effect a cure; but as soon as he had been paid four gold pieces he left for home without beginning the treatment. Four months later the Castilian sued for return of the fee plus the cost of pursuing the physician to Valencia.[62] Such cases, where it is inaction that is being criticized rather than anything concrete that the practitioner has done amiss, again suggest high public expectations for health care. When the Jew Bencet was accused of neglecting a patient (1294) there was evidently no thought of criticizing his skill, for he was offered the choice of giving back his fee or returning to Lerida to complete the cure.[63]

More fundamentally, however, criticisms of medical and surgical practice may have been rare simply because patients and practitioners defined their relationship by a contract. Today, medical malpractice is for us not a breach of a written contract but a "tort of negligence" that violates certain general rules and foundations, expectations and assumptions, that physicians or surgeons are, as professionals, presumed to share.[64] In a pre-professional age, patients bargained over the details of a contract; if a practitioner did not meet its terms – and here, as we have seen, other physicians or surgeons might be called in to decide the point at issue – he would not be paid, but no blame attached to him. Circum-scribed by contractual precision, therefore, patients could not easily imagine a further appeal to unwritten norms – nor, indeed, could their doctors. I know of only one case in the Crown of Aragon where unwritten standards of practice were invoked, and then as regards whether a would-be healer was justified in practicing at all, in a manner suggestive of the growing public interest in licensing. In Llançà (Catalonia), in 1308, when Ponç de Roca was accused of wounding Joan Gibern and causing him to lose his hand, he defended himself by blaming his victim for having gone for treatment to a veterinary (*menescalcus de animalibus*), Romanyan Ferrarius of Castelló d'Empúries "qui non est medicus." This man, Ponç argued, had bound the wounded arm so tightly that the hand had withered away, and Ponç added that two other practitioners from Castelló, called in on the case later, had claimed that a good *medicus* could have cured the wound.[65] Here it was not the patient who complained but his attacker, and Ponç

---

[61] ARV, Just. Val. 32, 11 kls. June 1320.
[62] ARV, Just. Val. 38/112 (26 March 1321).   [63] C 100/25 (19 Aug. 1294).
[64] I was first led to think about this distinction by its formulation in Kenneth De Ville, *Medical Malpractice in Nineteenth-Century America* (New York, 1990), pp. 156–9.
[65] "Ponit et intendit . . . quod posito quod idem Pontius vulneraverit Johannem . . . quod tamen non concedit immo diffitatur ex dicto vulnere dictus Johannes non fuit debilitatus nec etiam perdidit manus sed pocius per impericiam medicorum perdidit manum, et per malam curam.
  "Item ponit et intendit probare quod dictus Johannes fuit vulneratus in manu sinistra a parte interiore per longum et non a travers ita quod pars superior manus tam in ossibus quam in nervis quam etiam in pella remansit sincera.
  "Item ponit quod dictus Johannes post vulnus eidem illatum movebat manum et digitos et si habuisset bonam curam et peritum medicum curatus fuisset nec manum perdidisset.

was not accusing Romanyan of malpractice so much as denying Joan's right to consult him, hoping thus to escape a penalty for the consequences of the original assault; while the two local *medici* can more reasonably be understood as defending occupational self-interest than as maintaining internal standards of practice. Such a case – and an isolated one, at that – is far removed from the systematic appeal to other practitioners for a professional, third-party opinion that, on what seem to me somewhat insubstantial grounds, has been supposed to be in England "an expected type and process of adjudication" by 1354.[66]

Contract or no, the one thing that a patient might have felt entitled to expect was that he survive his doctor's attentions, and it is almost exclusively in instances of sudden and unexpected death that we find charges of incompetence brought to the justices to be resolved – for it was lay opinion rather than peer review that decided the matter: it was a personal expectation that had been violated, not a professional standard. Two such cases have been preserved in particular detail. In the first, Jaume de Fonts of Barcelona charged that Samuel, *fisicus*, had promised to cure his son Bernat, who was suffering from scabies (*gratella*); the physician had given the boy a syrup and had spread an ointment on his hands and feet, promising that Bernat would be cured in a few days. Instead, Bernat began to suffer pain, his body began to swell, and he soon died.[67] In the second case, María Egidii came all the way from Báguena (south of Daroca in Aragon) to Alagón (north of Zaragoza), a distance of a hundred kilometers or more, seeking treatment for her daughter, who was suffering in her right foot. María had no money for a fee, but the surgeon Mayl Abenforna agreed to cure the child for free at the request of the town authorities. María subsequently protested that Mayl had applied realgar to the girl's foot, opening wounds in it that led to her death.[68] These two complaints follow the same

---

"Item ponit quod dictus Johannes eligit sibi in medicum En Romanyan Ferrarium de Castilione qui est menescalcus de animalibus et qui non est medicus.

"Item ponit quod dictus Romanyan ligavit et astrinxit brachium et manum eidem Johanni in tantum quod fecit ea dessicari manum.

"Item ponit quod dictus Romanyan non est medicus nec erat tempore quo pensavit de dicto Johanne et per impericiam dicti Romanyan dictus manus fuit dessicata.

"Item ponit quod iamdicta manu dessicata et debilitata per malam curam fuit vocatus En Vilar ad dictam curam et etiam P. Vitalis medici de Castilione qui dixerunt quod propter malam curam dicta manus erat dessicata.

"Item ponit quod dicti medici cognoverunt quod si bonus medicus fuisset adhibitus ad dictam curam quod fuisset curatus et non debilitatus nec manum perdidisset." ADG, Sèrie C (procesos), new 16/old 53 no. 2 (Dec. 1308).

66 For the English procedure on which this generalization is based, see Cosman, "Malpractice," pp. 25–6, and Cosman, "Third Party," where the 1354 case report is reproduced as fig. 10. Its language suggests that it may have originated in the desire of a guild of surgical "masters" to eliminate an unauthorized competitor; as in the Llançà instance just discussed, the patient does not appear as a plaintiff.

67 Letter of 16 April 1330 (C 438/111v); summarized in Mutgé Vives, *Ciudad de Barcelona*, pp. 143–4.

68 C 593/32v (5 Nov. 1337); C 597/173r–v (30 Dec. 1338), reregistered at C 598/175 (but there dated 19 Dec.).

pattern: they involve a specific diagnosis and an unexpected death after an incautious promise of success for a particular remedy. Arnau de Vilanova's students at Montpellier would have learned better than to make such confident assurances.

But the complaints against Samuel and Mayl Abenforna share one other feature that we might not have foreseen: both men were Jews. In fact, the rare accusations of incompetence or bad practice that have survived from the Crown of Aragon are leveled, proportionally, far more often against Jews than against Christians, and this is of a piece with our earlier observations about the disadvantages suffered by Jewish practitioners.[69] Social and cultural pressures meant inevitably that a Jewish physician would find it difficult to exercise control over a Christian patient, to keep him psychologically (or for that matter legally) *in posse suo*. To some extent the Christian was predisposed to suspect his Jewish physician; he might well feel some guilt in consulting him contrary to ecclesiastical edict, and might experience some relief in denouncing him.[70] In such a situation a patient would find it easy, even perhaps proper, to challenge his physician's authority and to assert his independence – like the outspoken patient who aggressively warned Bonjuha Astruc (of Santa Coloma) that he had not visited his client as a physician should, that he had not done what was medically necessary for the illness, and that therefore his fee would be promised to other physicians if he, Bonjuha, did not effect a cure soon – if indeed he really could.[71] It may be that when, as we saw earlier, Jewish physicians were told they would only be paid if they brought about a complete cure, patients were in effect expressing the reservations and fears they felt when submitting themselves to treatment by a Jew.

The authority of the Muslim healer – similarly suspect because of his religion, and lacking the Jew's reputation for learning – must have been even weaker. The exodus of so many learned Muslims after the *reconquista* had left

---

[69] In the documentation from Manosque, two-thirds of suits for incompetence are against Jews (Shatzmiller, *Médecine et justice*, p. 27). Shatzmiller, "Doctors' Fees," pp. 206–7, cites a number of somewhat similar cases also involving Jews rather than Christians; in all of these, too, the practitioner was accused of the death of a patient rather than of malpractice (that is, of a failure to meet more general standards of practice).

[70] Danielle Jacquart expresses something of this when she writes of medieval France that "Il est ... possible que dans les procès professionels ... ce soient davantage des sentiments antisémites, que le constat d'un échec thérapeutique, qui aient poussé certains patients à poursuivre un practicien [juif] maladroit" (*Milieu médical*, p. 167).

[71] "Idem medicus promiserit curare antedictum venerabilem quantitate sibi promissa, et nunc dictus venerabilis non curetur culpa et necligencia dicti medici, eo quia ipsum non visitat ut medicus visitare tenetur infirmos quos imparaverit, nec facit ea ... que ad dictam infirmitatem pertinunt et pertinere debent ... Et ideo notificat dicto medicho ... quatinus continue curet antedictum venerabilem si ipsum curare poterit, alias quod habebit ... providere in salariis et aliis necessariis aliis medicis ipsum curantibus de quantitate eidem medico promissa": AHPT 3842, loose leaf (6 kls. Aug. 1330).

mostly empirics and charlatans to practice in the Crown of Aragon, and this could only have heightened Christian suspicion of their practice. In 1302 a citizen of Valencia, wounded by an arrow, was approached by a "sarracenus . . . qui dicebat se esse medicum" and swore that he could extract the point. According to the patient's later account, the Muslim made an incision and then by sleight of hand produced something glittering that he claimed to have taken from the wound; the patient's pains persisted, however, and only when surgeons removed the real arrow-point did he realize that he had been tricked.[72] Whether a deceit had actually been practiced is less important than recognizing how the combination of religious hostility with skepticism about the level of Muslim medical skills made it easy for Christians to believe that an unsuccessful treatment by a Muslim practitioner was somehow the latter's fault.[73]

Public and private confidence

The image of medicine conveyed by this "public" documentation, then, is one in which the typical Christian practitioner enjoyed considerable authority over his patients. It seems to portray a general public confidence in medicine, apparent in such things as the relative absence of complaints against practitioners as well as the widespread reputation for skill of certain individuals, which served to establish physicians and surgeons in a position of psychological as well as practical control over their patients. This is not easy to substantiate from the patients themselves, however. Precisely because the documentation is "public," formalized in language, it largely lacks any spontaneous character. Only rarely – as when in 1326 the town of Camprodon voluntarily took its surgeon's side in his suit against the abbot of Ripoll because "he is good and very useful and necessary to this town, especially for his skill [*propter sui artem*]"[74] – do we find breaking through the formalisms an expression of this conviction that medicine really does work. We have almost none of the "personal" documentation – letters, diaries – that has been used so successfully by historians to illuminate the feelings of individuals from the seventeenth century to the present about the medical culture of which they are a part, about their healers, health, and illness.[75]

---

[72] Joseph Ma. Roca, "Notes medicals històriques: Frau quirúrgich," quoting C 124/163v.

[73] Note too the case of Ali de Lucera (above, p. 52), who was not an empiric left behind in Spain but an immigrant; his patient's son accused him of killing his mother by using charms and sigils, though Christian physicians certainly used similar procedures.

[74] "Bonus et valde utilis est ac necessarius dicte ville et precipue propter sui artem": letter of 27 Nov. 1326 (C 188/106v).

[75] The essays in Porter, *Patients and Practitioners*, show how revealing such material can be for pre-industrial European society.

The principal exception to this is the material that survives in such remarkable quantity for King Jaume II and his family, which has already allowed us to reconstruct something of their medical histories and has been particularly revealing of the king's own assumptions, attitudes, and expectations regarding health and medical care (above, chapter 1). These tend to bear out the "public" image we have constructed for society as a whole. For at least the last twenty-five years of his life, Jaume II showed a willing dependence on physicians and surgeons. He sought their advice avidly, even for minor complaints – and not indeed merely advice, but instructions.[76] He obediently did as he was commanded, sometimes refusing to act in a particular physician's absence, because he was convinced that the skill, knowledge, and effort of medical practitioners was really useful in the maintenance or restoration of health – he was the model, in many respects, of a "compliant" patient. It would not do to over-generalize from a single case, and this one in particular, but in some respects the king may not be a bad sample of medical consumers. Exposed to all the cultural forces shaping the urban environment in which most medical activity was centered, he eventually decided what he wanted from health care, and his wealth and authority allowed him to realize impulses that his subjects might share but could not always act upon so easily. Cautiously we may say again that the inhabitants of the Crown of Aragon viewed medicine as an activity that had proved its effectiveness to the sick and wounded.

Moreover, even when the public admitted that self-professed *medici* might be ineffective or, worse, dishonest or frauds, they were still ready to believe that their own physicians deserved unqualified trust. King Jaume's son-in-law, Don Juan Manuel, repeated commonplace warnings against the tactics of unscrupulous doctors in his *Libro de los estados* (*c.* 1330): their bills can cause more pain than the disease they claim to cure; they prolong a disease and inflate the costs of medicines; they pretend to be better and more skillful than they really are; they give away their patient's secrets.[77] Yet Juan Manuel had absolute faith in his own physician, and it is this faith rather than any cynicism that he passed on to his son Ferrando in his *Libro infinido* (*c.* 1335): "Whenever you become ill, take care of yourself and do everything the doctors tell you to, because you will get well better that way. Trust the doctor who looks after you and don't give up on him, whatever he may tell you, even though it may not seem that he's doing much, because doctors often know a lot of things of great value

---

[76] A particularly marked instance is Jaume's dead-of-night appeal to Joan Amell, requiring him to come to Barcelona immediately from Mataró, thirty kilometers away (Martínez Ferrando, "Correos," pp. 105–6); cf. the tone of the king's summons to Amell on another occasion, brooking no excuses, published in MF, II:318, doc. 437.

[77] Don Juan Manuel, *Libro de los estados*, I.96 (pp. 201–2).

to health which appear trivial or stupid to those who don't understand."[78]
Patients simply did not *want* to mistrust their own physicians, once they had
committed themselves to their care.

---

[78] "Vos consejo que si alguna vegada enfermades . . . vos guardedes et fagades todo lo que los físicos vos mandaren, porque mas aina et mejor podades guarescer. Et del físico que de vos pensare, fiat bien et de su física, et non vos partades dél, qualquier cosa que vos digan, aunque vos semeje que non vos da grand física; ca sabed que algunas cosas menudas saben los físicos que á los que non lo entienden parescen que non son nada, que aprovechan ó empescen mucho para la salud del cuerpo": Don Juan Manuel, *Libro infinido*, pp. 266–7. Juan Manuel went on to extol his own physician: "yo vos digo verdaderamente que fasta el dia de hoy nunca fallé tan buenos físicos et tan leales, tan bien en la física como en todos sos fechos." His own fortunate experience as a patient is also reflected in his will (1339): Giménez Soler, *Don Juan Manuel*, pp. 699–700, 702.

7

Medicine's social role

The growing faith in medicine manifested by individuals was paralleled at other levels of society in the early fourteenth century. Town authorities developed an active interest in institutionalizing medical attention, as their readiness in the 1330s to adopt licensing procedures has already shown; for at least a generation before that, however, they had been appointing municipal physicians and surgeons, trying to ensure the continuing availability of medical advice to their citizens. This is one of the earliest signs of a swelling social conviction that medical learning carried authority and could be trusted, as from about 1300 on the community began to transfer jurisdiction over various forms of social behavior to the independent authority of physicians and surgeons. Today we label this process "medicalization," when aspects of human behavior that had previously been judged normal or deviant, good or bad, by the lay public are assigned to medical control and are redefined as health or illness, shedding their moral overtones. We are accustomed to think of contemporary medicalization as driven, if not by reformers who want to redefine behaviors like drug addiction as physical rather than moral states, then by the profession's own interest in extending its power. In the Crown of Aragon, however, "medicalization" seems to have originated in a growing public confidence in medicine that pre-dated the appearance of a self-conscious community of physicians.

A municipal role for the medical practitioner

By at least the second decade of the thirteenth century, municipal authorities in northern Italy were beginning to appoint town doctors, *medici condotti*: first in Bologna and perhaps Reggio, then in Perugia, and by the end of the century in half a dozen other cities, large and small, from Venice to Florence to Orvieto and Imola. The practice became well-nigh universal during the fourteenth century. At first these municipal *medici* seem to have been exclusively surgeons, charged

190

with caring for wounds and fractures among the citizenry, but by 1300 the Italian towns were contracting with physicians as well.[1] Vivian Nutton has plausibly suggested that these developments were triggered by the law schools' study of the Roman law, which had codified the rights and privileges of municipal doctors in the later empire, but were made possible by "the more advanced social organization" of the north Italian cities. In turn, Danielle Jacquart has remarked that the municipal practitioner was apparently a relatively late phenomenon in France, and again she has linked its spread to the increasing power of town government (in the troubled times of the late fourteenth and early fifteenth centuries).[2]

Municipal development in the Crown of Aragon – particularly in Catalonia – took place early, and as might be expected there too we find towns contracting for a physician's services well before 1300, nearly as soon as in Italy. Whatever the practice's roots, in Roman law or elsewhere, to institutionalize it was to give a new recognition to "public" health, by acknowledging that a healer (physician or surgeon) deserved to be allotted a civic role and official status. Such appointments necessarily bespeak not only public confidence in the power of medicine, but also a belief that it should somehow be possible to single out the more competent practitioners – the same belief that underpins the contemporary legislation in some Catalan towns requiring physicians and surgeons to meet a qualifying standard. In effect, the towns were trying to define what they believed physicians should be and do, well before practitioners themselves had developed a common understanding of their nature and role, and the agreements made by towns with their *medici* reveal certain fundamental elements of that definition.[3]

The series of contracts that happens to survive from Castelló d'Empúries is particularly full and rich in detail. The first town physician we meet there is Bernat de Cremis, who came to Castelló from Roses in May 1307 for a salary of 200 *sous* annually, but who seems almost immediately to have moved across the Pyrenees to the diocese of Carcassonne.[4] Bernat de Berriac, contracted in December of the same year (for 300 *sous*), had left for Barcelona by 1309.[5] Jaufridus Rubeus of Milan, who signed on in March 1314, had by October been succeeded by João of Portugal, and João was soon followed (in 1316) by Abraham des Castlar (at a salary of 600 *sous*), and Abraham in 1317 by Alfonso

---

[1] Nutton, "Continuity or Rediscovery?" pp. 26–9.

[2] Jacquart, *Milieu médical*, pp. 131–4.

[3] Naso, *Medici*, pp. 32–55, 97–101, 193–201, gives an account of municipal contracts with physicians in late-medieval Piedmont that closely resembles the practice in Catalonia, though its detail is drawn almost entirely from fifteenth-century examples.

[4] AHPG/CE, 4–A no. 1, 5 non. May 1307, and 4–A no. 4, 10 kls. May 1312, record the contract and his departure, respectively.

[5] Published by McVaugh, "Bernat de Berriacho," pp. 250-2.

de Burgos (at 500 *sous*).[6] The town achieved stability of health care only in 1326, when Maurat Vitalis arrived in Castelló and covenanted to remain there at an annual salary of 500 *sous*, raised to 800 *sous* in 1335; he died there in 1346.[7] His successor, Guerau de Castro Viridi, had already practiced in Banyoles and Besalú before moving to Castelló.[8]

In its contracts with these men we can see how the town was defining the niche its official physician was to fill. When Abraham des Castlar agreed to serve the town in 1316, he committed himself to certain conditions: "I will look at and assess all the urines brought to me by the citizens, whom I will advise as to bloodletting and diet, and generally as to their manner of life, and I will visit two or three times all the sick of the town who ask me to attend them."[9] The treatment of illness was something of an afterthought in this statement: the town's first concern in providing for its common life was to supply its citizens with someone who could knowledgably advise them on how to maintain their health.

But how did a community decide who was knowledgable enough to fill the niche, at a time when no "professional" criteria existed? Though there seems already to have been a sense that academic preparation did qualify a practitioner, even a limited amount of university training was still unusual in the early fourteenth century; and because the few medical students or graduates in practice had something of a competitive advantage in the municipal marketplace, they rarely stayed in one town very long. Only two of Castelló's first six appointees had demonstrable medical training: Bernat de Berriac, who was still working on his degree at Montpellier while practicing in Castelló and who left as soon as he completed it, and Jaufridus Rubeus, who called himself "medicine professor" and stayed in town less than six months.[10] Abraham des Castlar, as a Jew, could not have obtained a degree from a *studium* and instead had learned medicine from his father; as far as we know, the others too had received only a practical education. Yet, education aside, the town evidently still felt it could discriminate between good and bad, between "true" and "false" physicians, as

---

[6] For Jaufridus Rubeus, AHPG/CE 86, 4 non. Mar. 1313/14; for João of Portugal, AHPG/CE 87, 4 id. and 3 id. Oct. 1314; for Abraham des Castlar, AHPG/CE 89, 3 non. Mar. 1315/16, and 90, non. Sept. 1316; for Alfonso de Burgos, AHPG/CE 92, 3 non. Aug. 1317, and 5–F no. 4, f. 11 (26 April 1319).

[7] On Maurat, see McVaugh, "Bernat de Berriacho," pp. 244–6.

[8] AHCO, B–3 (no. 5), 73v, 4 non. Aug. 1323, for Banyoles; AHCO, B–22 (no. 42), 17 kls. Nov. 1334, for Besalú. His contract with Castelló is at AHPG/CE 177, 141v (23 May 1346).

[9] "Videbo et iudicabo omnes urinas que mihi apportabuntur per omnes habitatores dicte ville, et ... dabo eis consilia tam super flebotomiis quam eciam dietis, et generaliter regimina et consilia, et . . . visitabo bis vel ter illos infirmos habitatores dicte ville de quibus fuero requisitus": AHPG/CE 89, 3 non. Mar. 1315/16.

[10] Jaufridus had a professional reputation as well as a degree: he had served Alfons II in 1286–90 and Jaume II in 1313, immediately before taking the position with Castelló (C 151/211v). From Castelló he returned to King Jaume II, to whom in 1315 he complained of non-payment of a stipend by the count of Empúries; he died before the year was out (C 158/182v).

it were. The position fell vacant again in 1323, when there were three men in Castelló calling themselves physicians, as well as two surgeons, five apothecaries, and four barbers – and this time the consuls passed over all the *medici* to contract with one of the apothecaries, Bernat de Llampaies, to read urines and to give medical advice.[11] The appointment of Maurat Vitalis three years later at last gave the town the security of an academically trained physician who was prepared to settle there permanently.

Plainly in these early years the people of Castelló were caught between what they had come to see as the necessity of having health advice available and their sense that some advisors would prove more satisfactory than others. This tension meant that the terms of individual contracts tended to fluctuate, depending on whether town or practitioner was more anxious for the position to be filled. As we saw, between 1307 and 1335 the town physician's salary quadrupled, no doubt responding to forces in a wider market;[12] João of Portugal was given a stipend more than three times what he had earned in Manresa seven years before, yet the increase was not enough to keep him in Castelló.[13] But money was not the only contractual element that could be a subject for bargaining. Most of Castelló's official physicians agreed, like Abraham des Castlar, that two or three free visits to the sick would be covered by their salary from the town; however, the two Montpellier appointees – Bernat de Berriac and Maurat Vitalis – managed to hold out for the promise that they would *not* be required to attend the sick free of charge, and this was no doubt a factor in the latter's decision to settle there permanently. Yet university physicians were not always in such a good bargaining position, especially after their number began to increase in the second quarter of the century. Ramon de Tesarach, also Montpellier-trained, was anxious for employment when he agreed to a contract with Castelló in 1347 that set no limits at all on his duty to give free care to the sick, and he left the post quickly after the plague created new opportunities for advancement.[14] It was a

11 Document of Aug. 1323 (AHPG/CE 113/34). Bernat owned Teodorico's *Chirurgia*, so he clearly had pretensions to the role of healer (see above, chapter 3, n. 103).

12 In addition to his town salary, Maurat received 900 *sous* more every year from other quasi-public sources (the count of Empúries [AHPG/CE 12–F, no. 3, 10 kls. April 1330] and the Jewish community); such supplementary payments were occasionally made to earlier physicians, but it may be that they too increased in response to the market for able physicians.

13 C 143/126v (25 Feb. 1309), for João of Portugal's Manresa salary. He went to Vic from Manresa and then went back to Vic when he decided against Castelló, practicing until at least 1316 (ACFV 64, 8 id. May 1316).

14 Ramon de Tesarach, master of arts and medicine, came from the diocese of Elne in Roussillon, Mallorcan territory restored to the Crown of Aragon in 1344. In 1345 he tried to get a position with the bishop and chapter of Mallorca but was unsuccessful, despite a recommendation from the bishop of Gerona (see two letters of 2 Dec. 1345 in ADG, Sèrie U [Regesta litterarum], 9/132v–133). He remained in Gerona until he contracted with Castelló, where his salary from the town was supplemented by another 200 *sous* annually for serving the Jewish *aljama*; he stayed there two years (AHPG/CE 221/24v; document of 15 Jan. 1347, canceled 1349), and then moved to Barcelona. Now the bishop of Gerona offered him the position of physician to the

vital contractual point, for the right to charge the sick for treatment made a big difference to a physician's income: a typical year's salary from a town was less than might be made from a handful of private patients. At the same time that Guerau de Castro Viridi was receiving a retainer of 500 *sous* from Castelló, he was assured of one-tenth that sum for caring for just one patient in town, even if she died, while if she lived he was to expect a further reward.[15]

Castelló's situation was shared by the Crown's dozen or so other towns of the second rank, with perhaps 3,000–5,000 inhabitants (e.g., Puigcerdà, Manresa, and Cervera in Catalonia; Teruel and Calatayud in Aragon), that hoped to hire a town physician. They were large enough to present some opportunities to ambitious practitioners, but not large enough to be decisively attractive, and they thus could not count on holding onto the most successful individuals, who tended to move from town to town in an attempt to improve their situation. The case of Manresa shows the power that physicians enjoyed and the various ways in which towns tried to respond. In 1293 the municipal authorities paid an unspecified sum to master Pere, *fisicus*, to convince him to return to Manresa to practice – he had practiced there in the early 1280s but had left the town to try his luck in the much larger Tarragona, and now he had to be wooed back.[16] He stayed this second time only until 1295, when he accepted a new contract to serve Vilafranca del Penedès, a town comparable in size to Manresa. This time 107 citizens of Manresa each promised to pay him 5 *sous* if, after his contract with Vilafranca expired, he would return once again and treat them and their households.[17] Though Pere did return, he died almost immediately, and for the next two decades Manresa had to depend for medical care on practitioners whom chance brought temporarily to town and whom disenchantment or ambition took away: João of Portugal moved on after only a year, unable to collect his salary.[18] One such casual arrival was Pere de Gostemps, who had come to Manresa by

cathedral chapter of that city, left vacant by the death of Guerau de Sant Dionis (ADG, Sèrie U, 12/128v; letter of 30 Sept. 1349), but Ramon chose instead to stay in Barcelona, where in March 1350 he signed a ten-year contract as municipal physician (ACB, manual de Pere Borell, Mar. 1343–Dec. 1344, 20v, and AHCB, Llibres de Consell I–18/33; the second of these documents was transcribed by Roca, *Medicina catalana*, pp. 135–6, and marks the first appearance of a physician in the lists of the city's salaried personnel).

    Ramon seems to have died in 1362. A codicil to his will, dated 2 April of that year, left "de bonis meis universitati studii medicine Montispesulani 80 s. convertendos in utilitate eiusdem universitatis" (AHPB, manual de Ramon Morell, II Capibrevium 1355–62; the will is at ff. 21–22v, the codicil at f. 23r–v).

[15] The private contract, of 8 Sept. 1345, specifies that Guerau has been providing "varias et diversas curas et prestare consilia super dietis et regimine sanitatis infirmitati quam . . . Caterina . . . patitur" (AHPG/CE 220/13); the report of his town contract (AHPG/CE 177/141v, of 22 May 1346) refers to "salario sive pensione quam ego quolibet anno recipio racione officii mei super universitate dicte ville."

[16] AHCM 13, 5 kls. May 1292.

[17] AHCM 6, 4 kls. April 1296; Pere's will is AHCM 24, 15 kls. Mar. 1297.

[18] C 143/126v, 25 Feb. 1309.

1308 and built up a good reputation as a physician. In 1322 he hinted broadly that he was thinking of moving on to Barcelona, and the town council hastily promised him an appointment at 400 *sous* yearly if he would contract to remain in Manresa – which he did until his death *c*. 1345.[19] Thereafter Manresa once more became a target of opportunity for ambitious practitioners, like the Jew Maymo Bonjuha; trained by his physician father in Vic in the 1320s, Maymo had gone to Gerona in 1343 but moved to Manresa in 1347 when he heard there were no *metges* there.[20]

Because such towns of the second rank had much more limited resources than a Barcelona or a Valencia they often lagged behind in the payment of salaries, and this was another reason why their physicians (like João of Portugal) might soon move on. Communities tried to make the deficit up by promising the physician freedom from taxes,[21] but this was not always an effective inducement to stay. Once established in a community, a physician might be willing to put up with a salary always somewhat in arrears; he would have developed roots as well as other sources of income. But someone just starting his career was naturally more insistent upon his rights – like the young Pedro Cellerer, Arnau de Vilanova's disciple, who complained to Jaume II in 1316 that Teruel had paid him only a part of the 300 *sous* agreed upon for a year's residence there.[22] It must be admitted, too, that towns tried to spread their limited resources as thinly as possible. Vic and Montcada tried to share a municipal physician: Ramon Ardey was to interpret urines brought to him from either town, but he was to live in Vic, and Vic therefore undertook to pay two-thirds of his salary of 400 *sous*.[23] Tàrrega hired Gaufridus de la Foresta as its physician in 1320 for four years at

---

[19] AHCM, Llibres de Consell 2, 13 kls. Mar. 1322.

[20] Corbella, *Aljama*, p. 210, doc. 63; ACFV 276, 4 non. Mar. 1343; R[ubió] y B[alaguer], "Metges," p. 495 (citing C 651/66, of 22 Dec. 1348).

[21] For example, the Catalan surgeon Ramon de Molins was promised (perhaps in lieu of salary) that he need not contribute to "talliis questiis prestitis aut aliis quibuscumque exactionibus regalibus vel vicinalibus" as long as he lived in Manresa, which he did until he died (after 1345): AHCM, Llibres de Consell 2, 4 kls. Feb. 1334. The same terms were promised in 1332 by Calatayud in Aragon to Pedro Cellerer (C 861/229r–v). Rarely, physicians claimed as a principle that "consuetudo antiqua et approbata ubique terrarum sit quod sciencie liberales faciant peritum et phisicum exemptos ab omnibus . . . exaccionibus sive serviciis regalibus et vicinalibus" (letter of 28 Dec. 1295; C 89/148v), perhaps recalling Roman law (cf. *Digest* 27.1.6), but the rule does not seem to have been generally recognized.

Jewish communities do not seem to have given salaries to physicians drawn from among themselves, but they did offer them the same sort of enfranchisement to keep them from moving away: the *aljama* of Valencia promised to free Abraham Tahuell of all financial demands, "in remuneracionem salarii curarum per eum faciendarum," when he indicated that the *aljama* of Morvedre had made the same offer to him on condition that he relocate there (C 434/120v; 23 May 1329).

[22] C 159/108v (22 Nov. 1316).

[23] ACFV 225, 3 non. Oct. 1334, where Ramon described himself as "bacallarius in artibus." It is not immediately obvious why Montcada thought it was advantageous to participate in this arrangement, for it must have been far less than half the size of Vic and was seventy-five kilometers away, almost a suburb of Barcelona.

400 *sous* yearly; in the fourth year of his residence, however, they found only 200 *sous* for him – and spent the remainder of his stipend to keep a second physician in town.[24]

The actual contracts agreed to by physicians tend to follow a broadly common form and to be expressed largely in generalities, but on two points (apart from the amount of salary to be paid) they are always careful to go into detail; these, we can probably assume, were the main points of negotiation when a practitioner entered municipal service. One, already touched on above, was the amount of care the physician was expected to give to the citizens in return for his salary. The other concerned the amount of time that the physician was required to spend in the town. It was invariably understood that he was to make his permanent residence there as a condition of receiving his salary, and a town might insist that he deposit his books with them as a safeguard against desertion.[25] But could a physician leave his town for a short period of time, for personal or even professional reasons? Once again, physicians in a stronger bargaining position could hold out for greater independence: Bernat de Berriac was conceded four days' absence at a time from Castelló whenever he might be called away to treat the sick, whereas Alfonso de Burgos was forced to agree that if he were treating anyone in Castelló he could stay away from town only overnight, and that he would need to seek the town's permission for longer absences.[26] In Puigcerdà, town physicians were typically allowed only two days' absence from town at a time, and might have their salary docked if they overstayed their leave.[27] The first concern of the town consuls was to ensure their physicians' availability; defining the care they should provide or the fees they might charge was necessarily a secondary issue.

Towns sometimes contracted for the permanent presence of other health

---

[24] CRD Jaume II 7818 (1 Oct. 1324) and C 184/186v (8 Nov. 1324). The other 200 *sous* were being paid to Bernat Oller, who had been living in Tàrrega for at least two years (ACB, manual de Bernat de Vilarrúbia May 1322–July 1322, f. 56v). Another financial trick was that practiced by the town fathers of Cervera on Pere d'Odèn, whom they had enticed away from Huesca with the promise of freedom from taxation – a promise withdrawn after he had been serving the town for forty years and had perhaps begun to seem too old to be of use to its citizens any longer (C 616/115v; 6 Aug. 1341); the town played the same trick six days later on another physician who had long practiced there, Domènech de Aquilario (C 616/130r–v).

[25] Thus Calatayud tried to insist that Pedro Cellerer leave his books behind when he went off in 1326 to attend the infante Joan, to ensure that he would come back (C 249/195v).

[26] Bernat's predecessor in Castelló, Bernat de Cremis, could absent himself from town for three days when seeing patients. See nn. 4–6 above for specific references.

[27] Miquel Roger was allowed to leave Puigcerdà for two days on trips elsewhere in Cerdanya, or eight days outside the territory, but in both cases he had to seek the town's permission first (AHCP, Mateu d'Alp Liber extraneorum 1322, 7 id. Sept. 1322); Berenguer Aurer could leave for two days, but if he stayed away longer his salary was reduced proportionally (AHCP, Guillem Bernat de Santfeliu, Lib. debit. et firmit. 1324–5, 3 kls. Nov. 1324); while Jaume Puyoll was forbidden to leave town at all without permission, and if he did the consuls were empowered to discharge him immediately (AHCP, Mateu d'Alp Liber firmit. 1327–8, 7 id. Oct. 1327).

practitioners besides physicians, but much less often. There was never any need to assure the presence of barbers, for theirs was a common and easily learned craft, carried on as a sideline; no one could hope to make a living from barbering alone. Apothecaries could be expected, similarly, to appear anywhere that commerce was carried on; their trade, like barbering, was not an exclusive function of health needs. One of the very few known town contracts with an apothecary is from Cardona in Catalonia and is perhaps to be explained by Cardona's relative isolation in the mountains northwest of Manresa. In this case it was certainly not the salary that kept the man in town: induced by the promise of 100 *sous* yearly, Bernat Baldrich carried on as an apothecary for seventeen years in Cardona before moving to more populous Cervera in 1338 and suing for the entire 1,700 *sous*, still unpaid.[28]

Contracts with surgeons, to be sure, are not quite so uncommon as those with the minor occupations. They seem to have endured longer, on the whole, than those with physicians – and this, like the generally higher salaries paid to municipal physicians, suggests that surgeons did not enjoy as much public competition for their services. Manresa contracted with Berenguer de Acuta to act as its surgeon in 1322 for only a quarter of the salary it offered simultaneously to a physician, yet Berenguer stayed for twenty years;[29] Jaume Metge served as surgeon to Reus (outside Tarragona) from at least 1323 to 1332, and his son Ramon subsequently took his place.[30] Because such municipal contracts with surgeons are relatively scarce, it is difficult to generalize about the responsibilities involved; once more, however, physical presence seems to have been the prime concern of municipal authorities – though in Reus the town not only insisted that its surgeon could leave just one day per week, it also made him promise to provide first aid (*prima guarda*) free to all except for certain wounds of the stomach and genitals and broken arms and legs.[31] One's overriding impression is, nevertheless, that municipalities were not much interested in guaranteeing anything to their citizens beyond the presence of a practitioner whom they might consult; care itself had to be paid for individually by the patient concerned.

Broadly speaking, the pattern traced here is similar to that described by Nutton for the towns of late-medieval Italy, in which the town's principal concern was, again, to ensure the presence of a physician – who might be expected always to be on the lookout to better his situation.[32] But there are

---

[28] AHCM 154, 3 id. Mar. 1338; 700 *sous* on account were paid him within the week.
[29] AHCM, Llibres de Consell 2, 13 kls. Mar. 1322.
[30] Jaume was hired by the town in 1323 for 300 *sous* annually; his son's salary fifteen years later was apparently only 200 *sous*, but it was raised to 300 *sous* by 1340 (Vilaseca Anguera, *Metges*, pp. 21–2, 53–5, 59–61).
[31] Vilaseca Anguera, *Metges*, p. 21.
[32] Nutton, "Continuity or Rediscovery?" pp. 31–2.

certain striking differences. In Italy, great cities and small towns issued such contracts; in the Crown of Aragon, they are almost invariably entered into by these middle-sized, "second-rank" towns. Moreover, these towns hired at most one physician and one surgeon at a time, while in Italy multiple contracts were not unheard of, at least in the biggest cities: in 1324 Venice was feeling the strain of paying salaries to eleven physicians and seventeen surgeons.[33] In contrast, neither the Crown's richest and most populous urban centers, the capitals Barcelona and Valencia, nor the largest provincial cities, Zaragoza and Gerona (population *c.* 10,000), seem to have felt the need to contract for medical care before mid-century, and it may be that they had recognized from the beginning what the great Italian cities discovered later: that ordinarily no particular inducement was needed to cause physicians to gravitate towards the wealthiest communities.[34] Contracts are almost never found in the smaller towns of the third rank and below, either – in this case presumably because they could not hope to pay enough to attract or keep the man of their choice. Exceptionally, Santa Coloma de Queralt (population *c.* 900) managed in 1334 to convince a new *bacallarius in medicina* from Montpellier, Berenguer de Torroella, to stay in the town for two years at a salary of 300 *sous* per year, a sum scraped together by the Christian community with the assistance of the Jewish *aljama* and probably of the town's lord as well.[35] But within a few years Berenguer had left for Montblanc (population *c.* 2,200),[36] and by the end of the 1340s he seems to have established himself in Zaragoza. Santa Coloma did not try to hire a replacement, perhaps because there were still two experienced surgeons and a Jewish physician practicing in Santa Coloma in that decade.[37]

---

[33] Monticolo, *Capitolari*, I:354.

[34] Barcelona contracted briefly about 1320 with a *surgeon*, Bernat de Pertegaç, to make his residence in the city in exchange for a salary of 300 *sous* (C 184/102v–103; 1 Oct. 1324). Bernat had been practicing in Sant Celoni, forty kilometers northeast of Barcelona, when he joined the crusade to Almería in 1309; from this point until his death he was regularly in the employ of the royal family, and in 1323 he went with the infante Alfons on the conquest of Sardinia, where he died in 1326 (above, chapter 6, n. 34). He had changed his residence to Barcelona by 1315, and there he not only enjoyed royal patronage but came to receive a yearly retainer from the bishop and chapter of Barcelona as well as what he was given by the city. What seems to have been the first Barcelonan contract with a municipal physician comes two years after the plague (above, n. 14). The largest Catalan cities for which I have found clear-cut evidence of a contract with a *medical* practitioner are Tarragona, which had hired Berenguer ça Coma as municipal *fisicus* before 1342 (C 617/75), and Tortosa, on which see below. On the Italian experience, see Nutton, "Continuity or Rediscovery?" pp. 33–4.

[35] AHPT 3855/24v (26 April 1337) says the original contract with the town was signed 16 May 1334; an agreement on the latter date with the lord is at AHPT 3849/49v. The arrangement with the *aljama* is described in AHPT 3851/66 (7 April 1336).

[36] AHPT 3860/14v–15 (10 April 1340).

[37] The physician was Bonjuha Astruc, who had lived in Santa Coloma 1323–6 but subsequently moved to Valls. Santa Coloma tried to woo him back from Valls in 1330, promising him a salary of 100 *sous* annually (Seguar, "Aplech," p. 176, quotes an unidentified document to this effect), but Bonjuha was still resident in Valls in March 1331 (AHPT 3842/241) and may not have accepted the offer. By 1333, however, he had returned to Santa Coloma, and he lived there until

A final point of difference between Italy and the Crown of Aragon is that, while in both cases the two parties to the contract might agree to a variety of contractual requirements besides residency, only in Italy did these include restrictions on fees for medical treatment. Both societies provided free consultation to all citizens who cared to come to the practitioner, but in Italy the municipal authorities often went further and laid down how much a physician or surgeon might charge for actual treatment, depending on the illness or the wealth or status of his patients; it was often stipulated that the poor were to be treated free. In contrast, in no Spanish contract I have yet seen is there any attempt to regulate a town practitioner's fees: he seems always to have been free to charge what his clients would agree to pay. Towns of the second rank in the Crown of Aragon, trying to keep their best physicians from escaping to a wealthier market, were naturally in no position to restrict the practitioner's financial opportunities; at most, they might compel their physician to agree that he would not establish a partnership with one particular apothecary.

The exception to some of the preceding generalizations is Tortosa, a city of perhaps 8,000 that guarded the mouth of the largest river in Catalonia, the Ebro, which linked the city to Zaragoza and Aragon in the interior of the peninsula. Already by 1339 Tortosa had contracts with three different practitioners: a physician (paid 400 *sous* annually), a surgeon (300 *sous*), and a *herbolarius* (200 *sous*). No details (other than the normal residence requirement) are available about their responsibilities until 1346, by which time the number of physicians and surgeons contracted by the city had doubled: now it is specified that their principal duty is to treat the "malaltes des espital." The apothecary, too, "is obliged to go daily to the hospital of the city and make up the clysters, juleps, and ointments that he knows how to prepare for the hospital, with his own hands, free and for no payment."[38] This exceptional employment of a large municipal medical staff was evidently the consequence of something else equally exceptional, a public hospital demonstrably for the sick. As we will see below, our evidence for most other pre-plague hospitals in Catalonia shows only facilities for housing and feeding the poor, with no medical component whatsoever. Is this a result of the Catalan port's good communications with Italy? More needs to be known about the peculiarities of the Tortosan situation.[39] Still, the unusual extent of the practitioners' responsibilities to Tortosa and the remarkable care with

at least 1357 (Secall i Guell, "Metges i cirurgians"). Santa Coloma's resident surgeons were Pere Ritxart (active 1329–52) and his nephew Guillem Arnau (active Santa Coloma 1329–43, Cervera 1344–8).

38 AMT, Provisions I (1338–9), ff. 7v, 69, 70; Provisions III (1345–8), ff. 8, 49r–v, 56, 115v, 118.

39 Bayerri y Bertomeu, *Historia*, VII:346, 356, suggests Tortosa's close commercial ties with Sicily and Italy, with Genoa and Pisa in particular. Much of its municipal documentation has disappeared in the twentieth century: d'Alós, "Viatges," p. 110, listed nearly two dozen notarial manuals from pre-plague Tortosa, including a virtually complete sequence from the cathedral chapter after 1330, but none were to be found on a visit to the archive in 1989.

which they are spelled out are, if anything, additional signs that the towns in the Crown of Aragon had come to define and to realize their own conceptions of what a true "physician" should be and do, well before physicians as a community had defined their own identity.

Sexual behavior and anatomy

At the same time that municipal authorities in the Crown of Aragon were creating a quasi-professional niche for physicians, the wider society was coming generally to believe that medical personnel ought to possess a special expertise, entitling them to exercise public authority over certain aspects of ordinary life that were not nominally medical in character. In three quite different spheres where lay opinion, the assessment by *probi homines* or *matronas honestas*, had previously been sufficient as a basis for judgment – ecclesiastical tribunals, criminal law, and community policy – we find evidence of this acceptance of medical authority over social relationships. In each case the change seems to be taking place in the period 1275–1325, and to be responding to lay values rather than to the "medicalizing" ambitions of a professional community that was in any case not yet in being.

Perhaps the earliest of these changes involves the church's emerging tendency to appeal to the secular physician as an expert authority over certain problems in the canon law.[40] Christian tradition had long insisted that the health of the soul had to take precedence over that of the body, but it had not automatically questioned the usefulness or the authority of physicians: after all, the Bible itself represented the medical practitioner as the agent of God (Ecclesiasticus 38). Moreover, inasmuch as the church itself had been the principal source of medical expertise in the early Middle Ages, there had been little need to distinguish so sharply between spiritual and physical healing. But in the latter part of the thirteenth century medicine was moving towards autonomy, and it was assisted in this by ecclesiastical restrictions on clerical involvement in secular activity. Though these restrictions, embedded in the *Decretales* of Gregory IX (1234), did not absolutely forbid the study or practice of medicine by all clerics, they certainly discouraged it, and they thereby helped create a market for would-be secular practitioners; moreover, the prohibitions cut clerics off from medical training at the universities just before a new medical learning took shape there. The earlier restrictions were softened in 1298 to allow most parish priests (and, with the permission of their abbots, monks) to undertake formal medical study, but few clerics seem to have availed themselves of the

---

[40] The material that follows was presented in a slightly different form as "The Medicalization of Sexual Behavior in the Middle Ages: Two Case Histories" to the annual meeting of the American Association for the History of Medicine, Cleveland, Ohio, 3 May 1991.

liberalized provisions, and in any case by now the medical art was firmly and widely established outside the church.[41]

One reflection of this separation of medicine from the church is the tendency during the thirteenth century for ecclesiastical communities to begin to look for medical care outside themselves to the secular world: increasingly, their sick were being tended by lay physicians who supplemented or even replaced the *infirmarii* of monasteries or cathedral chapters. However, the church's acceptance of the new medicine was not merely a pragmatic one. Not only did it look increasingly to lay physicians for health care, it accepted the principle that medical practitioners' opinions were to be sought and preferred in matters where their art made them specially competent, and it incorporated this expertise into its own policies and institutions – a process particularly visible in its effect upon the church's regulation of sexual behavior.

The texts of Greco-Arabic medicine that were beginning to circulate in the thirteenth century encouraged physicians to offer increasingly detailed explanations not only of physiological but also of psychological activity. Danielle Jacquart and Claude Thomasset have shown that Avicenna's *Canon* in particular led physicians to develop a naturalistic, non-moralizing interpretation of sexual behavior and sexual pathology, which they treated as the mechanical autonomous consequences of a humoral physiology applied to brain function.[42] One such pathology that began to attract the attention of learned medicine after about 1220 was *amor heroicus*, the obsessive love that causes its frustrated sufferer to lose his appetite and grow insomniac and melancholy. Apparently the first European treatise wholly devoted to this disease was Arnau de Vilanova's *Tractatus de amore heroico*, completed at Barcelona in the 1280s, which worked out in circumstantial detail the physical interdependence of humoral and qualitative imbalance, psychological state, and physical symptoms.[43] The joyous perception of a desirable object, Arnau explained, vigorously heats the spirits in the heart, and these in turn overheat the body and brain. In the midbrain they addle the estimative faculty in its judgment, in the forebrain they dry out the ventricle and ensure that the object is retained firmly in mind. The drying-out of the rest of the body accounts for the lover's sunken eyes and drawn features; one of the four humors, yellow bile (hot and dry), comes to predominate and leads to a jaundiced skin and wasted body, while the lover's characteristic sigh is the

---

[41] See above, chapter 3. Amundsen, "Medieval Canon Law," clarifies the legislation and its history and is an important corrective to historians' frequent assertions that medical (and surgical) practice was entirely forbidden to the clergy in the later Middle Ages. However, it does not make the point that the prohibition on formal study amounted, in the social circumstances, to a *de facto* exclusion of many clerics from the new medical world of the fourteenth century. Talbot, *Medicine*, pp. 50–5, examines specifically the secularization of surgery. See also Diepgen, *Theologie*, pp. 7–11.

[42] Jacquart and Thomasset, *Sexuality and Medicine*, pp. 130ff.; Jacquart, "Medical Explanations."

[43] Text in Arnau de Vilanova, *De amore heroico*, pp. 11–54.

expulsion of air drawn in strongly by the attraction of the spirits in the heart. The new mechanizing psychophysiology had thus made its way to the Crown of Aragon. The case of *amor heroicus* illustrates the physicians' belief that the new medical learning enabled them to understand and explain sexual behavior, normal and abnormal – a belief that the church accepted when it introduced medical judgment into its own investigations of sexual dysfunction.

Among the actual sexual dysfunctions that Jacquart and Thomasset consider, impotence may have been perceived as having the most serious social implications, to judge from the attention given it by canon law from Gratian onwards.[44] Canonists concluded from Saint Paul's statement of the conjugal debt (1 Cor. 7:3–6) that sexual relations were integral to marriage; furthermore, the procreation of children was one purpose of that relationship. The example of Mary and Joseph showed that a couple who chose not to have sexual relations were still validly married; but if such relations had always been and would forever be made impossible to them by causes beyond their control, they were not. As to what such causes might be, the canonists were largely silent. They distinguished first between permanent impotence, which was assumed to be "natural," and temporary or relative impotence, due to sorcery and witchcraft: a man might by enchantment be rendered incapable of intercourse with his wife, yet remain potent with other women. (Conformably with the latter model, Constantine the African's translation of the *Pantegni* – the great medical encyclopedia of the twelfth century – discusses evil spells and nothing more as a cause of impotence.)[45] As for permanent or natural *impossibilitas coeundi*, the *Decretales* of Gregory IX had recognized that it might be due to physiological *frigiditas* in the husband or to anatomical incapacity in either partner (*sectio*, castration, in men or *arctatio*, "narrowness," in women).

The problems involved in establishing either sort of *impossibilitas* led canonists continuously to alter their criteria of proof; by the early thirteenth century the sworn assurance of the married couple on this point was no longer sufficient, and canonists were calling for confirmation by physical examinations wherever possible. These examinations were at first performed routinely by the laity, who were already called upon to carry out inspections in cases of rape. The *Decretales* implicitly acknowledge that "matronas providas et honestas" are the appropriate judges of a woman's anatomical adequacy for intercourse. Moreover, by testifying to a woman's virginity, such *matronas* could give presumptive proof of her husband's impotence;[46] or, if their inspection was

---

44 The following summary is based on Esmein, *Mariage*, I:232–67; and Bullough and Brundage, *Sexual Practices*, pp. 135–40. Makowski, "Conjugal Debt," pp. 106–8, made clear to me why impotence but not sterility made marriage canonically impossible.
45 Jacquart and Thomasset, *Sexuality and Medicine*, pp. 169–70, 172–3.
46 *Decretalium Gregorii IX*, X.IV.15; *Corpus Iuris Canonici*, II, ed. Friedberg, cols. 704–8.

inconclusive, the husband himself could be examined by a jury of men (or women).[47]

By the 1250s, however, the dependability of lay judgments on physiology and anatomy was in turn coming into question. Canonists repeated the warning of the *Decretum* that "the hand and eye of the midwife often make mistakes,"[48] and the *Summa* on the *Decretales* composed in 1253 by Henry of Susa (Hostiensis) shows that to some, at least, the secular medical tradition was coming to seem a possible alternative source of expertise. Discussing anatomical incompatibility for intercourse, Hostiensis says:

> Avicenna [presumably the *Canon*] says that sometimes, though a woman isn't narrow, her husband does not fit her nor she her husband, and each of them needs to change. On the other hand, I have heard from an expert woman that this rarely or never happens. Some say that these questions should really be left to the judgment of expert women; I would appeal to the pope in such a case.[49]

Hostiensis was still evidently unsure whether the medical texts of the *studium* – in particular Avicenna's *Canon*, which in the 1250s was just beginning to find university acceptance as authoritative[50] – really deserved to be set above the practical experience of lay observers.

Fifty years later, quite possibly encouraged by the naturalistic treatment furnished in the *Canon*, a much more thoroughgoing medicalization of impotence had taken place. Indeed, the dysfunction was a subject of particular attention at Montpellier as one aspect of the more general problem of sterility, during the career there of Arnau de Vilanova and for a generation thereafter.[51] Two discussions of the condition still have Arnau's name attached, the shorter

---

[47] Esmein, *Mariage*, I:254–5, n. 4, quotes Henry of Susa: "Quid si mulier dicit quod vir non potest eam cognoscere, allegans super hoc defectum membri viri, in hoc casu dic virum inspiciendum per homines expertos et honestos, sicut dixi de muliere arcta . . . Hoc expertus sum in duabus causis in quibus inspici feci virum nedum per laicos sed etiam per clericos."

Murray, "Origins and Role," considers only male impotence and so presents it implicitly as a condition administratively different from female incapacity for intercourse. Furthermore, by overlooking the evidence for male examination of males she perhaps makes the use of "wise women" more general, more deliberate, and more legally self-conscious than it was: "By swearing the wise women to examine, and possibly to excite, the man, the courts were . . . giving women an important and authoritative role in the legal system, an area in which their participation had traditionally been limited" (p. 247).

[48] "Manus obstetricum et oculus sepe fallatur" (Gratian, *Decretum* II.27.I.4.1; *Corpus Iuris Canonici*, I, ed. Friedberg, col. 1048), referring to their fallibility in determining virginity; repeated by Bernard of Parma (after 1240; Esmein, *Mariage*, I:262, n. 2).

[49] "Dicit Avicenna quod mulier quandoque non est angusta sed non convenit ei suus par et iterum non convenit pari, et indiget unusquisque eorum permutatione. Audivi tamen a muliere experta quod hoc aut vix aut nunquam accidere potest. Dicunt aliqui talia relinquenda esse judicio expertarum. Ego tamen papam consulerem in hoc casu": quoted by Esmein, *Mariage*, I:248–9, n. 4.

[50] Jacquart, "Réception."   [51] Demaitre, *Bernard de Gordon*, pp. 85–9.

of which is almost certainly correctly ascribed: it makes use of Arnau's characteristic doctrine of *proprietas* – a *forma mixtionis* that can be known only by experience, not reason – and it sets out the causes of sterility in the tabular form so congenial to him.[52] These causes all result from physiological defects – of the organs, of the semen or menstrua, or in the act of emission; there is no allusion whatsoever to witchcraft or enchantment. The other text *De sterilitate* often attributed to Arnau is, if not his, assuredly a product of early fourteenth-century Montpellier,[53] and is not merely a nosology but a therapeutics. The author acknowledges in passing that some couples may be made sterile by witchcraft, "and their cure must be left to God alone," but his main purpose is to explain naturalistically the physiology of intercourse and sterility, and to describe the precautions and medicines that can ensure conception. The Montpellier physicians were asserting their expert ability to recognize, classify, explain, and treat the dysfunction, which thereby became a medical one.

Yet it was not only the academic physicians who were asserting a control over impotence, as contemporary Catalan documentation makes clear. Between the thirteenth and fourteenth centuries practices seem to have changed in Catalonia, giving the physician the decisive role in pronouncing on impotence and allowing a spouse to escape from a childless marriage into a productive one. Early in 1245 the bishop of Seu d'Urgell instructed the abbot of Bellpuig to hear the case of Barquinona, a woman of Camarasa who claimed that her husband of three years was impotent. Barquinona maintained her claim under oath, and her husband Bernat confirmed it, though he insisted that he was capable of sexual relations with other women; he suggested that perhaps Barquinona "wasn't equipped like other women [*non habebat instrumentum ut alie mulieres*]." Then the abbot called two *honeste mulieres*, who examined Barquinona and asserted that not only was she still a virgin, she was "well built for receiving a man," "as well as any woman in the world." Two more lay witnesses were summoned and testified that they had spent three nights in the same room with the couple, had heard them "giving themselves to the task," with no sign of resistance from

---

[52] This is the text beginning "Maris et femine commixtio causa est," printed in the 1520 *Opera* at ff. 213[misnumbered 212]v–214 and surviving in four manuscripts; Paniagua, *Arnau de Vilanova*, p. 59, gives other reasons for accepting its authenticity. On Arnau's concept of *proprietas*, see *AVOMO* II:118, 250–1; III:61–2, 84–7. Arnau recommends that the physician set out his knowledge in tables in, e.g., his *Repetitio*: "quia mens humana vagari non cessat et distrahi per diversa solitis sensibus nisi freno detineatur vel occupetur" (f. 279rb).

[53] The work is published in sixteenth-century editions of Arnau's works – e.g., *Opera* (1520), ff. 211–13[misnumbered 212]v; the first half was edited by Karl Arlt in a Berlin dissertation of 1902 and the second published by Pagel, "Raymundus de Moleriis." In manuscript, the work is ascribed sometimes to Arnau and sometimes to Jordan de Turre, but most often to Raymond de Moleriis, chancellor at Montpellier in 1335. Paniagua (*Arnau de Vilanova*, p. 59) believes the attribution to Raymond is most probable.

Barquinona.[54] No specifically medical testimony was given or asked for. Bernat was not given a physical examination; local women evidently were called on to pronounce upon Barquinona's anatomy only because Bernat had originally raised the question of her formation; and villagers and family spoke to the attempt at intercourse. All this is very much according to the *Decretales* of Gregory IX.

Less than a century later we find that a new basis for judgment has come into operation: in a similar case in 1332, Maria, a woman of Valls, alleged to the archbishop of Tarragona that her husband Pere Reig was impotent. The archbishop's response was first to command Pere to submit to an examination, not by a layman, but by his own physician Berenguer ça Coma, *magister in medicina*, to test Maria's claim; then, two months later, Maria herself was summoned to Tarragona – her trip too may have been made for purposes of physical examination.[55] Evidently master Berenguer's judgment went against Maria, for the following month she was appealing the archiepiscopal decision that she continue to live with her husband, offering in support of her appeal a hearsay account of Pere's own admission of impotence. By now the ecclesiastical authorities had decided to seek a medical rather than a lay verdict on impotence, in what amounts to an acknowledgment of "professional" expertise.

---

[54] "Ad ista duo probanda introducte due honeste mulieres fuerunt que inspicerent eam et taliter dixerunt. A[nton?]ia Rotunda {testis} iurata dixit quod ipsa inspexit dictam Barquinonam diligenter et est virgo ut sibi videret. Interrogata si ipsa Barquinona habebit instrumentum abtam ad recipiendum hominem respondit quod sic secundum quod aliqua alia mulier de mundo. Bernarda den Vives {testis} iurata dixit quod inspexit diligenter et vidit naturam prefate Berengarie et est virgo et incognita ut sibi firmiter videret. Interrogata si ipsa Barquinona habebat instrumentum abtum ad hominem recipiendum respondit quod sic et est ita bene bastada ad illud officium secundum quod ipsa vel aliqua alia mulier.

"Isti alii duo testes producti fuerunt ad probandum quod prefatus maritus nisus fuit cognoscere dictam Barquinonam et quod ipsa non defendisset se. B. Irimam {testis} iuratus dixit quod fuit per tres noctes in eadem domo cum dicta Barquinona et B. Oldomarii et vidit quod ambo intraverunt lectum et postquam lumen fuit exteritum audiebat illos pulsantes et laborantes et operam dantes ad hoc quod possent se cognoscere et circa mediam noctem audivit illud iterum et credit quod dictus B. laborabat ad hoc quod posset dictam Barquinonam cognoscere et nunquam potuit intelligere quod dicta Barquinona defenderet se a marito suo. Requisitus de tempore respondit quod non recordatur": ACSU, parchment of 4 kls. Mar. 1244/5. I owe my knowledge of this document to the kindness of Paul Freedman.

[55] The very piece of paper that summoned Pere to submit to master Berenguer's judgment, dated 15 Sept. 1332, is still inserted loosely in AHAT, manuals de Valls, no. 26(d); it is transcribed on f. 12v of that volume. Later material on the case is in AHAT, manuals de Valls no. 52, ff. 1v, 7–8v. Berenguer ça Coma (or de Chumba) had studied at Montpellier, and there on 19 May 1332 he had defended *questiones disputate* on the *Aphorisms* of Hippocrates (the text is in MS Basel D.I.11, ff. 159–89v), so that his examination of Pere must have been one of the first responsibilities given him by his archbishop patron, the infante Joan. Joan died in 1334, but Berenguer had now begun intermittently to attend his royal brother, Alfons III; he was summoned to the dying king in December 1335. After Alfons' death Berenguer continued to live in Tarragona, where he was contracted as municipal physician; he left the town's service for that of Pere III in 1342, receiving an annual stipend from the king of 6,000 *sous* (C 873/150v and C 617/75, of 11 and 14 May). He died in 1348, presumably in the plague.

At Tarragona we have no actual account of the physical examination, but such a procedure is described in a case of virtually the same date from Perelada, near Figueres in northeastern Catalonia. To prove to the court that his wife Berengaria "could not fulfill her conjugal debt nor conceive nor bear a child," Guillem Castelló of Castelló d'Empúries called in, not a learned physician, but an experienced surgeon, Vesianus Pelegrini; in the presence of a matron of the town the surgeon "raised the knees of the said Berengaria and examined [her]" and declared on oath that

> she has a male penis and testicles like a man; and is so narrow that she can barely urinate through an opening that she has in a fissure that she has in the vulva, [a fissure] that lies beneath her penis; and has a flap stretched between her thighs like the wings of a bat, which covers the fissure in the vulva whenever she draws her knees toward her head; and she has more the aspect of a man than a woman, and there is no way in which Guillem or any other man can lie with her.[56]

The weight given here to the details of Berengaria's genital anatomy – full enough to allow us to conclude that she was probably a biological male with third-degree hypospadias[57] – anticipates the standards of judgment that would become articulated in Renaissance medicine. Michel Foucault notwithstanding, not only sexual behavior but sexual anatomy too had already become the province of medicine by the Middle Ages.[58]

Writing in southern France thirty years later, Montpellier-trained Guy de Chauliac commented explicitly on the examination for impotence in language that seems to suggest that he thought the physician's role in it was recent enough to need explanation:

---

[56] "Qui quidem medicus supradictus ad instanciam dicti Guillelmi vocavit dictam Berengariam una cum domina Cotona filia Guillelmi Bartholomei quondam de Castilione et in presencia dicte domine Cotone elevavit genua dicte Berengarie et recognovit et inspexit si ea que dicta erant et requisita per dictum Guillelmus erant vera quibus siquidem supradictam inspectis et recognitis per dictum medicum idem medicus dixit virtute iuramenti per eum prestiti in posse curie ville Perelate in principio sui regiminis quod dicta Berengaria habebat virgam virilem et testiculos ad modum hominis et est arta ita quod vix potest mingere per quoddam foramen parvum quod habet in fissura vulve quam habet suptus dictam virgam virilem et habet pellem inter crura sua stensam ad modum alarum vespertilionis que cohoperit fissuram dicte vulve tociens quociens ipsa Berengaria vertit genua sua versus faciem suam et quod habet formam virilem plus quam muliebrem, its quod dictus Guillelmus nec alter homo posse iacere secum nec habere rem carnaliter nec ipsa posset reddere ullatenus debitum coniugalis nec concipere nec infantare": AHPG/PL, manual de Bernat Sunyer 26 bis/52v (24 Aug. 1331). The practitioner referred to here, Vesianus Pelegrini, had practiced surgery in Perelada since 1310 and had often been called on by the court for forensic testimony; he died in 1336–7.

[57] Dr. Peter English of Duke University has offered this diagnosis.

[58] Foucault, *History of Sexuality*, I:36–49, seems to believe that the "medicalization of the sexually peculiar" began only in the nineteenth century. Daston and Park, "Hermaphrodites," have already pointed out that Foucault failed to recognize the evidence for the process in Renaissance France.

Truth to tell, since justice has adopted the habit of asking the doctor for an examination, the form the examination takes must be described. Once he has obtained permission from the court, the [doctor] must first of all examine the complexion and structure of the reproductive organs; then he must go to a matron used to such [procedures] and he must tell [the husband and wife] to lie together on several successive days in the presence of the said matron. She must administer spices and aromatics to them, she must warm them and anoint them with warm oils, she must massage them near the fire, she must order them to talk to each other and to embrace. Then she must report what she has seen to the doctor. When the doctor has been informed, he must bear testimony in all truth before the court.[59]

In the light of our case from thirteenth-century Urgell, Guy's outline suggests that the church had simply inserted medical personnel into the first stage of an older procedure, for the sake of their expertise in anatomy and physiology – the laity were still capable, if necessary, of testifying to the act of intercourse itself.[60] Secondary accounts of impotence cases elsewhere in Europe from the 1370s and 1380s suggest, however, that even this limited participation of the laity in the procedure dropped away.[61]

Medical testimony in criminal trials

In secular as well as ecclesiastical courts one can observe a growing European readiness in the last decades of the thirteenth century to concede a separate sphere of authority to medical expertise, a readiness particularly apparent in

---

[59] "Verum quia iusticia consueverit committere examen medicis, pro tanto ponitur hic modus examinandi; et est quod medicus, habita licencia a iusticia, examinet complexionem et compositionem membrorum generativorum, deinde habeat matronam in talibus consuetam et precipiat quod iaceant simul per aliquos dies, ipsa matrona presente cum eis, et det eis species et pigmenta et eos calefaciat et inungat cum oleis calidis et fricet iuxta ignem sarmentorum et iubeat eos confabulare et amplecti; deinde quod viderit refferat medico. Et quando medicus fuerit bene informatus coram iusticia de veritate deponere potest": Guy de Chauliac, *Cyrurgia Magna*, VI.iii.7; MS Bristol, City Reference Library 10, f. 227vb. The translation is that of Jacquart and Thomasset, *Sexuality and Medicine*, p. 172, who worked from the Latin text in Hoffman, "Beiträge," pp. 191–2.

[60] Murray, "Origins and Role," p. 245, comments: "Thus, the matron, while continuing to play a crucial role in establishing if the man were impotent, was moved out of direct participation in the court proceedings. This may be indicative of the increased legal disabilities that faced women at the end of the Middle Ages." It seems to me more illuminating to see this shift as further evidence of the growing social valuation of medical expertise than to look at it as a practice specifically disabling women – particularly since such lay juries had involved men as well as women (above, n. 47). Women continued to be called on to verify claims of virginity and of rape, as respectively in the cases published by Campillo, *Documentos*, p. 403, docs. 212–13 (from Daroca, 6 id. Feb. 1311, based on C 251/30v), and by Comenge, "Nuevos documentos," p. 294 (from Calatayud, probably in the 1320s; extracted from CRD Jaume II sin fecha 1369).

[61] Bullough and Brundage, *Sexual Practices*, pp. 138–40, citing English cases from 1377 and 1379; Jacquart and Thomasset, *Sexuality and Medicine*, p. 171, quoting a Parisian procedure of 1385.

some criminal proceedings.[62] It seems likely that the ground for these developments was laid by the parallel evolution of canon and civil law. The two legal
traditions are so entangled that it is not easy to distinguish early stages in the
process, but by the end of the thirteenth century both were in accord that it was
surgeons or physicians who could best judge the seriousness of wounds suffered
in an assault. Roman law originally gave no special forensic role to physicians,
but the medieval glossators of the civil law after Accursius (d. 1260) seem to be
acknowledging a new place for medical expertise.[63] In canon law the operative
statement was incorporated into the *Decretales*: if a man wounds another who
subsequently dies, he is not guilty of homicide if in the judgment of "skilled
practitioners" (*peritorum medicorum*) the wound would not of itself have been
fatal.[64] The *Speculum iudiciale* of Guilelmus Duranti (d. 1296) summed up the
conviction that medical expertise was superior to lay opinion in such cases: "A
wounded B, who subsequently died after contracting a fever, and A is accused
of murder but claims B died of the fever. Many lay witnesses brought forth
agree; yet a smaller number of physicians say the wound was the cause of the
fever. I answer: it is preferable to believe the few physicians, who better
understand the matter."[65] Such principles must have been known not only in
Italy but in the Crown of Aragon, not merely through the canon law (the editor
of the *Decretales*, the Dominican canonist Ramon de Penyafort, was a Catalan
and the confessor of Jaume I) but through the civil law as well, for the new
Roman law had penetrated there fairly quickly. Both canon and civil law were
taught at Lerida from the moment of its foundation in 1300.[66]

We find European practitioners called upon for expert testimony in criminal
proceedings already in the later thirteenth century, in accordance with these
principles. The earliest statutory provision for such testimony comes from
Bologna, which in the 1250s outlined the procedure to be followed by civic
authority when asking a surgeon to decide whether a wounded man was likely to
die from his injuries. The city statutes of 1288 and thereafter provide for the

---

[62] What follows was presented in a different form to the Institute of the History of Medicine, Johns
Hopkins University, and has profited from discussion there.

[63] For Rome, see Amundsen and Ferngren, "Forensic Role," p. 48. Searching the index to early
modern editions of the *Corpus Juris Civilis* (under "medicus" and "vulnus") yields several
marginal (post-Accursian) glosses that make plain that by now medical practitioners had the
legal task of determining whether a wound would prove fatal (e.g., "Ex *vulnere* an quis mortuus
sit, vel non sit, ut probetur, consilium est, ut statim mittatur medicus, qui referat an vulnus
mortale sit futurum"); so far, however, I have been able to locate only one of these glosses in the
text itself, at *Institutes* I.8 (*Corpus Juris Civilis*, V:44).

[64] *Decretalium* IX.v.xii, cap. 18; *Corpus Juris Canonici*, II, ed. Friedberg, cols. 800–1.

[65] Quoted from Ascheri, "'Consilium sapientis,'" p. 535, n. 4. Ascheri raises doubts as to the
Durantian authenticity of this passage (pp. 569–74) but leaves no doubt that the doctrine itself,
expressed in whatever language, had been established by this time.

[66] Coing, *Handbuch*, I:294–300; Hillgarth, *Spanish Kingdoms*, I:99–102, 276–7; Font y Rius,
"Desarollo," pp. 295–8. Miret y Sans, "Escolars catalans," shows that more than eighty Catalans
can be found at the Bologna *studium* in the single decade 1218–29.

selection (by lot, from a select pool) of two physicians whom the court could send to examine the victims of attacks, wounded or dead, and the first actual accounts of forensic testimony by Bolognese *medici* come from the same decade.[67] Joseph Shatzmiller has shown that a similar though procedurally less formal use of medical expertise was applied in the courts of Manosque (in Provence) at a still earlier date, from at least 1285;[68] much the same practice was followed in the Italian Piedmont by 1301 and is laid down in the Castilian *Leyes del Estilo* of *c.* 1310.[69]

It is at virtually the same moment that we begin to find references to a comparable procedure in Catalonia, the *desuspitatio*: a formal determination, accurate and objective, of the expected consequences of a wound. To be *desuspitatus* means, literally, to be pronounced out of danger, whether of death or of the loss, mutilation, or impairment of a limb; the term seems to have been peculiar to the region.[70] In the Catalan courts of the early fourteenth century a medical opinion of this sort was critical in resolving cases of assault: when one man was accused of wounding another, the court had to determine not only whether he was guilty but also how serious the wound was. If the injured party should eventually die, for example, did death result directly from the wound? The verdict might be of the utmost importance to the attacker.[71] What affected the court's decision in such cases was the medieval conviction that every individual bears some responsibility for maintaining his own health – even the victim of an unprovoked attack is still required to act sensibly and responsibly while recovering, must not (for example) overexercise recklessly or eat too

---

[67] Ortalli, "Perizia medica," and Simili, "Beginnings." The latter source quotes (p. 97) a report of 1287 in which two *medici* appointed by a judge visit a patient and declare his wound not to be fatal; Kantorowicz, "Cino da Pistoia," p. 287 n. 2, describes the 1289 forensic examination of a dead body, enumerating its wounds and distinguishing between mortal and non-lethal wounds. Fischer-Homberger, *Medizin vor Gericht*, pp. 31–8, provides a sense of the broader intellectual and professional context in which the Bologna developments took place.

[68] Shatzmiller, *Médecine et justice*, pp. 30–43.

[69] Naso, *Medici*, p. 200 n. 52; Ruíz Moreno, *Medicina*, pp. 165–7. Park, *Doctors*, p. 96, makes clear that similar procedures were being used in Florence by 1314.

[70] "Desuspitari de morte vel membri perdicione seu mutilacione aut debilitacione"; the list is from a letter of Alfons III setting a limit to surgeons' charges for the procedure (C 488/21v; below, p. 216 at n. 99). I have found one interesting passage employing the word in a different sense: when a woman in Santa Coloma de Queralt fell from a wall, accidentally injuring her head, and feared that her husband might be blamed, she formally "desuspitavit et desuspitat predictum virum suum": AHPT 3860/90–90v, 29 June 1340.

[71] This emerges, for example, in a Cervera case of 1347. Abram Bendit Deus Logar, struck in the head with an axe by Jaume de Peracamps, complained bitterly that the royal bailiff was preparing to let Jaume off with a fine; Abram argued that he had been wounded *letaliter* or at least risked mental impairment, and insisted that Jaume be punished "pena capitali ad ungem." The bailiff replied that Abram had been *desuspitatus* by two surgeons, who had declared that he was virtually cured, and that in that case it was perfectly permissible by Catalan custom and the *Usatges* of Barcelona to settle for a fine from Jaume: AHCC, manuals de Pere de Salvanera 11, binding (parchment of 5 kls. Mar. 1347/8).

much.[72] Thus a court was normally forced to determine how serious a wound originally had been, and how the patient had behaved thereafter. Obvious difficulties arose in trying to take testimony on these matters when a standard of occupational expertise had not yet become generally admitted; the *fueros* of Monzón (1289) had required practitioners to swear to testify truthfully on such matters, but they had not insisted upon a particular level of competence from such witnesses.

The earliest example of a Catalan *desuspitatio* I have found so far is from March 1297, though the technical term does not appear: two surgeons of Santa Coloma de Queralt (one Christian, one Jewish) were summoned to court and took their oath that three victims of an attack "are not in danger of dying from their wounds and have nothing to fear, in fact are cured, so long as they stay away from women and God preserves them from other mishaps."[73] The practice was at least a decade older, for it was undoubtedly the *desuspitatio* that the *cortes* of Monzón had had in mind in trying to enforce the truthfulness of physicians and surgeons.[74] It established itself only gradually, however, for there are still cases early in the fourteenth century where courts treat lay opinion as no less credible than medical judgment.[75] The technical term *desuspitatio* was in use by 1307.[76]

Systematic documentation of criminal cases is quite rare in the early fourteenth-century Crown of Aragon; the otherwise rich judicial archive of Valencia, for example, has almost no criminal records for the years before 1320.[77] We are fortunate that the series of *crims* from the municipal archives of Lerida is relatively full and can provide a picture of the evolution of the surgeon's role in this process that is probably valid for Catalonia generally. Already in its earliest stages the Leridan justices showed themselves well aware of the dangers of accepting casual and inexpert testimony. In 1313 Ramon Gili,

---

[72] As expressed by Baldo Ubaldi at mid-century, glossing *Digest* 9.2.52: "Imperatia medici vel negligentia infirmi, non imputatus percussori, nec auget delictum" (*Corpus Juris Civilis*, I, col. 1050).

[73] "Non erant in periculo mortis propter vulnera nec timebant aliquod, imo erant curati, tantummodo quod caverent se a mulieribus et deus caveret eis de aliis casibus": AHPT 3806/188v (7 March 1297).

[74] Above, chapter 3.

[75] As when a lay witness was questioned (1302) "si dictus Jo. Pictoris obiit propter dictum vulnus, et dixit se credere quod sic; credit tamen quod si medici qui eum tenebant in cura fuissent peritiores et fecissent curam dicto vulneri congruentem, dictus Johannes non obiisset propter dictum vulnus": ACA, Cancillería, procesos in quarto, 26/20.

[76] Bernat de Pertegaç of Sant Celoni (on whom see above, n. 34) "desuspitavit secundum suam consciencienciam et discrecionem quam habet in arte susurgie": AHMA 336/13 (28 March 1307).

[77] ARV, Just. Val. 36/136, 137v, presents a case (1321) where the surgeon Bernat Molla reports to the court on the extent of a victim's injuries, but strictly speaking it is not a *desuspitatio* since Bernat gives no prognosis; he states that the patient's legs are disabled at present, but he will say nothing about his prospects for recovery. The case is extracted in Roca Traver, *Justicia de Valencia*, p. 467, doc. 132.

accused of attacking Miquel Monso (who subsequently died), based his defense partially on the testimony of a bystander that the wound "was not and did not appear to be mortal, and he said it seemed to him that the aforesaid Miquel did not care for the wound and did not abstain from those foods that wounded men are accustomed to avoid."[78] The court evidently found this lay assertion of Miquel's irresponsibility inadequate, for it insisted on asking the *prohomens* of the village where the attack had taken place to confirm from the attending *metge* whether Miquel had died from the wound or from some other cause. The villagers reported that the local healer, Vicent, had sworn that "he had had the said Miquel de Monso under his care for a blow from a stone, which wounded him on the head and cut him so that blood and pus came out, and according to the signs [*senyals*] he didn't die from the said wound but rather from another illness or fever, and he believes that Miquel died from some such cause, not from the wound" – thus giving an expert's confirmation of what the lay observer had only guessed at.[79]

Except that in this instance the court took testimony by correspondence rather than in person, this case well represents the direction in which Leridan (and Catalan) practice would develop. As time went on, in cases of assault the court would ask a practitioner, almost invariably a surgeon (and usually the one attending the victim), to assess the state of the wound and the patient's compliance with norms of healthful behavior. The surgeon gave his testimony not merely on oath but "according to his *enteniment*," his understanding of the "art" or "science" of surgery: the frequent appeal to *sciencia* in particular, with all its overtones of a learned subject based on rational first principles (which many physicians would probably not have conceded was applicable to surgery), was an obvious device to emphasize that practicing surgeons could appreciate the consequences of wounds in ways that the laity could not.[80]

The summary Leridan reports give the conclusions reached by the surgeons – "the said Maria . . . is not in danger of death or loss of a limb, but she will lose the use of the little finger of her right hand"[81] – but not the medical reasoning that lay behind them. To the court, however, the surgeons had probably explained the *senyals* (as Vicent of Estadella called them) that led to their conclusion, and in

---

78 "Non erat nec aparebat mortale, [et] dixit se vidisse quod de predicto vulnere dictus Miquel non plagebat et nec cavebat sibi ab aliquo cibo quod homines vulneratos facere consuetum est": AML 764/112r–v (the case begins on f. 105).

79 "Ell tingues en sa cura al dit Michalet de Monson d'una nafra que era estat ferit en lo cap de pedra e acli atayllar e sanar de los e exien brach, e segons los senyals no's devia perdre per raho de la dita nafra mas somach(?) altra malaltia de febre, per la qual cosa era son enteniment que fos mort e no per la nafra": ibid., f. 112. The town wrote for information on 17 Jan. 1313, and the village replied two days later.

80 For surgery as "art," AML 768/54v (1328); as *sciencia*, AML 767/186v (1325) and 769/101v (1330).

81 AML 767/186.

desuspitationes from elsewhere in Catalonia one occasionally finds an explanation of the surgeon's reasoning.[82] A particularly thorough account has
survived from Gerona and is worth quoting at length.

> Guillem Guerau, a recognized surgical practitioner, <was> brought before the
> presence of the honorable Guillem de Rexach, justice of Verges, to judge or
> determine whether the wounds or blows inflicted on the person of Guillem de Foix
> . . . were mortal or involved the risk of death or loss of members. And having first
> sworn an oath, he declared that he had the said wounded man under his care, and
> that he had a moderate wound of the head without any effusion of blood that he had
> seen, and another moderate one to the left arm and to the little finger of the right
> hand. And the aforesaid wounded man ought not to die from these blows (which
> appeared to have been made with a club) or sustain any damage to his members
> – so long as he adhered to a proper regimen – inasmuch as neither in the head
> nor the arm did he have a broken bone and he had only good signs: he didn't
> have a swelling of the head, he wasn't vomiting or suffering from collapse
> [?*stratimentum*], which are all ominous indications. Therefore he stated that the
> patient was in no danger of death or disability and declared him *desuspitatus*.[83]

Here, beyond the essentials we have already found in more succinct documentation, we are given observational and interpretative detail as to the probable

---

[82] These explanations vary greatly, as does the evidence they draw on (though I have no reason to
think that they were ever based on actual autopsies). Margarita Babonera of Banyoles was
adjudged not to have died of her head wound because "craneus non erat fractus, et quando ipsam
Margaritam medebatur . . . de vulnere predicta, aliquociens ipsum vulnus reperiebatur turpe,
aliquociens pulcrum, et illud ut verisimiliter apparebat eveniebat sibi propter malum regimen
corporis ipsius Margarite": ADG, Sèrie C (procesos), old 55 fasc. 1 (of Aug. 1327). The surgeon
was Ramon Cerdà of Banyoles, active 1323–30 (ACA, Cancillería, procesos in cuarto, 22/5,
where he is found treating another head wound). A little fuller reasoning is given in a case where
"dictus Poncius est mortalis et debet mori propter multam effusionem et amissionem sanguinis
vulneris sibi facte in tibia et racione doloris quod idem Poncius patitur in utroque latere et propter
febrem quod similiter in suo corde patitur": AHPG/PL 22/54v (29 July 1324). The surgeon was
Vesianus Pelegrini of Perelada, on whom see above, n. 56.
[83] "Guilelmus Geraldi medicus cisurgie constitutus in presencia discreti G. de Rexacho iudici
ordinarii de Virginibus adhibitus seu auductus ad iudicandum seu discernendum an vulnera seu
percussiones que fuerunt illate in personam G. de Fuxiano al. vocati en Loberi' de Virginibus die
beati Nicholay de sero proxime preteriti sint mortalia sive mortis periculosa vel deterioracionis
membrorum. Et prestito prius per eundem iuramento, dixit quod ipse tenet in cura dictum
vulneratum et est vulneratus in capite modicum sine sanguinis effusione quod ipse viderit et
modicum in brachio sinistro et in digito minoris manus dextere. Et ex predictis percussionibus,
que apparent esse facte cum baculo, dictus vulneratus non debet mori nec sustinere
debilitacionem membri sui – dum tamen velit stare regimini medicine – ex eo quia non habet in
capite nec in brachio aliqua effrectione ossi et habuit omnia bona signa in persona sua, quia non
habet tumorem in capite nec sustinuit vomitum nec eciam stratimentum in persona sua, que
essent signa periculosa. Quare dicit quod ipse est sine suspicione mortis vel debilitacionis et sic
desuspitavit eundem." My translation alters tenses so as to maintain grammatical consistency.
The document quoted here, embodying the formal *desuspitatio* by Guillem Guerau and dated
14 Dec. 1338, is inserted loosely into ADG, Sèrie U (Regesta litterarum), 6, at f. 66v, which
reports the case of "P. Vitalis sacristi ecclesie de Virginibus . . . diffamatus quod percusserat
vulneraverat seu al. maletractaverat G. de Fuxano." Guillem was a surgeon of Ullà as late as 1342
(ADG, Sèrie C [Marmessories], Ant. C 5 no. 19).

cause of the wounds and their character. Guillem does not quote academic authorities, as the physicians of Manosque sometimes did in explaining their reasoning,[84] and his enumeration of the symptoms that render a skull fracture more sinister may be based simply on experience, but they are perfectly in keeping with the surgical texts of the day.[85]

Though more knowledgeable than a layman, an attending surgeon was not necessarily more trustworthy. His honesty might be questioned,[86] and his testimony therefore often included an oath not to accept a bribe from plaintiff or defendant. But personal considerations could also affect his conclusion. The surgeon's reputation for practical and theoretical expertise was in the balance in a *desuspitatio*; in difficult cases he might ask for extra time in which to consider his judgment.[87] After all, if he predicted that a patient would die of his wounds, and he did not, he risked having it said that he had been fooled (*enguanyat*); if he announced that a patient would not die, and he did, he could be accused of both "negligenciam et impericiam artis cirurgie," as Guerau de Sant Dionis was in Gerona.[88] On balance, however, the latter decision was professionally the less risky. By qualifying his assurances – "the said Astruch will not die of his wound," ran one typical declaration, "unless he accidentally incurs a fever or some other illness, as happens to men every day, or thinks the wrong things, or lies with a woman, or eats the wrong foods"[89] – the surgeon could throw the blame on a patient who did not recover. The claim that "he should have survived, but he chose not to follow my advice," allowed the practitioner to evade most accusations of incompetence. Something of this attitude is apparent in the testimony delivered by the Geronan surgeon Berenguer ça Riera, asked by a court at the beginning of the century to comment on the death of a young

---

[84] They appeal to "Galianus in libro natomie" (Shatzmiller, *Médecine et justice*, p. 237; the text in question cannot be further identified), Hippocrates' *Aphorisms* (ibid., pp. 163, 198), Gilbertus [Anglicus?] (ibid., p. 64) and, less specifically, the "actores artis sirurgie" (ibid., p. 234).

[85] E.g., Henri de Mondeville, *Chirurgia* II.3.i.2 (Pagel, *Chirurgie*, 41:147–8), where Henri recommends giving the victim a drink to see if he vomits; if so, Henri says, it is a bad sign, since anatomy shows that brain and stomach are connected by many large nerves.

[86] As in C 173/42 (1 May 1321), where the king reviews a *desuspitatio* and appears to question the background and judgment of a "master Pere"; or C 572/141r–v (16 Nov. 1334), where the Geronan surgeon Guillem ça Riera is found innocent of having falsely claimed that Jaume Vidal could recover from his wounds.

[87] Thus in Perelada the surgeon Vesianus Pelegrini asks for eight days rather than five in which to come to a decision because the wound "est multum suspectus et periculosus iuxta experienciam artis mee": AHPG/PL 26 bis/15 (1 May 1331).

[88] Guerau had pronounced *desuspitatus* a patient who died the next day; he was absolved at the plea of the king and queen of Mallorca (C 576/101r–v). It should be pointed out that Guerau was a physician, and that the accusation against him was probably encouraged by his intrusion upon what was normally a surgical prerogative.

[89] "Dictus Astruch Vidal ex dicto vulnere non timet mortem . . . nisi accidenter ei evenerit febris vel aliqua alia infirmitas sive morbi ut aliis hominibus quotidie evenit vel eciam propter malum pensamentum sive costen [?] aut propter concubitum mulieris vel malas et contrarias comestiones sive cibos": AHPT 3828, 11 kls. Jan. 1321.

apprentice who, struck accidentally on the head by a stone, had run about the town and eaten totally inappropriate things before dying two weeks later. Berenguer blamed the death on the youth's own thoughtlessness; if he had acted and eaten sensibly (and if he, Berenguer, had had care of him), the youth would certainly have lived.[90]

It was not long before defendants began to realize that, all things being equal, there was an excellent chance of the attending surgeon's giving a judgment favorable to their side; in such a situation, if the patient did then die, for whatever reason, the accused having already been freed of guilt for the death would pay no further penalty.[91] Before the *desuspitatio* came into use, we find defendants trying to throw the blame for their victim's death on the "clumsiness and carelessness of the practitioners who treated him for his wound"; the advent of the new procedure meant that in a doubtful case the defendant had more reason to unite with the surgeon against the victim than to challenge his competence.[92] Hence friends of the accused often demanded independently that the court call for a *desuspitatio*;[93] or they might seek out the surgeon and ask him for it directly – occasionally, as a precaution, even when no charge had yet been leveled.[94] A cautious surgeon who requested extra time in which to come to a

[90] The case is described in McVaugh, "Royal Surgeons." Or see the Barcelona case of 1313 in which the court used medical testimony to decide that a victim who had died even though he had been *desuspitatus* did so "non solum ex dictis vulneribus sed alio superveniente caso et malo sui regimine": C 210/45v, of 21 May 1313. The case cited above in n. 73 shows that surgeons had recognized the need to protect themselves as far back as the procedure can be traced ("they are cured so long as they stay away from women, and God preserves them from other mishaps").

A much more positive assessment of patient compliance is found in the case of Poncius in n. 82 above, where the surgeon pronounced the wound mortal but insisted that the victim was faithfully following doctor's orders, "stetit in dieta quod idem medicus sibi dedit, nec habuit malum regimen in se." But here the surgeon had apparently been summoned by the plaintiff's family, and was perhaps expected to fix guilt *on* the accused rather than free him of it.

[91] As in the case of Antoni Paschasii of Bell-lloc, who hit a woman over the head with his staff. She died, but Antoni was declared innocent of her death because the surgeon who cared for her, Salomon Abrahe of Arboç, had already formally pronounced her cured (C 866/42; 29 April 1339).

[92] See the two cases in AHCP, Jaume Ripoll Liber extraneorum 1285–6, f. 7 (24 July 1285) and f. 21 (25 Oct. 1285).

[93] In a particularly clear example of 1330, the procurator of two friends accused of injuring a couple in Montbrió asked the bailiff of Santa Coloma de Queralt that, because "que . . . vulnera (ut ego audivi) letalia non existunt, et forte mala cura vel culpa dictorum vulneratorum mors probabiliter sequi posset . . . cum medicis sçirurçie certificetis vos an dicta vulnera sint letalia vel non, et an secundum scienciam medicine vel scisuzie predicti debeant evadere mortem vel non, et quod predictis factis de hiis que in veritate inveneritis faciatis mihi fieri publicum instrumentum ut possit veritas in posterum apparere": AHPT 3842, loose leaf. See also AHPT 3854/75 (15 Oct. 1339), where the surgeon Guillem Arnau pronounces a victim out of danger and the accused's representative, "ad cuius instanciam predicta fuerit facta in conservacionem iuris dicti A. Rubei [the accused], petiit fieri publicum instrumentum."

[94] See, for example, the formal statement made before a notary by the surgeon Pere Fontanet of Manresa, apparently independently of any criminal proceedings, that a patient had recovered from a stomach wound received a month before: AHCM 194, 2 non. May 1345. The woman who wanted to put it on record that her head wound was an accident may have been taking just such a precaution – perhaps at her husband's insistence (above, n. 70).

decision, when a wound seemed suspicious or dangerous, could come under considerable pressure from the attacker to prepare a *desuspitatio* while the victim was still alive.[95]

Naturally municipal authorities recognized that a surgeon's judgment was subject to a variety of influences, and they tried to respond to the problem in several ways. In some instances they required all *desuspitationes* to be performed, not by just one surgeon, but by two or more acting in concert – as in Barcelona in 1322.[96] They might also assign third parties, surgeons not involved in the patient's treatment, to evaluate his condition.[97] Where Jews were involved as plaintiffs or defendants, Jewish as well as Christian practitioners were occasionally asked for their opinion.[98] What courts did *not* do was abandon the *desuspitatio* and return to uninformed testimony, for they, like the public, now took for granted the need for expert surgical opinion in coming to a judicial decision.

The right to provide a *desuspitatio* carried with it certain economic rewards, some perfectly legitimate and some less so. No one questioned that a surgeon deserved a small fee for testifying, but he might also be offered a bribe by the defense to certify that the victim would have recovered had he behaved sensibly, that the victim's death was not the result of the attack; or he himself might demand an exorbitant sum to guarantee his appearance in court. The Barcelona councilors and *probi homines* complained to the king in 1334 that the city's surgeons routinely refused to respond to a judicial summons to perform the procedure until they had been paid an extortionate quantity by (typically) the defendant's friends; if the defense did not immediately meet these terms, it ran the risk that the victim would worsen and die, making a *desuspitatio* considerably more unlikely. The defendant was in effect being forced to pay a high fee if he did not want to risk a verdict that the plaintiff's wounds were mortal; the

---

[95] Jaume Pages of Vilafranca complained that although his victim – the cleric Francesc Guilaberti – "curatus fuerit et absque suspicione seu periculo, cirurgici qui eundem Franciscum curarunt ipsum desuspitare de ipsis vulneribus renuerunt, in favorem dicti clerici nec minus in dicti Jacobi et amicorum suorum preiudicium et non modicum nocumentum," and he asked that the *desuspitatio* be performed, "as is customary in such cases": C 603/195v (10 Sept. 1339).

[96] "Item que neguna dessuspitacio no pusca esser feta per .i. metge solament, [al]menys de .ii. metges": AHCB, Llibres de Consell I–7/35v (18 May 1322).

[97] So, apparently, in AML 773/215v (1340).

[98] Thus in Santa Coloma, 1321: one Jew and one Christian prepared the *desuspitatio* for a Jew (attacker unidentified): AHPT 3828/144v, 148. But such a precaution seems to have been unusual. In the same town in 1339, two Christians declared a Christian attacked by a Jew to be out of danger (AHPT 4336/30r–v), while in Cervera, in the case described in n. 71 above, it was two Christian surgeons who declared a Jew attacked by a Christian out of danger. In Zaragoza, in a case of assault between Muslims, the *desuspitatio* was prepared by the Christian practitioner (Sancho Oliver, active 1319–37) who had successfully treated the victim: ANZ, manual de Frances Martínez de Teruel, Jan.–Nov. 1325, ff. 44v–45 (12 April 1325).

potential for bribery was obvious, and the king in his response set the maximum fee that might be charged as 10 *sous*.[99] Similar attempts to free surgeons from temptation were made in other communities, often enough to suggest that surgeons continued to enjoy a hidden income from their manipulation of the procedure.[100]

The surgeons should not be judged too harshly for pursuing the opportunities provided by the *desuspitatio*, however: the procedure gave them a sure fee, whereas payment for normal surgical care tended to be uncertain, sometimes conditional, and often difficult to collect. At the beginning of July 1335 the town of Vilafranca del Penedès was, like Barcelona before it, granted a royal privilege restricting to 10 *sous* the charge made by surgeons for forensic testimony, and in this community the practitioners seem to have counterattacked; it is surely no coincidence that they immediately complained to the king that their patients routinely refused to pay for medical and surgical services rendered.[101] They won, six weeks later, an order from the king to his vicar and bailiff in Vilafranca to distrain on the goods of anyone who had received treatment from surgeons and physicians (or had obtained medicines from apothecaries) and had failed to pay.[102]

The model of the *desuspitatio* suggested the possibility of seeking the surgeon's expert testimony on other medical issues before the court where lay opinion risked introducing partisan interests. At the beginning of 1332 Arnau Esteve was accused before the justices in Lerida of having killed Bertomeu de Castelló in a brawl in which Arnau himself had been wounded in the side and shoulder. Arnau claimed that his wounds rendered him incapable of coming to court, and the justices consulted a series of surgeons to see whether this was so. Master Bertran de Miralles declared on 17 February that Arnau was still *en peryll*, more than at first, and could not attend; Bertran repeated his statement six days later after consulting a colleague, master Thomas, and finding him in agreement. The next month the plaintiffs protested that by now Arnau was cured, but master Thomas and a new surgeon, master Francesc Garrigues, replied that he was still in danger from an abscessed wound (*enpustemada e enfistolada*). A further protest by the plaintiffs led master Bertran and yet another surgeon, master Pere de Segons, to agree in June that Arnau could at last come to court, and after three days he reluctantly appeared, complaining however that his wounds were bursting open. Two days later master Thomas and a *fifth* surgeon,

---

99 C 488/21v (25 May 1334), and AHCB, Llibre vert, v. 2, f. 250r–v. Mutgé Vives, *Ciudad de Barcelona*, pp. 38, 128, does not fully bring out the significance of the document.

100 As, for example, in Lerida in 1344, when the town decreed that only 5 *sous* were to be paid to the surgeon who prepared the *desuspitatio*, and that if two shared the responsibility they were to divide that sum – "e si fer non volen quen sien forçats": AML 397/43 (17 Sept. 1344).

101 C 472/270r–v (1 July 1335).   102 C 469/75 (10 Aug. 1335).

master Johan de Solsona, were back again warning that Arnau's wound was still "ulcerating and deeply abscessed [*enpustemada e enfistolada e dins lo cors*]."[103] The *desuspitatio*-model obviously underlies the court's attempt here to use the experts' prognosis as a way of mediating between the two opposing parties.[104] Judge, plaintiff, and defendant alike sought a definite judgment on Arnau's condition from Lerida's community of surgeons – "community" in a very real sense, for, six months after the original brawl, every surgeon in the city must have examined Arnau's wounds, alone or in consultation with a colleague – even though obviously they were not in agreement on his condition.

The Catalan use of medical practitioners as expert witnesses differs in several points of detail from comparable practices being introduced elsewhere in Europe at this time. Most striking, perhaps, is the more limited function they appear to have had in Spain. In Bologna (and Manosque) they were not only charged with performing what are in effect *desuspitationes*, they were also required to carry out *post mortem* examinations for the court;[105] in Venice they had been made responsible since 1281 for reporting to the authorities all wounds brought to them for treatment, and when their patients died they were expected to certify the cause of death.[106] In these societies they were more nearly agents of the court than witnesses for a party to a suit, as in the Catalan *desuspitationes*, and in Italy this is reflected in the fact that they and their fees were formally regulated by municipal government. Perhaps it was the more nearly public character of their authority in Bologna that explains why that city tried to ensure that all qualified surgeons would participate equally in these forensic

---

[103] AML 770, ff. 118–131v. "Thomas" is probably Thomas Anglici, on whom see McVaugh and García Ballester, "Medical Faculty," pp. 12–13 n. 12.

[104] Note, however, that legislation establishing virtually the same procedure can already be found in the *Assises* of the kingdom of Jerusalem of 1265/6, where someone claiming a medical excuse for inability to come to court is to be examined by a physician or surgeon, who will then declare on oath whether the excuse is medically valid: Wickersheimer, "Organisation," p. 695.

[105] When surgeons are first found giving expert testimony in Bologna (1288), their role is to examine corpses to see how many wounds would have proved mortal, and whether any of the wounds might have been inflicted after death; however, the regulations of 1335 describe something sounding much more like a *desuspitatio* ("declarare teneantur qualitatem vulnerum, signa omnia et causas ex quibus iudicent seu referant ea esse vel non esse mortalia"), though the inquiry is initiated by the plaintiff rather than the defendant: Fasoli and Sella, *Statuti de Bologna*, pp. 172–3; Ortalli, "Perizia medica," pp. 234–5. Garosi, "Perizie," calls attention to instances of both functions being exercised in a number of other Italian towns in the later Middle Ages, but does not always date the texts he cites. In Catalonia (or at least in Lerida) it was not surgeons but the city fathers (*pahers*) who were expected to certify that wounds had caused death (e.g., AML 773/228v, of 1340); the testimony of surgeons was apparently thought necessary only when survival was still a possibility.

[106] Ruggiero, "Cooperation," p. 159 n. 11; Monticolo, *Capitolari*, I:267–381, provides fuller documentation. I have found no evidence of these practices in the fourteenth-century Crown of Aragon, though something similar seems to have existed earlier at Montpellier under Jaume I (Huici Miranda and Cabanes Pecourt, *Documentos*, pp. 204–5).

tasks, rather than leaving their selection to a judge or to the interested parties.[107]

Neither in Italy nor in the Crown of Aragon were such surgeons drawn only from those with municipal salaries. The new appeal to surgeons for expert testimony before the law was a separate, independent force helping to shape a social role for medical practitioners. And once again a lay impulse had preceded professional self-awareness – the surgeons, indeed, did not even have the opportunity to develop the common sense of narrow disciplinary identity that academic training was beginning to give to some physicians. The quick success of the *desuspitatio* in the Crown of Aragon expressed public belief that craft knowledge and expertise carried special authority in certain matters of community concern.

The medicalization of leprosy

Perhaps the most convincing instance of the way in which ordinary society was providing a public role for medicine can be seen in the evident medicalization of leprosy early in the fourteenth century. The change is particularly significant because leprosy was, beyond all others, the disease most invested with social meaning. In a society in which it was accepted that physical sickness could be the consequence of sin,[108] leprosy was routinely held up as the manifestation of moral corruption, as it had been since ancient times: the extremes of bodily disfigurement that can be associated with what is now distinguished as lepromatous leprosy marked the sufferer as a source of moral as well as physical infection. It was thus easy and tempting for a community to use the category as a weapon against its disliked or mistrusted members, to seize upon signs of skin disease as justification for labeling them as "lepers" without trying to distinguish from minor conditions a disease that even today is notoriously difficult to diagnose.[109]

---

[107] The regulations of 1288 speak simply of "medici periti in arte medicandi," which might seem to include physicians, but in 1292 they are specified more closely as "de sapiencioribus et dignioribus cirexie et medicine," "fidedignos et expertos in arte cirexie et medicine"; a hundred years later physicians were insisting that this label had excluded them (Ortalli, "Perizia medica," pp. 256–9). Certainly individual documents regularly identify them as surgeons (e.g., "Medico in ciroia" – ibid., p. 249 n. 65) when specification is made. Ortalli (pp. 243–8) suspects that by 1335 some practitioners had obtained the privilege of being selected more than once before the pool was exhausted. As for Manosque, Shatzmiller (*Médecine et justice*, pp. 36–7) argues that there was no attempt made there at objectivity and random selection – again more like Catalonia.

[108] Diepgen, *Theologie*, pp. 48–58; and see above, chapter 6, p. 171.

[109] Brody, *Disease of the Soul*. Jacquart and Thomasset (*Sexuality and Medicine*, pp. 180–2) suggest that much of what was called leprosy in the Middle Ages was really *lymphogranuloma venereum*, in order to explain their finding of a medieval association of "leprosy" with venereal contact; on this association, however, see below n. 121.

Indeed, for Robert Moore the Middle Ages' response to leprosy is like its reaction to heresy and Jewishness in testifying to the formation of a "persecuting society" in the twelfth century. He describes a surge in the establishment of leper houses at that time, peaking at the end of the twelfth century, noting at the same time a change in popular attitudes from compassionate to coercive – the latter embodied in the canon of Lateran III (1179) that insisted on the segregation of lepers. Though at one point Moore suggests that perhaps "heresy, leprosy and Jewishness lay . . . in the eyes of the beholders," in the end he does accept the existence of a twelfth-century epidemic of lepromatous leprosy that burnt itself out at the end of the thirteenth (when foundations of leper houses begin to decline). Nevertheless, he still argues that the power to make the diagnosis (through juries of townspeople, sometimes incorporating lepers as well) remained an important tool of social control: it offered "a far-reaching and flexible principle upon which almost anybody might be excluded from the community."[110]

This is why it is so surprising to find in the documentation from the early fourteenth-century Crown of Aragon evidence for a steady change in public attitude towards both the disease and the authority over it of the physician. By the second decade of the century, while the decision was still often in the hands of laymen,[111] there existed a sense that physicians might overrule the decision of a lay jury – though which judgment was final was not yet clear. When a woman of Gorga (Valencia) was labeled a leper by her neighbors in 1310, she appealed to the king and was pronounced free of the disease by two of the leading physicians in the kingdom; the neighbors, however, were not convinced.[112] Bernat Cubells of Ontinyent (Valencia) was similarly accused of leprosy in 1318 by the local justiciar and was committed to the lazar house in the capital; the hospital's administrator doubted the diagnosis, and when Valencian physicians agreed with him he sent Bernat back to Ontinyent – whereupon straightway the justiciar remanded him to the leprosary again.[113]

---

[110] Moore, *Formation*, pp. 45–80; the passages quoted are from pp. 67, 79.

[111] Thus in 1311 the people of Cervera feared that one of their number was a leper and might infect them, and the king instructed his bailiff to make a decision and expel the man if leprous; the instructions say nothing about seeking medical advice (C 148/59v; 13 Aug. 1311). "Expulsion" would presumably have been to Cervera's leprosary, founded by the mid-thirteenth century (Duran i Sanpere, *Llibre de Cervera*, pp. 213–14).

[112] The text, of 12 April 1310 (C 144/197), is quoted in Demaitre, "Description and Diagnosis," p. 343 n. 107.

[113] "Barcelona uxor Bernardi Cubells vicini de Ontinyen . . . exposuit reverenter quod Francischus Constantini olim iustic. dicti loci asserendo indebite dictum Bernardum Cubells fore leprosum expulsit eum a loco predicto . . . et duci fecit eum apud hospitale Sancti Lazari Valencie in quo leprosi recipi consueverunt et cum dictus Bernardus Cubells fuisset in dicto hospitali administrator eiusdem videns predictum Bernardum non pati egritudinem supradictam habito super hoc consilio medicorum Valencie qui eundem viderunt fecit eum reduci ad locum predictum de Ontinynen predictus que justic. hoc non obstante fecit eum iteratus reduci in civitate Valencie ipsoque existente in ea medici eiusdem civitatis ad instanciam predicte

In the middle of our period falls the great "lepers' plot" of 1321. In the spring of that year the story arose in France that the lepers of the kingdom had conspired to put powders and poisons into the water everywhere, in order that the healthy, drinking this water, would contract the same disease. The story spread quickly and led to the seizure and burning of lepers, first in individual communities and then more systematically throughout France, and in June King Philippe V gave orders for their general arrest, examination, and execution.[114] Word of the supposed plot and of the French reaction came to Jaume II almost immediately, together with the news that French lepers were fleeing into his realm. His first reaction was to command that all strangers in the kingdom should be apprehended and expelled if they were found to be leprous, but he soon adopted a tougher policy, ordering that suspected lepers be seized and their powders destroyed, that they be questioned under torture and burnt if they confessed to the plot. Local inquisitions of this sort are known from Huesca, Ejea, Tarazona, Manresa, Montblanc, and Barcelona in the summer of 1321, though in Aragon as in France the disturbances lasted only a few months.[115]

Most if not all of these examinations for leprosy must have been carried out by a frightened populace, not by learned physicians, and the likelihood of diagnostic error may have led to a reaction and encouraged (at some levels) a gradual recognition that leprosy should be established as a specifically medical condition. Just a year later, Amonant, a physician from Gascony who had decided to move to Aragon, was seized in Huesca as he was making his way south and was accused of being a leper and of planning to poison the water. Amonant appealed to the infante Alfons, who arranged for a tribunal of Huescan physicians and *homines fidedignos* to certify that the Gascon physician was free of the disease. Amonant was frightened enough to ask for a more general certificate three weeks later, and in the end he apparently decided not to stay in the Crown of Aragon.[116] It seems not impossible that episodes like this encouraged a wider realization of the dangers inherent in permitting leprosy to be determined by the lay public, and favored a dependence on purely medical criteria to diagnose it.[117]

At the beginning of the century, therefore, while there was already some sense

Barcelone viderunt virum suum predictum et cognoverunt eum predicta egritudine minime detineri sicque ipsi medici ipsum Bernardum cum litteris eorum et cur. Valenc. ipsorum sigillis sigillatis in quibus prefatum iusticiam certiorarunt plenarie de predictis ad dictum locum de Ontinynen protinus remiserunt": C 164/200v (26 Jan. 1318).

[114] Barber, "Lepers"; Beriac,"Persécution."

[115] C 246/227–239, passim; the king's first letter on the subject to his officials is dated 10 June 1321.

[116] C 370/228v (28 June 1322) and C 371/5 (20 July).

[117] Certainly in the immediate aftermath of the persecutions there are signs of both official and public reaction, as the baselessness of many accusations became recognized: see the royal provision for restitution of the citizens of Huesca and Jaca who had been unjustly imprisoned for the disease (C 283/20; 21 Nov. 1321), or Tarazona's request for the release of two women it had forced into a leprosary during the scare (C 221/242v; 24 May 1322).

that physicians should make the final determination, the lay public still exercised some control, skeptical of medicine's claim to be capable of deciding who was leprous and who was not. Yet a quarter-century later that claim was widely accepted. In 1327 the town of Teruel acted upon its suspicion that one of its citizens was a leper by appealing directly for a medical examination and diagnosis so that he could be segregated if he had the disease;[118] Cervera took similar action the next year.[119] By 1330 both the public and the afflicted were coming to look to physicians as arbiters.

The case richest in detail is that of Pere Teixidor of Oristà, west of Vic, whom neighbors denounced as a leper before the vicar's court there in 1333. They argued that because Pere mingled freely with the healthy, who might not know that he was sick, and because "leprosy naturally passes from a leper to healthy people by *participatione et conversatione*," he should be committed to a leper-house. Pere surrendered himself to the vicar, but begged that he should be examined by physicians to see whether he had leprosy. Thereupon the court summoned physicians, in particular Martí de Soler – "physician to the cathedral chapter and to the city of Vic, and bachelor in medicine" – to inspect Pere. Martí reported back to the court that he had examined Pere and, as far as human frailty permitted, he was able to exonerate (*desenculpavit*) Pere and affirm that he was healthy and free of the disease; furthermore, he insisted, the public ran no risk in its contact with Pere inasmuch as "there is no leprosy in his body now, and therefore it cannot pass from him to anyone else." Thereupon, on the express principle that a physician's judgment is decisive in medical matters – that "medico est credendum in sua arte" – the court commanded that Pere be free to return home and that no voices be raised maliciously against him.[120]

There are a number of particularly interesting features about this text. First of all, perhaps, might be emphasized the public acknowledgment of medical authority: Pere's appeal to physicians may have been merely an act of desperation, but the court's presumption that "medico est credendum in sua arte" is a studied generalization of great significance. Probably courts found it easy to

[118] "Ex parte universitatis ville Turolii fuit expositum coram nobis quod licet Andreas de Salamone vicinus dicte ville ut ex eius aspectu aperere dicitur sit lepra percussus et propterea mortuus fuerit sepius, ut se a cohabitacione aliorum separaret ne ipsos a dicto morbo qui contagiosus existit inficiat, attamen hoc ipse facere denegavit, quod redundat in non modicum detrimentum eorum omnium qui cum ipso habent necessario conversari. Quare ad supplicacionem humilem propterea nobis factam vobis dicimus et mandamus quatenus si per fisicos de infirmitate predicta noticiam habentes iudicatum fuerit prefatum Andream leprosum fore, ipsum a cohabitacione aliorum separari faciatis, ut cum aliis eodem morbo laborantibus cohabitet vel per se ipsum solum": C 380/35r–v (25 Aug. 1327).

[119] C 428/261v–262r (26 April 1328): Bertholinus d'Escales is to be examined by *medicis probis hominibus et personis in hoc expertis* and if found leprous is to be expelled to a suitable place.

[120] "Natura ipsius infirmitatis sit quod ex participacione et conversacione cum persona leprosa . . . ipsa lepra transivisse in personas sanas . . . In corpore suo lepra non erat nunc, et sic ab ipso in alium transire non poterat": ACFV 260, 3 kls. Feb. 1333.

accept a medical verdict in such cases because the diagnostic task was so like a *desuspitatio*, where medical testimony had long been essential to judgment; the actual word used, *desenculpare*, suggests strongly that Pere's examination by physicians before the vicar and his justiciar was an extension of trial procedures. We should also remark, in passing, that there is no allusion here to sexual congress as a favored mode of transmission, although it is often argued that leprosy was seen as venereal in character.[121] And finally we should note that the court emphasized the academic qualifications of its expert. Martí de Soler had practiced in Vic since 1328, and would continue to do so into the 1340s, but he does not insist upon his title elsewhere – in legal documents, for example – though he might have done so had he gone on to become a master. In the court's eyes, however, an academic preparation no matter how brief was evidently an important testimonial to Martí's professional standing. And given that background, certain features of his testimony are worth bringing out: the naturalistic character of his diagnosis, based on discrete, visible *signa lepre*, and the materialist view of transmission that he appears to assume ("if you don't have it in your body, you can't give it to anyone else").

The documentation from the Crown of Aragon tends to support the conclusions of Luke Demaitre about changing attitudes towards leprosy in the early fourteenth century. Demaitre has studied with great care a set of treatises from this period, all deriving from the Montpellier tradition (including one often assigned to Arnau de Vilanova), which offered accounts of the etiology and symptomatology of the disease. He has shown that these academic writers had adopted a "non-moralizing or naturalistic stance" towards leprosy, arguing that this helped to diminish the irrationality of the social response to it. In particular, he has emphasized the growing care with which these works – all from the years 1300–35 or so – attempted to define and tabulate the signs that would make possible a quick and unequivocal diagnosis specific to leprosy, and has concluded – as our documents, a different form of evidence, seem to confirm – that the establishment of such diagnostic criteria encouraged public willingness to accept "professional" rather than lay judgment.[122]

The scholastic physician's principal authority for such criteria (as in so much

---

[121] Jacquart and Thomasset (*Sexuality and Medicine*, pp. 177–93) believe that since "lepra" was seen as venereal in transmission it cannot have been true leprosy; Demaitre, "Description and Diagnosis," pp. 334–9, argues that a belief in its venereal nature "was more in tune with folklore than on the level of scholarly debate."

[122] Demaitre, "Description and Diagnosis." Jeanselme, "Comment l'Europe," pp. 33–62, collects scattered fourteenth- and fifteenth-century evidence on leprosy examinations elsewhere in Europe, some of which at least show medical "professionals" beginning to have a role in the process before 1350. Garosi, "Perizie," quotes Italian texts of 1267 and 1281 instancing the use of physicians (in the earlier case, associated with laymen) to examine individuals who had been labeled as "lepers"; it would seem that as regards leprosy, as well as forensic testimony, the Italian towns were the first to "medicalize."

else) was Avicenna, but by the end of the thirteenth century medieval authors had enlarged upon the signs he had identified in the *Canon*.[123] A short work usually ascribed to Arnau de Vilanova, *De signis leprosorum*, lists five sets of accepted physical indicators of the disease, as of *c*. 1300:[124]

(1)   voice – harsh rather than clear;
(2)   urine – whitish, with little clots like bran that tinkle when the urinal is swirled;
(3)   pulse – weak;
(4)   blood – yields graininess when strained through a cloth; when allowed to stand and settle, salt will not dissolve in the supernatant;
(5)   members – thinning out or loss of hair and lashes, deformation of the face, ulceration of the nasal septum, roughened skin anywhere on the body, loss of sensation in the extremities.

We can easily imagine Martí de Soler using such a brief guide – or the *Canon* itself – in confirming that Pere was free of the disease. Loss of sensation in particular would have been a useful criterion for distinguishing leprosy in its early stages from other skin disorders.[125]

Unfortunately no certificate has survived from pre-plague Catalonia that would let us see whether these criteria were the ones actually employed. The earliest document I know of from the Crown of Aragon is dated 1372, from Seu d'Urgell, where the three practitioners (a physician and two surgeons) charged with determining whether Ramona Iserna was a leper reported that they

> had drawn blood from the said Ramona and had examined her entire body and had studied her urine . . . and they had found no sign of leprosy in any of these, as described in book IV of Avicenna; instead, the disease she has in her nose is a kind of cancer, which is specific to one part of the body, while leprosy is universal, so that leprosy should lead to some destruction or change in the hands, the feet, the nails, the hair, or the blood, none of which we have found in the said Ramona Iserna, as far as our own art and understanding can tell.[126]

---

[123]   Avicenna, *Liber canonis*, IV.3.iii.1–2; ff. 442v–443.
[124]   Inc., "Cognoscuntur leprosi . . . "; it is known in a dozen manuscripts and was published under Arnau's name in the sixteenth century (in, e.g., the edition of 1520 at f. 214r). The work is occasionally ascribed to Jordan de Turre, who continued to enjoy a reputation as a student of leprosy in the 1360s (Guy de Chauliac, *Chirurgia Magna*, VI.1.ii; Nicaise, *Grande chirurgie*, p. 403) and to whom another tabular *Signa leprosorum* is attributed in MS Basel D.I.11 (f. 97va). Whether the work is Arnau's or Jordan's (Paniagua, *Arnau de Vilanova*, p. 62, doubts Arnau's authorship), it was evidently composed by a member of the Montpellier faculty with links to the Crown of Aragon.
[125]   See Demaitre, "Description and Diagnosis," pp. 340–3, on medieval diagnostic techniques.
[126]   "Avien feta sagnar la dita Ramona Iserna, e que han vista e sguardada tota la persona de la dita Ramona, e la sua aigua, e colada la sua sagnia, e agut sguardament de tots los seus membres; e en totes aqueles parts senyall de messelia [= leprosy] no an trobat, segons que és posat en lo quart libre de Vincena, ans lo mal que ha en lo nas és speci de cranch, lo qual és particural [*sic*] en un

These practitioners did indeed use an examination of Ramona's blood and urine in coming to their judgment, guided by the *Canon*, but what they seem to have found particularly diagnostic in identifying her condition as cancer rather than leprosy was that it was confined to her nose and so could not be leprosy, which is a universal rather than a localized disease. In this distinction too, as it happens, they were following Avicenna.[127]

Perhaps it should be added that the leper hospitals – there was at least one in virtually every town in the realm – were not invariably cut off utterly from society, were not always prisons into which people would go only under compulsion; many institutions, no doubt, were grim, but others established a more comfortable environment for their residents.[128] The leprosary (*domus infirmorum*) in Barcelona was an ecclesiastical hospital closely supervised, after 1326, by an episcopally appointed administrator; admission was not conditional on the ability to pay, for most residents seem to have been impoverished.[129] Evidently quite different was the leprosary at Manresa, where Guillem de Pujol of Prats de Lluçanes was admitted as *frater et socius* and promised food, room, and a share in the alms donated to the hospital only after he agreed to pay his fellows an entrance fee of 70 *sous*.[130] Forty years later the *maior domus* of that same Manresa hospital, himself a leper, was kept busy investing its capital in land and rents with the municipality and local citizenry; he arranged for a procurator to collect benefactions to the leprosary, and paid his mother 30 *sous* to stay with him for a year in the hospital "tending to my concerns."[131] Though despite the general European decline of the disease there continued to be public alarm over leprosy in Catalonia (as late as 1341 a scare led the king to command the segregation of lepers in the Vall d'Aran),[132] there is little sign any longer of a sustained, widespread, unreasoning fear of individual sufferers.

The interest of this apparent medicalization of leprosy is not just that it made the disease less irrational, more "social," by bringing it under the authority of physicians. For the "authority of physicians" was, in this professionalizing age, something we have seen being gradually established at a number of different

---

membre, e meselia és universal, perquè's deu perseguir meselia en mans, en peus, en ungles e en pells, e en sanch, algun destrouiment o cambiament que en la dita Ramona no és stat atrobat de present, segons art e conexenza nostra, salva reverencia e coneixenza de maestre en medicina major nostre": I quote the transcription of Moliné, "Diagnòstic mèdic," pp. 5–6.

127 "Et cum cancer qui est lepra membri unius sit de illis quibus non est sanatio, tunc quod dicemus de lepra que est cancer corporis totius, verumtamen in lepra est res una et est quod egritudo spargitur in totum corpus": Avicenna, *Liber canonis*, f. 443rb.

128 Jeanselme, "Comment l'Europe," pp. 75–83, makes plain how widely conditions could vary in northern European leprosaries.

129 Pérez Santamaría, "Hospital de San Lázaro."

130 AHCM 33, 6 id. July 1304.

131 " . . . faciendo operas meas": AHCM 197, 16 kls. Mar. 1345.

132 C 1058/28v–29 (5 Oct. 1341).

levels. It was surely easier for university-trained canonists or civil lawyers to presume the expertise of physicians and surgeons, and to begin to assign responsibility to them in the courts, than it was for the community at large to believe in their special skills. General acceptance was speeded up as the public became able to identify the new symbols of that expertise, the academic degrees that become more frequent after the 1320s. It may not be by chance that in the few cases where we can identify the physician called on to decide whether a person is leprous, that physician can claim a medical degree. For the public to accept "learned medicine" as the best judge of whether someone truly had a dread disease meant acknowledging – at a broad social level – that texts and learning did confer an advantage, did contribute something beyond what *probi homines* might hope to know. Moore views the creation of medical juries to diagnose leprosy as a fifteenth- or sixteenth-century phenomenon, and hints that it should be associated, like changing tactics of repression against heretics and Jews, with the attempt by bureaucratic regimes to take over the powers of the community at large;[133] but in the Crown of Aragon, at least, this and other powers had been voluntarily delegated to medical practitioners by the community at a much earlier date.

The limits of medicalization

The tendency to defer to medical expertise, to turn over to physicians the responsibility for judgments with important social consequences, was of course by no means universal within lay society. The limits of such medicalization of daily life are suggested by the many situations where the medical verdicts we insist upon today were only rarely called for. A messenger who fell sick on royal service had merely to get a certificate of illness from civil authority in order to claim his expenses; a vassal writing to the king to excuse his absence from military attendance on the grounds of an *infirmitas arthetica* ordinarily needed to provide no medical certificate.[134] Even so, these limits are not absolutes: there

---

[133] Moore, *Formation*, pp. 78, 134.

[134] Martínez Ferrando, "Correos," p. 110. For military exemptions, see C 62/152 (May 1285); or C 860/90v (Nov. 1336), when a draper of Cervera is allowed to find a substitute for the army because of "quandam infirmitatem intrinsecam quam sepissime pati dicitur." When the royal vicar refused to accept that a man's claim of illness excused him from military service, Pere III commanded that "si eum tunc dicta infirmitate repereatis detineri, contra ipsum racione predicta nulla procedeatis . . . dicta enim infirmitas . . . reddit ipsum a dicto exercito totaliter excusatus," without suggesting that the excuse needed verification by a physician (C 613/116v; 21 July 1341). To be sure, a medical examination may have been passed over in silence. A member of the infante Alfons' household was permitted to leave the Sardinian army in 1323 when his illness was certified jointly by his surgeons – and the archbishop of Zaragoza (C 395/153r–v)! Lluis Cifuentes has suggested in private conversation that medical confirmation became more important to such excuses in the second half of the century, citing C 1400/170r–v (1354) and C 901/30 (1357).

are signs of the gradual penetration of medical authority into most of these spheres where it was not yet formally in place.

The non-medicalized character of medieval life seems particularly striking in certain institutions which we share with the Middle Ages – in public health, for example. Most communities of any size had introduced public health legislation of various sorts by 1300 and were continually tinkering with its details. Especially common were the restraints on butchers, forbidding them to sell the meat of diseased animals or to discard the blood of slaughtered cattle carelessly on the ground.[135] An analogous prohibition was imposed on barbers, who were forbidden to keep pails of blood at their door.[136] At the individual level, urban inhabitants were concerned with conditions that might breed disease, and they often appealed to the king for relief. The condition of water was a particular worry as a cause of illness: the inhabitants of Vilafranca complained that "infections were being produced by stagnant water and ordure and filth" in a certain street, "with ensuing illnesses and deaths," and asked that the street be kept clean.[137] The fouling of drinking water by industrial waste (as by the dyers of Berga in 1319) was another source of complaints.[138] Both levels of concern, public and individual, reveal a popular acceptance of an infection-model of disease, as arising from corrupted matter transmitted by the air. But none of this legislation displays any sense that medical practitioners are indispensable in determining how diseases arise, what conditions are and are not harmful to health: it was not the town's contracted physician but its *probi homines* who were assigned to investigate the contamination of Manresa's drinking water in 1340.[139] Physicians were not called in to advise the town council on its ordinances or to consider whether a particular tub of offal was a hazard; formally, these were still social rather than medical decisions.

In some cities certain matters pertaining to public health fell under the jurisdiction of an unusual official, the *mustaçaf*, an institution taken over by the Christians from Islamic life, where, as the *muhtasib*, he had been charged with regulating urban trades and market activity. In Islam, his specific duties had varied locally, but they could include verifying the honesty of drug-sellers and the qualifications of physicians and surgeons, as well as ensuring that water sources were kept free of pollution and public cookware kept clean. His was not

---

[135] Carreras y Candi, "Ordinacions urbanes," 11:306 (Barcelona 1301, on diseased meat) and 12:289–90 (Valls 1319, on discarding blood); C 102/72v (Valencia 1295, on diseased meat); AML, Llibre de consell 396/53 (Lerida 1340, on diseased meat).

[136] AHCB, Llibres de consell, I–1/6v (1301), 81 (1313), and regularly thereafter.

[137] "Quod ex restangnacione aque et fece ac inmunditis . . . insurgebant infecciones et sequebantur infirmitates et mortes": C 364/133 (23 April 1320). Again, in 1306 the men of Guardamar were permitted to unblock a stagnant pond so that water could flow through it because it was causing disease (C 203/155v). See also the concern over *aqua putrefacta* in Zaragoza, 1314 (C 352/83v).

[138] C 167/11v–12 (31 Jan. 1319).   [139] C 608/29v–30 (12 Sept. 1340).

a medical office, however, and indeed his right to inspect medical practice has been taken to suggest a "social disdain" for the physician.[140]

The first *mustaçaf* in the Crown of Aragon was established in Valencia immediately after its conquest in 1238; in that city he was selected annually by the king from among three names presented to him by the city.[141] The Valencian *mustaçaf* had responsibility for ensuring the accuracy of weights and measures, for preventing fraud in the production and sale of goods, and for keeping streets and public spaces clean and open – he was, as in Islam, an inspector and regulator of hygiene and economic life, though there is no evidence that he supervised such medical practice as there was, and the introduction of licensing in Valencia in the next century expressed a very different regulatory principle. The *mustaçaf* prosecuted the casual discard of filth, trash, and animal carcasses; blocked and stinking drains and sewers; and rotting meat and stale fish offered for sale. In Barcelona, these matters were controlled by the city council, not by a separate policeman, until 1339, when at the city's request Pere III granted them the same institution, with similar responsibilities, to be elected in much the same way.[142] But though such things are today perceived as health-related, the public authority of the *mustaçaf* seems to have fused with the expertise of the medical occupations only at the beginning of the next century.[143]

Yet the non-medical character of public health ought not to be over-emphasized, for one case from the late 1330s suggests that physicians were already understood as appropriate judges of a community's general healthfulness, even though they might not be charged formally with overseeing it. In 1337 a married couple from Reyal, in Valencia, quarreled bitterly over whether their town could be described as healthy or not: the wife wanted to leave the town (and probably her husband as well), complaining that Reyal was unhealthy and caused her regularly to fall ill, while her spouse insisted that his wife and his town were both equally sound. In the end, the couple hired medical experts, learned physicians from the capital, to come out and assess the situation. Anticlimactically, perhaps, the two patched things up before the physicians rendered their opinion – but the case makes plain that for some, at least, public

---

140 Hamarneh, "Origin," pp. 164–72; Dols, *Medieval Islamic Medicine*, pp. 33–4 and n. 172.

141 Sevillano Colom, "Institución del mustaçaf," is a comparative survey; his *Valencia urbana medieval* focuses on Valencia and is rich in textual detail. On the relation between the Islamic and Christian official, see Glick, "Case Study."

142 Manresa was granted a *mustaçaf* in 1337, by which time Lerida already had one (Fita y Colomer, *Llibre vert*, p. 10).

143 Sevillano Colom, *Valencia urbana medieval*, pp. 51–2, follows a secondary source in supposing that already in the thirteenth century King Jaume I had assigned the *mustaçaf* the task of joining with two apothecaries in examining all the drugs being sold in the city for their quality; this is in line with earlier practice in Islam, and if it were so it would push the medicalization of the office back in time. However, the text on which he bases this conclusion is a regulation issued, not by Jaume I, but by Martí I in 1403 (*Furs e ordinations*, p. 380).

health fell under medical authority, even if institutional sanction was still lacking.[144]

A second instance of apparent "non-medicalization," equally striking to modern eyes, is the scarcity of medical supervision in the hospitals of the Crown of Aragon. Historians have tended to imagine that hospitals must inevitably take on a medical role, and most today would probably agree that many medieval hospitals had become medical institutions by the fifteenth century, yet little attention has been given to the process of transition – for these hospitals originated as charitable institutions established to care for the poor, not merely the impoverished but the orphaned, disabled, and aged, healthy and ill alike. In the Crown of Aragon, documents from the early 1300s often describe hospital residents collectively as *pauperes et infirmi*, and we would probably be right to think of them as "the helpless" rather than as just "the sick" – that is, as still having primarily a social rather than a specifically medical identity.[145] Urban growth and economic decline in the early fourteenth century increased their numbers, which seemed to threaten public order. The bourgeoisie responded by founding new hospitals and assuming the responsibility for existing ecclesiastical foundations: in Valencia, three hospitals had been added by 1345 to the five (and a leprosary) that the city had already possessed in 1300.[146]

---

[144] "Saura dicebat se nolle habitare secum in Regali dicti Poncii in quo plures infirmitates sustinuerat ac male vixerat ac vivebat, dicto Poncio contrarium asserente ac dicente dictam suam uxorem sanam fore ac dictus Regali similiter esse sanum seu sanitas preservativum": C 591/128 (11 kls. Oct. 1337). The couple agreed to pay 200 *sous* to the *medici in fisica periti et experti* whose opinion they sought, so serious issues were evidently involved, and it may be that Saura was trying to find canonical grounds for separation, though by 1300 cruelty (*saevitia*) was the typical excuse; Bullough and Brundage, *Sexual Practices*, pp. 370–5, 453–5.

[145] Typical is Berga's hospital, 1347, described as a place "in quo pauperibus tam sanis quam egris in potu cibo lectu et aliis consueverant necessaria ministrari" (C 647/91r–v). By her will, Queen Blanca founded a hospital in Perelló (Coll de Balaguer), in which Jaume II's detailed instructions of 1314 made it explicit that both healthy and ill were to be accommodated; the overriding concern was that they be poor. The administrator (*hospitalarius*) should provide "pauperibus qui infirmi non fuerint una die, infirmis autem pauperibus provideat quousque convaluerint vel vires resumpserint recedendi": ACA pergaminos Jaume II 3236, of 16 June 1314; registered at C 211/177. On the founding of the hospital, see MF, I:162–3 n. 9. In 1354–67 it was still apparently feeding and sheltering the poor rather than the sick *per se*, to judge from its accounts (ACA, varia de Cancillería 360). (The recurrent phrase "casa dels malalts" means typically a lepers' hospital, where the categorization was definitely medical rather than social; see ACA pergaminos Jaume II 432, of 10 Nov. 1294, a will making bequests to "pauperibus infirmis" in three "hospitales" of Vilafranca as well as to the "domus infirmorum" there.) Naso, *Medici*, pp. 17–30, characterizes the hospitals of medieval Piedmont in the same way. Describing Languedoc in the mid-thirteenth century, John H. Mundy might have been speaking of Catalonia a hundred years later: "Other than leper-houses, it is hard to know what functions individual hospitals performed . . . In general . . . hospitals sometimes specialized in one or several of the following categories: poor transients, the sick, the aged, poor maidens, pregnant women, widows, orphans, and bastards" ("Charity," p. 254).

[146] Rubio Vela, *Pobreza*, pp. 13–74; Burns, "Hospitales"; Batlle, "Ayuda." Mollat, *Poor in the Middle Ages*, examines the medieval concept of poverty and the charitable responses of society. For a close look at hospitals in a related society, see Caille, *Hôpitaux*.

Hospitals were neither numerous nor large in the Crown of Aragon, even in the biggest cities, and there is little evidence that they made regular medical care available to their "infirmi." The Valencian hospital of En Clapers, founded in 1311, can have had no more than thirty-four beds, and the town's seven other hospitals seem to have been far smaller.[147] Barcelona had a leprosary and five hospitals (two of which had ten and sixteen inmates respectively at the beginning of the century);[148] Gerona had two (and a leprosary);[149] Zaragoza, six.[150] Typically, each would be staffed by an administrator (*hospitalarius*) and a small number of attendants, religious or secular.

Historians of the hospital point out, with reason, that such a staff could still provide effective care for the sick by offering rest and nourishment and conscientious nursing, that to highlight the appearance of "hospital doctors" narrowly defined is to misconstrue the central function of a medieval charitable institution.[151] But if our purpose is instead to measure the growing social significance of the *medicus*, it is important to identify the stages by which, for some hospital patrons, a specifically medical care – provided by *phisici* and *cirurgici* – came to be seen as of particular value. The "medicalization" of hospital care, so defined, seems to have taken place at different rates in various parts of medieval and early modern Europe: very late in England, where the first medical staff attached to even London hospitals is not found until the early sixteenth century; much earlier in Italy, where physicians are increasingly associated with hospitals after 1350, perhaps as a reaction to the arrival of the plague.[152]

In this respect the Crown of Aragon more nearly follows the Italian pattern. Occasional though it was, some medical or surgical care was certainly possible in Catalan hospitals of the late thirteenth century, as Llull's *Blanquerna* implies,[153] and after 1300 references to a physician attending the inmates become somewhat more common. The merchant Bernat dez Clapers provided

---

[147] This was its size in 1384 (Rubio Vela, *Pobreza*, p. 129), and it is more likely to have expanded than to have shrunk in the seventy years after its foundation.

[148] Batlle i Gallart and Casas i Nadal, "Caritat privada"; Pifarré Torres, "Dos visitas."

[149] Guilleré, "Assistance."

[150] Beltran, Lacarra, and Canellas, *Historia de Zaragoza*, p. 322; one ("para pobres") was established by a canon-physician, Guillermo Fuerte, in 1305 (ibid., p. 285). Burns, "Hospitales," p. 136, cites secondary sources to show that Tortosa had six hospitals. Miquel Parellada and Sánchez Real, *Hospitales*, describe just one hospital in Tarragona from the first half of the century.

[151] See the remarks of Horden, "Discipline of Relevance," pp. 366–7.

[152] For England, see Rawcliffe, "Hospitals," pp. 7–9, and Carlin, "Medieval English Hospitals," pp. 29–31. For Italy, see Henderson, "Hospitals," pp. 81–2, and Park, "Healing the Poor," pp. 27–32.

[153] Llull's novel of *c.* 1283 speaks of a "malalt qui havia menjuadura en la cama, e no.n pudia guarir," who was lying in the hospital founded by Evast, where Evast and a *metge* visited him; "e con lo metge li hac posada la pólvora que li sulia posar, Evast ligà e adobà la nafra al malalt": Llull, *Blanquerna*, I.17; I:112–13.

for a salary of 50 *sous* annually for "cuidam medico qui curet infirmos patientes" in his Valencian foundation of 1311;[154] Tortosa by 1345 had contracted with physicians, surgeons, and a *herbolarius* to visit the sick in its hospital as part of their responsibilities to the town poor.[155] In Barcelona, which apparently did not yet have contracts with practitioners, the town took a different tack, getting Pere III to command in 1336 that "all physicians and surgeons who practice their craft in this city . . . must visit all those lying ill or detained by some illness in the hospitals of the aforesaid city, and offer them their best advice, without charge"; the city hospitals seem to have had no regular medical care until then.[156] It is tempting to imagine that municipal assumption of responsibility for the poor, together with a growing sense of the efficacy of medicine, were about to effect the medicalization of the hospital, even though in 1345 that end was not yet clearly in sight. The first circumstantial evidence of systematic medical care in hospitals generally comes from the second half of the century.[157]

The fullest evidence of how the lines were still drawn between the medical and social spheres comes from the realm of psychiatry, where the claims of the medical community were not yet accepted by the general public. The learned medical tradition of the early fourteenth century recognized mental disturbances as illnesses, as conditions having a somatic origin and in principle curable by diet or medicines, and they had constructed a careful nosology. Most mental illnesses could be categorized as either *ablatio mentis* or *alienatio*. The former group included instances not only of the complete loss of mental faculties – syncope or apoplexy or epilepsy or *suffocatio matricis* – but also of loss or diminution of the individual faculties: of the imagination (*stupor*), of reasoning (*stoliditas* or *amentia*), or of memory (*oblivio*). *Alienatio* encompassed the various perversions or distortions of the same faculties: *alienatio scientiationis*, for

---

154 Rubio Vela, "Hospital medieval," p. 384.

155 Above, n. 38.

156 "Omnes fisici et cirurgici qui in dicta civitate utantur seu praticent dictis officiis . . . teneantur qualibet septimana visitare omnes infirmos iacentes aut infirmitate aliqua detentos in hospitalibus civitatis pretacte eis absque solucione aliqua sua bona consilia impensuri": C 862/101v (31 Dec. 1336).

157 For Valencia, Rubio Vela, *Pobreza*, pp. 128–53 and appendix II (for the period beginning 1374). For Barcelona, see Roca, *Ordinacions*, pp. 25-35 (for the period beginning 1378); Batlle i Gallart and Casas i Nadal concede of the situation there seventy years before that "l'assistència mèdica era gairebé nulla" ("Caritat privada," p. 162). The Tarragona hospital was still called the "hospitale pauperum" in 1346, and the first solid evidence of medical care given there comes from 1403 (Miquel Parellada and Sánchez Real, *Hospitales*). City hospitals probably became medicalized more rapidly than those in small towns. Looking more broadly at Europe, Mollat (*Poor in the Middle Ages*, p. 288) automatically assumes the medical role of the medieval hospital, but he too agrees that "it took a long time . . . for the idea to take hold that hospital personnel should have medical or paramedical training," and with one exception – the Paris Hôtel-Dieu in 1328 – his examples of medical staff are all from the second half of the century.

example, could manifest itself as *mania* or *melancolia* or *heroys* depending on whether it was accompanied by fury or fear or lust.[158] Such a classification is set out in Arnau de Vilanova's *De parte operativa*, which is in effect a monograph on psychiatry. The work's choppiness and apparently unfinished state suggest that it may have been assembled after Arnau's death, perhaps from notes he had designed for a practical counterpart to his *Speculum medicine*;[159] it begins by arguing generally that an illness to any member can be studied through the damaged function of that member, and the intention apparently was to illustrate this point by moving from head to foot, but it never really gets beyond the head.

Mental illnesses were not merely theoretical but clinical entities for Arnau, conditions he was prepared to identify and differentiate in his patients. In teaching his students at Montpellier, he discussed *ablatio mentis* to illustrate how the physician discriminates between superficially similar illnesses. If you are called to a patient said to have lost his mind, Arnau explained, you should review the possible illnesses from which he might be suffering, and what the specific symptoms are that distinguish one from another.

> In apoplexy, every sign of life has stopped except breathing; in syncope and *suffocatio matricis* breathing stops too, but in syncope the extremities become cold, the face is discolored and *mortificatur*, and the forehead is covered with cold sweat, while none of this occurs in *suffocatio matricis*. In epilepsy the visage, the eyes, and the lips are contorted, or at least the lips or the eyes, and not in the other conditions. In *stupor* a patient can respond to stimuli but has no fever; in lethargy he is feverish but cannot be aroused.[160]

There is nothing abstract about this procedure that Arnau is recommending to his students. What he is setting forth is in effect a technique of differential diagnosis, something that had always been a fundamental constituent of Galenic medicine considered as practical art.[161] The whole purpose of Galen's little treatise *De rigore* (translated by Arnau from Arabic into Latin in 1282), for example, is just that: to explain how the physician can discriminate among four

---

158 Jackson, "Unusual Mental States," outlines the psychiatric nosology of classical antiquity inherited by the medieval physician.

159 Paniagua, *Arnau de Vilanova*, p. 52.

160 "Recolere debet quod proprium est in appoplexia quod omnis manifesta vite accio cessat excepto anhelitu; in syncopi vero et suffocatione matricis etiam cessat anhelitus, sed in syncopi infrigidantur extrema, facies discoloratur et mortificatur, et frons sudore frigido irroratur. In suffocatione vero matricis nichil istorum apparet. In epilentia vero vultus et oculi et labia torquentur, aut saltem labia vel oculi tantum torquentur aut inversantur, et non in aliis. In stupore quoque patiens excitatus surgere potest et respondere <neque> febricitat, sed litargicus febricitat nec potest surgere nec respondere": Arnau de Vilanova, *Repetitio*, MS Munich CLM 14245, f. 28v; the passage has been omitted from the sixteenth-century editions.

161 See the stimulating article by García Ballester, "Galen as a Medical Practitioner"; he gives an example of Galenic "differential diagnosis" on p. 24 n. 86.

different types of involuntary motion (rigor, tremor, palpitation, and spasm) that his patients may display.[162]

Galenic medical theory characteristically tried to link nosology with clinical manifestations through a materialist physiology: thus the involuntary motions differentiated in *De rigore* were explained as variously produced by complexional factors, hot and cold, within the body. Medieval physicians were faithful to this program and indeed often developed extremely elaborate mechanisms to account for the etiology of diseases, including psychiatric complaints. As we have already seen, one such disease – *amor heroicus*, obsessive love or "lover's malady" – was attracting special attention in the thirteenth and fourteenth centuries.[163] As *heroys*, a variety of *alienatio*, Arnau de Vilanova included this disease among the psychiatric complaints he classified and treated in *De parte operativa*, but his discussion pays less attention to cure than to cause: he describes only psychotherapeutic measures against the disease, designed to distract the sufferer (sweet music, foreign travel, and so forth).[164] This is atypical of the approach usually adopted by *De parte* in its account of psychiatric illnesses, for there in most instances Arnau proposes treatments designed specifically to block the underlying physiological mechanisms responsible for pathological behavior. Mania, he tells us, arises when an excess of adust choler dries and especially heats the brain, thereby giving rise to the uncontrollable restlessness, noisiness, and aggression characteristic of those afflicted by the disease. It should be treated with its qualitative contraries: moistening, diuretic medicines – cold ones are permissible if temperate ones are not available, but hot ones must be avoided.[165]

Thus the medieval medical tradition believed that mental illnesses existed, that they could be diagnosed, distinguished, and treated. It is not clear, however, that the lay public shared that conviction. In all the evidence available from the Crown of Aragon there is very little to show that people thought of mental disorder as a medical problem – or at least as a problem that physicians could relieve. Arnau no doubt felt sure that he could identify and treat *amor heroicus*, but he nowhere refers to his direct experience with the disease, and indeed despite all the recent scholarly interest in the subject only one somewhat questionable reference to an actual sufferer anywhere in the West has been uncovered during the period here in question.[166] The sample of seventy cases

---

[162] The work is summarized in the introduction by Michael R. McVaugh to Galen, *De rigore*, pp. 12–13. An English translation of the Greek was published by Sider and McVaugh, "Galen *On Tremor*."

[163] Above, p. 201.

[164] Arnau de Vilanova, *De parte operativa*, f. 129ra.

[165] Ibid., ff. 127va, 128vb.

[166] The lone reference is in Bona Fortuna's *Tractatus super Viaticum*, composed in the early fourteenth century (perhaps at Montpellier; see above, chapter 3, n. 61): discussing psychotherapies, the author says "Mutatio igitur regionis est valde bona et hoc vidi prodesse, unde

recorded in the *Experimenta* attributed to Arnau includes just two complaints that might be called psychiatric: one of epilepsy (but epilepsy had a unique history), and one of forgetfulness – in the author himself.[167]

In the much wider sample of cases turned up in archival searches throughout the Crown, only one unmistakably reveals a psychiatric patient: a boy afflicted with "stulticia seu oradura" left by his father with a surgeon for a year, on the understanding that if the boy should happen to be cured the 50 *sous* fee would be quadrupled.[168] This could perfectly well have been the father's way of removing disruption from the household; no more than the other instances I have cited is it a convincing sign of public confidence in psychiatry. Indeed, a common familial response to madness was simply to treat it like habitual drunkenness: seize the victim and lock him away.[169] In 1326 Bernat Bisbe became *furiosus* (with occasional lucid intervals), wandering nude through Molins de Rei; his relatives took steps to sequester him lest they be blamed for anything he did.[170] Guillem Mascaró, a Barcelona apothecary who in 1315 likewise became *demens et quoddammodo furiosus*, was captured and sent home in chains to his father.[171] Such sufferers fared no better than the friendless or vagrant insane.[172] Any medical treatment that they may have received is passed over silently; if any was given, it had solved nothing.

Perhaps because there was no widespread conviction that medical expertise was relevant to madness, the determination of mental incompetence was not reserved to physicians. In the very years that leprosy was becoming a medical category, insanity remained fixed firmly as a lay one, even though – like leprosy – it was a label whose consequences were of the utmost importance to an individual or his family. (They were not always undesirable ones: a suicide's

---

feci quod quidam de consilio et consensu parentum suorum fuit <accusatus?> homicidii et compulsus fuit exulare a patria et sanatus est": Wack, *Lovesickness*, p. 262. It seems to me quite conceivable that the "patient" was an authorial invention introduced to reinforce Bona Fortuna's point.

167 McVaugh, "*Experimenta*," gives extracts from the work; Arnau's cure for his own forgetfulness can be found on p. 117. The cure for epilepsy is not transcribed here; in the sole manuscript, Salamanca Universidad 2089, it is numbered "6" on fol. 123va. Paniagua, *Arnau de Vilanova*, p. 62, doubts the authenticity of the separate treatise on epilepsy sometimes ascribed to Arnau. Temkin, *Falling Sickness*, pp. 118–33, surveys late medieval theories of the nature and cause of the disease.

168 AHPT 3847/242v (21 Feb. 1334); above, chapter 5 n. 114.

169 E.g., C 872/29 (27 June 1341), where a father and brother receive permission to put their insensate kinswoman *sub vinculis ferreis*, for fear of shame and scandal – though here drink too seems to have been a factor.

170 C 188/103v (5 Nov. 1326).

171 ADB, Notul. Comm. 3/36.

172 When Juan the son of Lopez became *furiosus et vexatur sepius a demonio cum infirmitatibus huiusmodi agravatur*, and went about attacking people indiscriminately in Daroca, the men of the town were empowered to seize and imprison him (C 454/101r–v; 15 June 1332. The man identified as *furiosus et pauper* in Cervera in 1343 was imprisoned for a time and then expelled (C 623/8).

goods were normally forfeit in law, but not if it could be argued that illness had caused a temporary madness.)[173] Furthermore, insanity was also an accusation that could be leveled out of jealousy or greed. It is impossible not to suspect, for example, that those who claimed that Dominicus Petri Luppi was "so weakened in reason and memory by age and sickness that he cannot administer his affairs" might have had a selfish interest in his estate;[174] or that the sister of Bernat de Piraria was right when she protested that their uncle had induced her dying brother to execute a new will while he was driven out of his mind with pain from an infection (*busayna*).[175] In none of the many legal cases I have found that turn on supposed insanity is there any sign that establishing mental incompetence required an expert and non-partisan medical determination; in the case of Bernat de Piraria, indeed, the king turned to canon lawyers rather than physicians to settle the issue.[176]

Yet in this sphere too medicalization was imminent. By 1375 the insane were being segregated within Barcelona's hospital of en Colom, chained separately in a *casa dels orats*, and the first European hospital created solely for the insane was established in Valencia in 1409.[177] Only three years later, when a Valencian delegate to the Compromise of Caspe (which settled the Aragonese crown on the Trastámara line) seemed mentally incapable of fulfilling his responsibilities, university-trained physicians were incorporated into the tribunal that took testimony from witnesses and pronounced the delegate incompetent to serve.[178] Public willingness to admit a learned medicine into more and more areas of

---

[173] C 39/166v (20 Feb. 1277).

[174] "Ex senectute et quadam valida egritudine qua fuit oppressus adeo defectum racionis atque memorie pateretur quod bona sua amministrare non possit": in Visiedo (Aragon), 1334 (C 467/163). See also the grandson who simply asserts to the king that his grandfather is squandering his wealth because he is *impotens et non compos mentis*, and is granted an administrator for the old man's goods (C 134/229v; 20 Feb. 1305).

[175] C 604/135r–v (11 Dec. 1339).

[176] It might be noted that Clement V at the council of Vienne declared that "Si furiosus aut infans seu dormiens hominem mutilet vel occidat, nullam ex hoc irregularitatem incurrit" (*Clementinarum* V.4.1; *Corpus Juris Canonici*, II, ed. Friedberg, col. 1184), but he did not specify how "furiosus" was to be established. When the niece of Na Barcelona asked that a trustee be appointed for her aunt on the grounds that she was paralyzed and unfit to manage her affairs, it was the judge, not physicians, who visited her and determined that the older woman was "mente capta ut per evidenciam persone sue constat nobis manifeste" (ARV, Just. Civil 19/5v; 20 Jan. 1326). In another case, a woman claimed that her husband "factus fuerit furiosus et ipsa infirmitate laboret in tantum ut de eius sanitatis nulla habetur suspectio, et iam antequam furor ipsum arriperet incepisset male uti bonis suis et in facultatibus minui, ex quo bonorum administratio fuit adiudicata dicte uxori" (C 593/208v–209); once again, a medical diagnosis is lacking.

[177] Cardoner, *Història*, p. 178; Rubio Vela, *Pobreza*, p. 66. The treatment of madness in this hospital still consisted of confinement, although medical attention was given to the patients' other illnesses (Rodrigo Pertegás, *Hospitales*, pp. 26–8).

[178] Ruiz Moreno, "Juicio de insanía." Even so, Peset ("Terminología," 11:82) doubts that the medical testimony weighed importantly in the final decision. Certainly in England lunacy determinations seem to have been made by lay juries (following common-sense views of biological

social life evidently continued undiminished throughout the fourteenth century and beyond.[179]

The irrelevance of collegiality

By the 1340s there are many signs that medical expertise was becoming incorporated into a broad range of social institutions for which, in the earlier Middle Ages, lay opinion had sufficed. It would seem natural that physicians as a group would have appreciated the advantages that these developments could bring and would have encouraged or at least capitalized upon them; we might expect physicians rapidly to have recognized that this expanded social role for the learning they could claim would allow them to profit collectively from the powers being extended to them. Yet in all this period there is no indication that practitioners perceived the opportunities provided by organization and corporate activity. Even in the Crown's largest and wealthiest cities, like Barcelona, where the most learned and ambitious practitioners settled, physicians and surgeons continued to function virtually as individual entrepreneurs. The establishment of licensing requirements in Catalonia and Valencia would have allowed them as a body to take control over the entry to practice, but there is simply no evidence that examinations were yet being used to screen out anyone – except perhaps Jews – from practicing in Barcelona or Valencia. Nor was there a guild structure to enforce internal barriers between the various health occupations; physicians made no collective effort to protect the border between medicine and surgery, which was thus constantly being crossed by surgical émigrés who wanted to associate themselves more closely with the prestige of learning. Despite occasions of cooperative practice often enforced by circumstances, despite the social niche being prepared for the discipline, a sense of occupational community or identity among physicians *as distinct from other kinds of practitioners* apparently had not taken shape by the middle of the century.

What has so far been presented as an argument *ex silentio* fortunately can claim direct support from the actions of the Barcelona physicians in the 1340s: given outright the opportunity of organizing into a *collegium*, thereby to defend their common interest against surgeons, empirics, and competitors generally, they ignored it and continued on their individual courses. This opportunity arose, indirectly, out of a medical response to the one surgical prerogative – a financially important one – that physicians did not have: the right to issue a

and psychological causation) down to early modern times, even though English insane were being admitted to hospital (Bethlehem, in London) by the 1370s; see Rawcliffe, "Hospitals," p. 11, and Neugebauer, "Medieval and Early Modern Theories."

[179] Peset, "Terminología," shows that a technical psychiatric terminology had entered vernacular Catalan literature by the first half of the fifteenth century – in the work of Ausiàs Marc (d. 1459) or Jaume Roig (d. 1478), for example.

desuspitatio, to receive a fee for testifying in criminal trials for assault involving injury or death. Here, though nowhere else, the border between the two occupations *had* become sharply defined by 1340: in only one of the innumerable Catalan *desuspitationes* so far known can a physician be found offering such testimony to a court, and that in a case where he was charged with incompetence and ignorance of surgery because his judgment turned out to be wrong![180] Incompetent or not, the fact that the witness could not claim to be a surgeon was evidently a useful weapon that the parties to the case might brandish if the victim died unexpectedly. In this situation, one might well expect physicians to have been envious of the surgeons' prerogative and to have tried to move in on it – and that did in fact happen; but it was as competing individuals that they pressed the claims of medicine, not as members of a community with disciplinary solidarity.

In April 1341 Pere III wrote to his vicar in Barcelona, instructing him that henceforth a suitable and competent (*bonum et idoneum*) physician was to be included in all *desuspitationes*: the reason for this, the king explained, was that "they have sometimes been performed by surgeons who do not understand illnesses and cannot make prognoses, and who besides are often corrupted by bribes, and therefore it is appropriate to add a suitable physician to the proceedings who will understand the illnesses and the consequences that arise from wounds and blows."[181] The bland presumption in the royal letter that physicians' intellectual formation gave them a broader competence than surgeons ignores the growing tendency of the latter to acquire medical learning; from the letter's tone, it might have been drafted by a physician.

Indeed, there is reason to suspect that it *was* a physician, not the king, who drafted this ruling. The original document had left it to the royal vicar to choose a suitable physician to take part in the procedure, but three days later King Pere wrote again to his vicar and took the choice out of his hands, nominating one Francesc de Pla of Barcelona as the suitable and competent physician who was now to advise the city's surgeons in their *desuspitationes*.[182] Francesc had been in practice in Barcelona for at least twenty-five years, and was (aside from Pere

---

[180] Above, n. 88.

[181] "Cum nonnulli in civitate Barchinone post percussiones et vulnera subsecuta petant et requirant desuspitari seu a suspicione mortis carere percussos sive etiam vulneratos, et hoc fiat aliquociens per aliquos cirurgicos qui infirmitates et eventus ignorant, et aliqui ex eis prece vel precio pluries corrumpantur, et sit decens et congruum ut aliquis phisicus decens et idoneus predicte dessuspitacioni addatur qui sciat cognoscere infirmitates et eventus qui pervenire possunt ex vulneribus et percussionibus supradictis, idcirco volentes super hiis tucius providere, vobis dicimus et expresse mandamus quatenus quociens contigerit quod petatur ut aliquis vulneratus vel percussus desuspitaretur in iurisdiccione vobis comissa semper cum cirurgicis per nos assumendis habeatis et eligatis unum bonum et idoneum phisicum dicte civitatis, qui una cum eis intersit dessuspitacionis predicte, et sine eius consilio qui eventum infirmitatis investiget non possit fieri dessuspitacio supradicta." C 1057/117v–118 (27 April 1341).

[182] C 871/190v–191 (30 April 1341).

Gavet, now inactive) perhaps the senior physician in the city. He had traveled to Sardinia with the infante Alfons' army in 1323, and he had treated both Jaume II and Alfons III in their last illnesses, so that he had long enjoyed the confidence of the royal family.[183] At least once (in 1333) he had taken part in a tribunal to assess the qualifications of an applicant to practice medicine, which again suggests his prominence in his craft, though he appears to have been practically rather than academically trained. Now in 1341 he was using his influence to persuade the king to let physicians move into the one area where surgeons had hitherto enjoyed total authority, thus extending the legal powers of physicians *vis-à-vis* surgeons but vesting these new powers in himself – making him, in practical terms, the head of his craft in Barcelona.

In May of the next year Francesc de Pla moved to consolidate his position and formalize his personal authority over the city's medical corps, physicians and surgeons alike. Two royal charters, both drawn up on 23 May 1342 *ex provisione facta in audientia*, express the realization of his ambitions. The first places Francesc and his presumable kinsman Pere de Pla in charge of examining all physicians and surgeons of doubtful competence; the appointment is presented as a response to the concern expressed by "the medical and surgical practitioners of Barcelona" over the ignorance of many now practicing in the city and the harm they were doing.[184] The second also cites the dangers inherent in medical practice as then being carried on in Barcelona, and responds by giving the city's *medici* (thereby apparently including surgeons as well as physicians) legal existence as a *collegium*, with the rights to elect a rector or prior and four councilors, to certify the competence of would-be practitioners by examination, and to expel incompetents from the city.[185]

Taken together, the three grants won by Francesc from the king in 1341–2 established a corporation of medical practitioners that would have control over its membership by supervising the qualifications of those who wished to practice, a corporation in which physicians were set at the top. Just as the *furs* of 1329 had given the physicians of Valencia city authority over medical activity throughout the kingdom, these documents of 1342 gave the new *collegium* supervisory power not merely over urban Barcelona but over the vicariates of

---

[183] For these biographical details, see RP 290/51v, C 883/71, C 500/226r–v, and RP 306/34. Francesc was in practice as early as 30 June 1316, when he witnessed a document as "fisicus": ACB, manual de Guillem Borrell VI–X 1316, f. 30.

[184] "Ex parte medicorum fisice et cirurgie civitatis eiusdem fuit nobis humiliter suplicatum quod, cum nonnulli in dicta civitate ipsis officiis abutentes inprovidi et ignari in offensam rei publice dampnumque irreparabile plurimorum inferant ob eorum ignoranciam a bonis curis et legitimis deviando personis diversis . . . dignaremur super hoc salubre remedium adhibere." C 617/98r–v; the original document (damaged) is preserved as CRD Pere III 1848. Pere de Pla had had no career of particular distinction, though he is known to have been practicing by 1328.

[185] The document is published by García Ballester, "Orígenes," pp. 148–9. This study briefly alludes (p. 141 n. 55) to the date of the previous document cited, but does not comment on the coincidence of date.

Barcelona and Valls and the bailiwick of Barcelona. But whereas in Valencia the medical community had been placed under the control of municipal authorities, the Barcelona group was left essentially independent: only in holding elections and drawing up regulations was it required to get "advice and consent" from members of the urban *consell* (three were sufficient). Superficially, these documents would seem to reveal the establishment of an autonomous medical profession in Barcelona, what one scholar has interpreted as "the product of the internal dynamic of the Barcelonan physicians."[186] Yet the evidence of the wider context now implies that the "dynamic" behind the royal privileges was not a newly self-aware medical community acting in its own (much less the public) interest, but one well-connected physician – Francesc de Pla – ambitious to advance his own career, and that personal control of the *desuspitatio* and therefore necessarily of surgery had been his original and perhaps principal objective.

Moreover, Francesc's colleagues too proved more interested in the goal of personal financial gain than in the advantages that autonomy and corporate status might bring them. They paid no attention to the powers inherent in the new *collegium*; instead, they wasted little time before attacking Francesc and the original privilege he had extracted from the king, his monopoly over the super-vision of *desuspitationes*. Six months after founding the *collegium* the king responded to a request from another Barcelona physician, Berenguer de Prat (perhaps a newcomer to practice in the city): emphasizing a title Francesc never claimed, "bacallarius in artibus et medicina," Berenguer complained that Francesc's monopoly worked against the public good as well as against the interests of physicians – not just his, Berenguer's, own interests, but those of every other physician in the city. The king's apologetic response withdrew the exclusive privilege and instructed his vicar from now on to allow any competent physician to take part in the procedure. "You have been denying magister Berenguer and other qualified physicians the right to take part in *desuspitationes*, much to the disadvantage of the public, and of those physicians . . . [but]" (the king concluded disingenuously) "it was never our intention that all *desuspitationes* should be carried out by magister Francesc alone."[187] The

---

186 García Ballester, "Orígenes," p. 139.
187 "Pro parte magistri Berengarii de Prato fisici, bacallarii in artibus et medicina, fuit reverenter expositum coram nobis quod . . . vos ipsum magistrum Berengarium necnon alios fisicos civitatis eiusdem sufficientes idoneos et expertos ad desuspitaciones ipsas admittere recusatis in dispendium rei publice necnon ipsius supplicantis et aliorum predictorum evidentem detrimentum. Sane cum intencionis nostre non fuerit nec velimus omnes desuspitaciones per dictum magistrum Franciscum fieri (cum ex hoc posset rei publice dampna varia suboriri), propterea vobis dicimus et mandamus expresse quod ad desuspitaciones ipsas admitatis prefatum magistrum Berengarium de Prato et alios etiam fisicos eiusdem civitatis sufficientes idoneos et expertos, illasque faciatis de et cum consilio eorundem, pretacta nostra littera non obstante." C 874/105 (26 Dec. 1342).

desuspitatio had acquired such social and economic importance that it, not the corporate control of admission to practice, was the real preoccupation of Barcelonan physicians in the 1340s; individual practitioners continued to look out for themselves, whatever they may occasionally have said about the public good.[188]

Indeed, as far as can be ascertained, Francesc's medical *collegium* had only a paper existence for the rest of the decade. There is no evidence that the Barcelona practitioners ever exercised or even asserted their collegial authority to hold examinations and to expel the unqualified. Pere de Soler, a young surgeon from a family of practitioners in Vic, arrived in Barcelona in early 1346 to try his luck in medical practice there. He was unsure enough of his welcome to appeal to Pere III for support, and he obtained from the king a letter commanding the Barcelona physicians to examine the young man and to grant him a license to practice if they found him capable.[189] King Pere addressed his letter, not to the *collegium*, not to a corporate entity, but to four individuals whom in effect he appointed as examiners: Pere de Martorell, who is otherwise unknown; Francesc de Castellar, who had been practicing medicine in the city since at least 1333 but was also a *clericus tonsuratus* and thus probably had some claims to learning; and two other men whom we have already met, Francesc de Pla and Berenguer de Prat – the two protagonists in the quarrel over the *desuspitatio*, four years before, who in this case were compelled to work together.

The impression given by this case that municipal practitioners had not yet come together as a body to control and restrict their craft is confirmed by the details of another examination, arranged a year after Pere de Soler's. This time it was a surgeon who asked to be examined, Romeu de Lirana of Barcelona, and again King Pere simply appointed an examining board: Berenguer Basset, Bernat Vives, Bernat de Pla, and Pere Sinola.[190] Not only did the king's action bypass the supposed *collegium*, ostensibly charged with licensing, but his appointees were not even all medical practitioners: the first two were citizens of Barcelona, representatives of municipal government – and, as it proves, the same two lay representatives had sat on the examining board for another would-be surgeon in 1338.[191] Apparently the licensing procedures of the 1330s remained unchanged a decade later, unaffected by Francesc de Pla's intrigues: the royal vicar, the city councilors, and *probi homines* chose surgical examiners, the town

---

[188] Another sign that the creation of the *collegium* was not responding to a pressing need felt by the city's medical personnel is the fact that five weeks after it had come into existence it was still not the new corporation but the king who was directing the investigation of incompetent practitioners: C 873/160v (1 July 1342).

[189] C 638/132v (12 Feb. 1346).

[190] C 882/141v–142r (2 Jan. 1347).

[191] C 869/158r–v, of 8 July 1340 (confirming the examination dated 22 Oct. 1338).

government selected its own representatives, and together they examined the qualifications of candidates who presented themselves. Evidently the powers conferred by a collegiate structure still seemed irrelevant to the practitioners who could have exercised them.

Conclusion

It does not seem too strong to say that during the first forty years of the fourteenth century the social role of medicine in the Crown of Aragon was transformed, particularly in the wealthier and more urbanized regions. Already in the late thirteenth century it was becoming widely accepted among the public that medical learning made for better medical care – though in most quarters there were not enough medical practitioners to meet the growing demand, and physicians in particular (most of whom can have had little or no academic training) were rare. Public support, from the monarch on down, favored the broad dissemination of at least the generalities of learned medicine at all levels of practice, and this, coupled with a steady increase in the number of secular practitioners as well as in the proportion of physicians who were university-trained, meant that by the 1340s a certain level of medical learning was being assumed as, in principle, a necessary prerequisite for practice.

The introduction of licensing requirements in the 1330s gave this assumption concreteness, even though such requirements were imposed irregularly and sporadically. These were expressions of municipal development and are not to be found in the smaller communities, where the supply of medical personnel with whatever qualifications was still inadequate, due to the practitioners' tendency to gravitate toward more populous and prosperous cities. When examinations were conducted, municipalities turned them over to tribunals in which physicians and surgeons played the preponderant, sometimes the only, role: this can be understood as a further example of the tendency to medicalization – the surrender of public responsibility for health to a medical corps – that in other spheres can already be seen in the late thirteenth century. The acceptance in principle of a system of medical licensing thus sets a seal on what might be called the triumph of a new medical practitioner.

It is superficially tempting to view this process as one of the "professionalization" of medicine. Some historians have indeed already sought to locate the origins of a medical profession in the early fourteenth century. By 1350, so runs the story, physicians had institutionalized a specialized body of knowledge

241

within the university and on that ground had won lay confirmation of their legal identity, the right to control entry into medical practice, and the power to supervise the auxiliary medical occupations.[1] Subsequent medical sociology has followed this outline, using it to elaborate a more nuanced understanding of the profession. Eliot Freidson has argued that while the medieval, university-trained practitioners did constitute a profession, it was merely a narrow "learned" one, one whose monopoly was dependent on state support and could never be wholly effective in excluding empirics and other healers from practice; only when learned medicine gained a scientific foundation in the late nineteenth century and began to have good practical results did it become a "consulting" profession, a monopoly resting not on governmental fiat but on a new public confidence in the effectiveness of medical learning.[2]

Yet neither the historians' nor the sociologists' model seems to conform to developments in the Crown of Aragon. Both assume unquestioningly that learned physicians aim instinctively at professional status and the exclusion of others from practice – that "the spontaneous coming together of the practitioners in associations" needs no further explanation than their common perception of self-interest[3] – and Freidson at least implies that the success of the learned "professionals" must inevitably have been achieved in spite of public resistance to their claims. However, as we have discovered, this was apparently not the case in Spain. There the laity seems in fact to have believed quickly in the promise offered by learned medicine, and to have tried to institutionalize that learning in various ways by delegating responsibility over matters of health to practitioners who might possess specialized knowledge. So far as the evidence goes, it was regularly the lay public – municipal governments, courts of law, patients themselves – who took the lead in the attempted institutionalization of medical knowledge, not the physicians. One might say, using Freidson's terms, that this lay public was trying to call a medical "*consulting* profession" into being, creating a new social role that a self-aware "*learned* profession" did not yet exist to fill.

For despite our modern expectations, early fourteenth-century physicians in the Crown of Aragon were far from conceiving of themselves as a disciplinary community with shared interests and goals. Instead, they were part of a more general community of practitioners in which clear-cut occupational distinctions did not yet exist, practitioners who had all begun to share to a greater or lesser extent in the new learned medical culture. Those who decided to practice as "physicians" had come to their knowledge by a number of different routes, most

---

[1] Bullough, *Development of Medicine*, esp. pp. 4–5, 108–9.
[2] Freidson, *Profession of Medicine*, chap. 1.
[3] A. M. Carr-Saunders and P. A. Wilson, *The Professions* (Oxford, 1933); quoted by Freidson, *Profession of Medicine*, p. 1.

of them still without formal medical education. Under these circumstances, professional association was not a natural instinct; it had to be learned.[4]

Moreover, in the first decades of the century the circumstances of their practice must have reinforced medical individualism and competitiveness. Physicians at the end of the 1200s were true solo practitioners, independent of their colleagues as well as of their clients; their numbers were small and each one served a captive population. As their number increased, however, their patients became able to choose among several physicians, dispersed though they might be over the countryside, and practices could be shaped by client wishes: if physicians did not give their patients what they wanted for the fee they wanted, there were now competitors who would.[5] It was just this sort of client-dependent tyranny that Henri de Mondeville decried so bitterly, and it could spark antagonism and competitiveness until the old assumptions of autonomous solo practice were broken.

On the other hand, the growing number of practitioners of all sorts also meant that they now had more occasion for interchange and for establishing common occupational ground, a process encouraged by the spread of the new medical learning among them, and this in turn fostered cooperative arrangements in practice. Such arrangements perhaps came most naturally to academics, who had acquired a certain solidarity by virtue of their schooling – Arnau de Vilanova's advice to his students took for granted the utility of informal cooperative arrangements among physicians – but practitioners at all levels were soon caught up in them, formally and informally. Nevertheless, the tension between competitive and cooperative tendencies remained unresolved as late as the 1340s; as the dispute over the Barcelonan *desuspitatio* shows, not even the *phisici* had arrived at a sense of shared occupational identity. Individual physicians still saw other members of their craft as the competition; they did not yet appreciate the advantages of organizing to protect and extend their collective interest against other competing health occupations. Personal rather than craft autonomy was still the goal. The physicians of the Crown of Aragon were approaching a sense of narrower community, but they had not yet adopted the "professional" role their society was preparing for them.

How far can the picture presented in this book be generalized to the rest of

---

[4] Park, "Medicine and Society," pp. 80–2, recognizes the existence of a common medical culture among various groups of practitioners in the later Middle Ages, but interprets it as developing *after* the learned profession had established itself as a monopoly, rather than before (as seems to me to have been the case in the Crown of Aragon).

[5] See Freidson, *Profession of Medicine*, p. 92 (and generally his chap. 5): "[such a] physician may neither count on the loyalty of his patient (with whom he has no contract) nor on that of his colleagues (with whom he has no ties and who are competing with him) . . . Under these circumstances, he is quite isolated from his colleagues and relatively free of their control but at the same time he is very vulnerable to control by his clients. To keep them, he must give them what they want – . . . or someone else will."

early fourteenth-century Europe? It will be impossible to be sure until we have systematic, close-grained studies of medicine and society elsewhere during this period. At the moment, the scattered data we have – usually regarding urban centers, or the role of elite practitioners – permit only restricted comparisons, leaving most of the important questions unanswered, but even so they suggest not so much markedly different patterns as different rates of development in different societies. It seems not improbable that the success of the new medical practitioner was originally a southern European phenomenon, encouraged generally by municipal evolution and growth. In the great cities of north-central Italy, like Florence or Bologna, medico-social and -institutional developments seem if anything to have anticipated similar events in the Crown of Aragon, where urban life was somewhat less precocious and medical faculties were markedly less prominent. But the contrast with lesser Italian towns is not so pronounced: Irma Naso's careful examination of medicine in late-medieval Piedmont reveals a medical culture that in most respects is by the fifteenth century remarkably similar to the Crown of Aragon a hundred years before – though she assumes that the presence of medical guilds there after 1400 and of a self-conscious academic profession were inevitable consequences of a professionalizing drive that she reads back into the largely undocumented fourteenth century.[6]

Further north, in England and in France, it is less clear that medico-social relationships kept pace. Certainly the temptation to generalize from metropolitan Paris to France (not to mention Europe) needs to be resisted firmly: the monopolistic control over practice already exercised by the Parisian medical faculty by 1300 was only possible in that particular academic setting, unique in the medieval West.[7] Nevertheless, Margaret Pelling's close studies of medicine in sixteenth-century England depict a medical culture that could be the lineal descendant of the one I have presented: each exhibits a high demand for services in rural as well as urban areas, great occupational diversity in a weakly stratified medical corps, and a variety of financial arrangements reflecting cooperative as well as client-dependent practice.[8] What most differentiates her early modern England from the fourteenth-century Crown of Aragon is a diminished and much less general public enthusiasm for medical learning *per se*, as well perhaps as a self-conscious defensiveness in academic physicians that is quite different from the self-confidence that the earlier Spanish practitioners seem to display. Whether this contrast is due to the passage of time or to the effect of regional peculiarities remains to be seen.

---

6 Naso, *Medici*; this interpretation (which is not a central theme of her study) is reflected at, e.g., pp. 33 and 219.
7 Kibre, "Faculty of Medicine."
8 Pelling, "Medical Practice"; Pelling, "Occupational Diversity"; Pelling and Webster, "Medical Practitioners."

Regional peculiarities there certainly were. The fourteenth-century Crown of Aragon, for example, provided unusual opportunities for Jewish physicians to practice, and we might wonder whether their medical activity helped to retard the emergence there of a sense of occupational identity, since the fact that Jews would have been excluded from cooperative arrangements in their practice meant that competition and the tyranny of the client could never be entirely eliminated. For the moment, however, such speculations await further research, as do questions about changing European attitudes to medicine over time. More than one historian has been willing to suppose that the plague of 1348 must decisively have altered the meaning and character of health care, but there is by no means agreement on how or even whether it did so.[9]

Perhaps this account of an emergent learned medicine in a *pre*-plague society will make it possible some day to decide what lasting medico-social effects the epidemic had, for it can provide a benchmark for future investigations and seems to me to raise at least one new question that deserves to be explored. In the 1340s the lay public in the Crown of Aragon – and perhaps elsewhere – was eager to confer authority on a discipline it had come to perceive as peculiarly knowledgeable as well as trustworthy, a community capable of making dispassionate judgments in the public interest, though the medical practitioners themselves tended to remain autonomous entrepreneurs motivated by self-interest with little if any sense of collective identity and shared purpose: society did not yet recognize that its expectations for medicine had outstripped the reality. Is it too far-fetched to wonder whether this disjunction affected how doctors and patients reacted to each other when, at the end of the 1340s, the promise of the new medical learning was suddenly confronted by the grim reality of the Black Death?

---

[9] Among recent writers, for example, Park sees it as weakening public confidence in medicine and encouraging professional reform among physicians (*Doctors*, pp. 34–42) and as focusing a new attention on public health ("Medicine and Society," p. 87); Gottfried, *Doctors*, makes an extreme claim for its importance in the rise of surgery; while Siraisi ("Physician's Task," p. 108) suggests that it left the medical profession "essentially unchanged." Getz, "Black Death," argues that the trend of recent historical writing is to cast doubt on the disruptive effect of the plague, whether on psychology or on institutions.

Appendix

The reader may find useful an account of the basis on which certain tables in this book have been constructed, an account longer than was feasible in the text proper.

Table 2.3 is based on my systematic search in the archives of Barcelona (ACA, ACB, ADB, AHCB, AHPB), Valencia (AMV, ARV, ACV), and Zaragoza (AMZ, ANZ, ASZ) for named practitioners of the four health occupations, a search virtually exhaustive for the years 1285–1348. I have found relatively little archival material from the years 1348–50, and though I have examined much documentation from the 1350s, my search of that decade is far from complete. These limitations to my investigation make my counts of practitioners more questionable towards the beginning and end of the period studied in this book. I have assumed that a practitioner identified as active in Barcelona in 1324 and 1331, say, was also in the city during the intervening years, and I have so counted him in making up this table. However, practitioners whom I can last identify alive in 1339 (for example) but who actually lived on another fifteen years, unrecorded in the confusion of the plague and overlooked by me in the 1350s, would be missing from my counts for the 1340s, and their disappearance would give rise to an apparent decline that would grow more pronounced as the decade goes on. (This artificial effect does not seem to me to be a full explanation for the gradual shrinkage in number of practitioners already apparent in the 1330s, especially since this contraction is not apparent in the other, smaller communities analyzed in the same way in table 2.4). Because a *reverse* decline effect of this sort may also have influenced the earliest years of my count, I have chosen to begin my year-by-year analysis of urban practitioner levels twenty-five years into the records I have examined, by which time the practitioner population revealed there was more or less stable.

Table 2.5 lists in order of size, as measured by number of hearths, all Catalan towns for whom practitioners have been identified in the ACA, together with the numbers of practitioners of each kind I have found there. I have included Valls in this list even though no practitioners from that town turned up in the archives, so as not to pass over the existence of an important small community. The practitioner from Pallerols was a "healer" and does not fall into any of the four occupational categories. The number of hearths has been taken from the *fogatge* of 1365 published by Iglesies ("Fogaje," pp. 317ff.), with some values missing from that list supplied from the *fogatge* of 1378 printed in *Cortes*, II:55–134, and marked in the table with an asterisk (Pons i Guri, "Fogatjament," pp. 264–7, shows that the date 1378 rather than the traditional one of 1359 is correct). Two other towns boasted a practitioner but were omitted from both *fogatges*: Sant Vicenç dels Horts (a physician) and Arbúcies (a surgeon).

The hearth-counts for the largest Catalan cities in the *fogatge* of 1365 apparently surveyed more than the narrow urban limits and thus already included a part of the "catchment areas" for physicians in those communities. Iglesies (pp. 308ff.) shows that this is the reason why Tarragona, with 1,366 hearths in 1365, was given only 860 in 1378, when her suburban communities were counted separately; similarly, Tortosa fell from 2,006 to 991, Lerida from 2,234 to 1,213, and Montblanc from 601 to 457. I have used these 1378 values (marked with a double asterisk) in order to make the series more nearly consistent internally; if, as Russell argues, the Catalan cities were losing population at this time, the 1365 values might have been 10 to 15 percent higher than those obtained in 1378. Russell (*Medieval Regions*, pp. 166–75) attempts to offer a fuller list of populations in cities and towns throughout the Crown of Aragon at mid-century.

Bibliography

Abulafia, David S. H. "The End of Muslim Sicily." In *Muslims under Latin Rule, 1100–1300*, ed. James M. Powell. Princeton, 1990.

"Monarchs and Minorities in the Late Medieval Western Mediterranean: Lucera and Its Analogues," In *Christendom and Its Discontents*, ed. Peter Diehl and Scott L. Waugh. Berkeley/Los Angeles, forthcoming.

Agrimi, Jole, and Chiara Crisciani. "Medici e 'vetulae' dal duecento al quattrocento: Problemi di una ricerca." In *Cultura popolare e cultura dotta nel seicento (Atti del Convegno di Studio di Genova [23–25 novembre 1982])*, pp. 144–59. Milan, 1983.

d'Alós, Ramon. "De la marmessoria d'Arnau de Vilanova." In *Miscel.lània Prat de la Riba*, I:289–306. Barcelona, n.d.

"Viatges d'investigació a l'Arxiu i Biblioteca Capitular de Tortosa: I. L'Arxiu Capitular de Tortosa." *Butlletí de la Biblioteca de Catalunya* 5 (1918–19): 103–19.

Amundsen, Darrel W. "History of Medical Ethics: Medieval Europe." In *Encyclopedia of Bioethics*, III:938–51. New York/London, 1978.

"Medieval Canon Law on Medical and Surgical Practice by the Clergy." *Bulletin of the History of Medicine* 52 (1978): 22–44.

"The Medieval Catholic Tradition." In *Caring and Curing*, ed. Ronald Numbers and Darrel W. Amundsen, pp. 65–107. New York/London, 1986.

Amundsen, Darrel W., and Gary B. Ferngren. "Evolution of the Patient-Physician Relationship: Antiquity through the Renaissance." In *The Clinical Encounter: The Moral Fabric of the Patient-Physician Relationship*, ed. Earl E. Shelp, pp. 1–46. Dordrecht/Boston, 1983.

"The Forensic Role of Physicians in Roman Law." *Bulletin of the History of Medicine* 53 (1979): 39–56.

Arnau de Vilanova. *Antidotarium*. In *Arnaldi de Villanova . . . Opera* (1520), ff. 243v–262.

Aphorismi de gradibus. Edited by Michael R. McVaugh. *AVOMO*, vol. II. Granada/Barcelona, 1975.

Consilium sive cure febris ethice. In *Opera* (1520), ff. 209v–210.

Contra calculum. In *Opera* (1520), ff. 305-307v.

De cautelis medicorum. In *Opera* (1520), ff. 215v–216v.

De intentione medicorum. In *Opera* (1520), ff. 36–38v.

De ornatu mulierum. In *Opera* (1520), ff. 267v–271v.

248

De parte operativa. In *Opera* (1520), ff. 123–130.

De sigillis. In *Opera* (1520), ff. 301v–302.

De simplicibus. In *Opera* (1520), ff. 233v–243v.

De vinis. In *Opera* (1520), ff. 262–265v.

Epistola de dosi tyriacalium medicinarum. Edited by Michael R. McVaugh. *AVOMO*, III:55–91. Barcelona, 1985.

Medicationis parabole. Edited by Juan A. Paniagua. *AVOMO*, vol. VI, part 1. Barcelona, 1990.

Obres Catalanes. Edited by Miquel Batllori. 2 vols. Barcelona, 1947.

Opera. Lyons, 1520.

Opera Medica Omnia (AVOMO). Ed. Luis García Ballester, Michael R. McVaugh, and Juan A. Paniagua. Granada, 1975; Barcelona, 1981– .

Regimen sanitatis ad regem Aragonum. In *Opera* (1520), ff. 82–86.

Repetitio super canone vita brevis. In *Opera* (1520), ff. 275v–281.

Speculum medicine. In *Opera* (1520), ff. 1–36.

Tractatus de amore heroico. Edited by Michael R. McVaugh. *AVOMO*, III:1–54. Barcelona, 1985.

Tractatus de consideracionibus operis medicine sive de flebotomia. Edited by Luke Demaitre. *AVOMO*, vol. IV. Barcelona, 1988.

Arribas Palau, Antonio, *La conquista de Cerdeña por Jaime II de Aragón*. Barcelona, 1952.

Ascheri, Mario. "'Consilium sapientis,' perizia medica e 'res iudicata': Diritto dei 'dottori' et istituzioni comunali." In *Proceedings of the Fifth International Congress of Medieval Canon Law*, ed. Stephan Kuttner and Kenneth Pennington, pp. 533–79. *Monumenta Iuris Canonici* Series C: Subsidia. Vol. VI. Vatican City, 1980.

Assis, Yom Tov. "Juifs de France réfugiés en Aragon (XIIIe–XIVe siècles)." *Revue des Etudes Juives* 142 (1983): 285–322.

Avezou, Robert. "Un prince aragonais archevêque de Tolède au XIVe siècle, D. Juan de Aragón y Anjou." *Bulletin Hispanique* 32 (1930): 326–71.

Avicenna. *Liber canonis*. Venice, 1507; rpt., Hildesheim, 1964.

Baer, (Yitzhak) Fritz. *A History of the Jews in Christian Spain*. 2 vols. Philadelphia, 1961.

Die Juden im Christlichen Spanien. Part 1, Urkunden und Regesten. Vol. I, *Aragonien und Navarra*. Berlin, 1929/1936; rpt., England, 1970.

Barber, Malcolm. "Lepers, Jews and Moslems: The Plot to Overthrow Christendom in 1321." *History* 66 (1981): 1–17.

Barthélemy, Louis. *Les médecins à Marseille avant et pendant le moyen âge*. Marseille, 1883.

Batlle i Gallart, Carme. "Els apotecaris de Barcelona en el món dels negocies pels volts de 1300." *Cuadernos de Historia Económica de Cataluña* 18 (1978): 97–109.

"La ayuda a los pobres en la parroquia de San Justo de Barcelona." In *A pobreza e a assistência aos pobres na península ibérica durante a idade média*, 1:59–71. Actas das 1as Jornadas Luso-Espanholas de História Medieval. Lisbon, 1973.

Batlle i Gallart, Carme, and Montserrat Casas i Nadal. "La caritat privada i les institucions benèfiques de Barcelona (segle XIII)." In *La pobreza y la asistencia a los pobres en la Cataluña medieval*, ed. Manuel Riu, pp. 117–90. Anuario de Estudios Medievales, anejo 9. Barcelona, 1980.

Bautier, Robert-Henri. "Un nouvel ensemble documentaire pour l'histoire des pestes du XIVe siècle: L'exemple de la ville de Vich en Catalogne." *Comptes Rendus de l'Académie des Inscriptions et Belles-Lettres*, 1988 (April–June), 432–55.

Bayerri Bertomeu, Enrique. *Los codices medievales de la catedral de Tortosa.* Tortosa, 1962.

Historia de Tortosa y su comarca. 8 vols. Tortosa, 1933–59.

Beaujouan, Guy. "Manuscrits médicaux du Moyen Age conservés en Espagne." *Mélanges de la Casa de Velázquez* 8 (1972): 161–221.

Beltrán, Antonio, José María Lacarra, and Angel Canellas. *Historia de Zaragoza.* Vol. I, *Edades antigua y media.* Zaragoza, 1976.

Benton, John F. "The Birthplace of Arnau de Vilanova: A Case for Villanueva de Jiloca near Daroca." *Viator* 13 (1982): 245–57.

Berica, Fr. "La persécution des lépreux dans la France méridionale en 1321." *Moyen Age* 93 (1987): 203–21.

Bernard Gordon. *Lilium medicine.* Venice, 1498.

Bertran i Roigé, Prim. "El menjador de l'almoina de la catedral de Lleida. Notes sobre l'alimentació dels pobres Lleidatans al 1338." *Ilerda* 40 (1979): 89–124.

Bisson, T. N. *The Medieval Crown of Aragon.* Oxford, 1986.

Blue, Catherine Ann. "Ermengaud Blasi, Medieval Physician and Scholar." M.A. thesis, University of North Carolina, 1978.

Bofarull y Sans, Francisco, ed. *Gremios y cofradías de la antigua corona de Aragón*, vol. II. In *Colección de documentos inéditos del archivo general de la corona de Aragón*, ed. Bofarull y Sans, vol. XLI. Barcelona, 1910.

Bonnassie, Pierre. *La organización del trabajo en Barcelona a fines del siglo XV.* Anuario de Estudios Medievales, anejo 8. Barcelona, 1975.

Boswell, John. *The Royal Treasure.* New Haven/London, 1977.

Brezzi, Paolo, and Egmont Lee, eds. *Sources of Social History: Private Acts of the Late Middle Ages.* Toronto, 1984.

Brody, Saul Nathaniel. *The Disease of the Soul.* Ithaca/London, 1974.

Brown, Judith C. "A Woman's Place was in the Home: Women's Work in Renaissance Tuscany." In *Rewriting the Renaissance*, ed. Margaret W. Ferguson, Maureen Quilligan, and Nancy J. Vickers, pp. 206–24. Chicago/London, 1986.

Bullough, Vern L. *The Development of Medicine as a Profession: The Contribution of the Medieval University to Modern Medicine.* Basle/New York, 1966.

Bullough, Vern L., and James Brundage, eds. *Sexual Practices and the Medieval Church.* Buffalo, 1982.

Burns, Robert I. "Los hospitales del reino de Valencia en el siglo XIII." *Anuario de Estudios Medievales* 2 (1965): 135–54.

"Muslims in the Thirteenth-Century Realms of Aragon: Interaction and Reaction." In *Muslims under Latin Rule, 1100–1300*, ed. James M. Powell, pp. 57–102. Princeton, 1990.

Society and Documentation in Crusader Valencia. Princeton, 1985.

"Spanish Islam in Transition: Acculturative Survival and Its Price in the Christian Kingdom of Valencia, 1240–1280." In *Islam and Cultural Change in the Middle Ages*, ed. Speros Vyronis, Jr., pp. 87–105. Wiesbaden, 1975. (Reprinted in Robert I. Burns, *Moors and Crusaders in Mediterranean Spain.* London, 1978.)

Bylebyl, Jerome J. "The Medical Meaning of *Physica*." *Osiris*, 2nd ser., 6 (1990): 16–41.

Caille, J. *Hôpitaux et charité publique à Narbonne au Moyen Age*. Toulouse, 1978.

Calvanico, Raffaele. *Fonti per la storia della medicina e della chirurgia per il regno di Napoli nel periodo Angioino (a. 1273–1410)*. Naples, 1962.

del Campillo, Toribio. *Documentos históricos de Daroca y su comunidad*. Zaragoza, 1915.

Cardoner i Planas, Antoni. "Ejemplos de especialización médica durante los siglos XIV y XV." *Anales de Medicina* 42 (1956): 201–3.

———. *Història de la medicina a la Corona d'Aragò*. Barcelona, [1973].

———. "El linaje de los Cabrit en relación con la medicina del siglo XIV." *Sefarad* 16 (1956): 357–67.

———. "El médico judío Benvenist Samuel y su parentesco con Samuel Benvenist de Barcelona." *Sefarad* 1 (1941): 327–45.

———. "Nuevos datos acerca de Jafuda Bonsenyor." *Sefarad* 4 (1944): 287–93.

Cardoner i Planas, Antoni, and Francisca Vendrell Gallostra. "Aportaciones al estudio de la familia Abenardut, médicos reales." *Sefarad* 7 (1947): 303–48.

Carlin, Martha. "Medieval English Hospitals." In *The Hospital in History*, ed. Lindsay Granshaw and Roy Porter, pp. 21–39. London/New York, 1989.

Carreras Artau, Joaquim. "La llibreria d'Arnau de Vilanova." *AST* 11 (1935): 63–84.

Carreras y Candi, Francesch. "Ordinacions urbanes de bon govern a Catalunya." *BRABLB* 11 (1924): 292–334, 365–431; 12 (1925–6): 37–62, 121–53, 189–208, 286–95; 13 (1927): 368–80, 419–23, 520–33.

Carreras Valls, Ricard. "Introducció a la història de la cirurgia a Catalunya: Bernat Serra i altres cirurgians Catalans il.lustres de segle XIV." In *Tres treballs premiats en el concurs d'homenatge a Gimbernat*, pp. 1–63. Masnou, 1936.

Cartulaire de l'Université de Montpellier. Vol. I. Montpellier, 1890.

Chabás, Roque. "Inventario de los libros, ropas y demás efectos de Arnaldo de Villanueva." *Revista de Archivos, Bibliotecas y Museos* 9 (1903): 189–203.

The Chronicle of San Juan de la Peña. Translated by Lynn H. Nelson. Philadelphia, 1991.

Cifuentes i Comamala, Lluis. "La medicina i els professionals de la sanitat en les expedicions militars a Sardenya de 1323–24 i 1354–55." Tesi de llicenciatura, Universitat Autónoma de Barcelona, Facultat de Ciències, Seminari d'Història de les Ciències, 1990.

Coing, Helmut, ed. *Handbuch der Quellen und Literatur der neuren Europäischen Privatrechtsgeschichte*. Vol. I, *Mittelalter*. Munich, 1973.

Comenge y Ferrer, Luis. "Formas de munificencia real para con los archiatros de Aragón." *BRABLB* 2, año 3 (1903): 1–15.

———. "Historia de la medicina en Cataluña (Continuación)." *Revista de Ciencias Médicas de Barcelona* 22 (1896): 177–90.

———. *La medicina en Cataluña (bosquejo histórico)*. Barcelona, n.d.

———. *La medicina en el reino de Aragón, siglo XIV*. Valladolid, 1974.

———. "Nuevos documentos relativos a la historia de la medicina en el reino de Aragón." *Gaceta Médica Catalana* 28, no. 670 (31 May 1905): 289–94.

———. *Receptari de Manresa (siglo XIV)*. Barcelona, 1899.

Conde y Delgado de Molina, Rafael. "Análisis de la tipología documental del siglo XIV: Fuentes del Archivo de la Corona de Aragón." In *La mutación de la segunda mitad del siglo xiv en España*, ed. Federico Udina Martorell, pp. 47–69. Cuadernos de Historia, no. 8. Madrid, 1977.

"Fonts per a l'estudi del consum alimentari en els temps medievals." In *Alimentació i societat a la Catalunya medieval*. Anuario de Estudios Medievales, Anex 20. Barcelona, 1988.

Contreras, Antonio. "La difusión de la Cyrurgia de Teodorico Borgognoni en los paises de habla catalana." Tesis de Licenciatura en Medicina, University of Cantabria, 1986.

Corbella, Ramon. *La aljama de juheus de Vich*. Vich, 1909.

Corpus Iuris Civilis Iustinianei. Lyons, 1627; rpt., Osnabrück, 1965.

Cortes de los Antiguos Reinos de Aragón y de Valencia y principado de Cataluña, vol. I, part 1. Madrid, 1896.

Cosman, Madeleine Pelner. "Medieval Medical Malpractice: The Dicta and the Dockets." *Bulletin of the New York Academy of Medicine* 49 (1973): 22–47.

"The Medieval Medical Third Party: Compulsory Consultation and Malpractice Insurance." *Annals of Plastic Surgery* 8 (1982): 152–62.

Crisciani, Chiara. "History, Novelty, and Progress in Scholastic Medicine." *Osiris*, 2nd ser., 6 (1990): 118–39.

Daems, Willem F. "Ermengald Blasius' Tabellen zum 'Antidotarium Nicolai.'" *Pharmaceutica Acta Helvetiae* 4 (1979): 1–6.

Daston, Lorraine, and Katharine Park. "Hermaphrodites in Renaissance France." *Critical Matrix* 1, no. 5 (1985).

Delmas, Bruno. "Médailles astrologiques et talismaniques dans le Midi de la France (XIIIe–XVIe siècle)." *96e Congrès national des sociétés savantes, archéologie*, 2:437–54. Toulouse, 1971.

Demaitre, Luke E. "The Description and Diagnosis of Leprosy by Fourteenth-Century Physicians." *Bulletin of the History of Medicine* 59 (1985): 327–44.

Doctor Bernard de Gordon: Professor and Practitioner. Toronto, 1980.

"The Idea of Childhood and Child Care in Medical Writings of the Middle Ages." *Journal of Psychohistory* 4 (1977): 461–90.

Diepgen, Paul. "Arnalds Stellung zur Magie, Astrologie und Oneiromantie." *Archiv für Geschichte der Medizin* 5 (1911–12): 88–115. (Reprinted in Paul Diepgen, *Medizin und Kultur*, pp. 150–72. Stuttgart, 1938.)

Die Theologie und der ärztliche Stand. Studien zur Geschichte der Beziehungen zwischen Theologie und Medizin im Mittelalter, vol. I. Berlin/Grunewald, 1922.

Dols, Michael W. *The Black Death in the Middle East*. Princeton, 1977.

Medieval Islamic Medicine. Berkeley/Los Angeles/London, 1984.

Dossat, Yves. *Saisimentum comitatus Tholosani*. Collection de documents inédits sur l'histoire de France, octavo ser., vol. I. Paris, 1966.

Dufourcq, Charles-E. "Prix et niveaux de vie dans les pays catalans et maghribins à la fin du XIIIe et au début du XIVe siècles." *Le Moyen Age* 20 (1965): 475–520.

Dufourcq, Charles-E., and Jean Gautier-Dalché. *Historia económica y social de la España cristiana en la edad media*. Barcelona, 1983.

Dulieu, Louis. *La pharmacie à Montpellier de ses origines à nos jours*. Avignon, [1973].

Durán Gudiol, Antonio. *La Judería de Huesca*. Colección Basica Aragonesa, vol. 46. Zaragoza, 1984.

Duran i Sanpere, Agustí. *Llibre de Cervera*. Barcelona, 1977.

Duran y Sanpere, Agustín, and F. Gómez Gabarnet. "Las escuelas de gramática en Cervera." *BRABLB* 17 (1944): 5–77.

Dureau-Lapeyssonnie, Jeanne-Marie. "L'œuvre d'Antoine Ricart, médecin catalan du XVe siècle." In *Médecine humaine et vétérinaire à la fin du moyen âge*, by Guy Beaujouan, Yvonne Poulle-Drieux, and Jeanne-Marie Dureau-Lapeyssonnie, pp. 171–364. Geneva/Paris, 1966.

Edelstein, Ludwig. *Ancient Medicine*. Baltimore, 1967.

Emery, Richard W. "Jewish Physicians in Medieval Perpignan." *Michael* 12 (1991): 113–34.

The Jews of Perpignan. New York, 1959.

Esmein, A. *Le mariage en droit canonique*. 2 vols. Paris, 1891; rpt., New York, 1968.

Evans, Joan. *Magical Jewels of the Middle Ages and the Renaissance*. Oxford, 1922; rpt., New York, 1976.

Faraudo de Saint-Germain, Luis. "El 'Libre de Sent Sovi': Recetario de cocina catalana medieval." *BRABLB* 24 (1951–2): 5–81.

Fasoli, Gina, and Pietro Sella, eds. *Statuti de Bologna dell'anno 1288*. Studi e Testi, vol. 73. Vatican City, 1937.

Finke, Heinrich. *Acta Aragonensia*. 3 vols. Berlin, 1908–22; rpt., Aalen, 1966.

Aus den Tagen Bonifaz VIII. Munich, 1902.

"Nachträge und Ergänzungen zu den Acta Aragonensia Band 1–3." In *AA*, III:585–768; reprinted from *Spanische Forschungen der Görresgesellschaft*, ser. 1, 4 (1933): 355–536.

Finucane, Ronald C. *Miracles and Pilgrims: Popular Beliefs in Medieval England*. London/Melbourne/Toronto, 1977.

Fischer-Homburger, Esther. *Medizin vor Gericht: Gerichtsmedizin von der Renaissance bis zur Aufklärung*. Bern/Stuttgart/Vienna, 1983.

Fita y Colomer, Fidel. *Lo llibre vert de Manresa*. Barcelona, 1880.

Flinn, Michael W. *The European Demographic System, 1500–1820*. Baltimore, 1981.

Font y Rius, José María. "El desarollo general del derecho en los territorios de la Corona de Aragón (sig. XII–XIV)." *7 Congrés d'Història de la Corona d'Aragó*, 1:290–326. Barcelona, 1962.

Foucault, Michel. *The History of Sexuality*. 3 vols. New York, 1980–6.

Fournier, Marcel. *Les statuts et privilèges des universités françaises depuis leur fondation jusqu'en 1789*. 4 vols. Paris, 1890–4; rpt., Aalen, 1970.

Franco Sánchez, Francisco, and María Sol Cabello García. *Muḥammad aš-Šafra, el medico y su época*. Alicante, 1990.

Freedman, Paul H. *The Diocese of Vic: Tradition and Regeneration in Medieval Catalonia*. New Brunswick, 1983.

The Origins of Peasant Servitude in Medieval Catalonia. Cambridge, 1991.

Freidson, Eliot. *Profession of Medicine*. New York, 1971.

Freitag, Robert. "Die katalanischen Handwerkerorganisationen unter Königsschutz im Mittelalter insbesondere Aufbau und Aufgaben im 14. Jahrhundert." *Gesammelte Aufsätze zur Kulturgeschichte Spaniens* 24 (1968): 41–226.

Friedberg, Aemilius. *Corpus Juris Canonici*. 2 vols. Leipzig, 1879; rpt., Graz, 1959.

Fullana Mira, Luis. "La casa de Lauria en el Reino de Valencia." *III Congreso de Historia de la Corona de Aragón*, 1:65–164. Valencia, 1923.

Furs e ordinations fetes per los gloriosos reys de Arago als regnícols del regne de Valencia. Valencia, 1492; rpt., Valencia, 1976.

Galen. *De rigore: Translatio libri Galieni de rigore et tremore et iectigatione et spasmo.* Edited by Michael R. McVaugh. *AVOMO,* vol. XVI. Barcelona, 1981.

———. *On Examinations by Which the Best Physicians Are Recognized.* Edited by Albert Z. Iskandar. *CMG* Supplementum Orientale, vol. IV. Berlin, 1988.

García Ballester, Luis. "Arnau de Vilanova (c. 1240–1311) y la reforma de los estudios médicos en Montpellier (1309): El Hipócrates y la introducción del nuevo Galeno." *Dynamis* 2 (1982): 97–158.

———. "Galen as a Medical Practitioner: Problems in Diagnosis." In *Galen: Problems and Prospects,* ed. Vivian Nutton, pp. 13–46. London, 1981.

———. *Historia social de la medicina en la España de los siglos XIII al XVI.* Vol. I. Madrid, 1976.

———. "Medical Science in Thirteenth-Century Castile: Problems and Prospects." *Bulletin of the History of Medicine* 61 (1987): 183–202.

———. "Los orígenes de la profesión médica en Cataluña: El 'collegium' de médicos de Barcelona (1342)." In *Estudios dedicados a Juan Peset Aleixandre,* I:129–49. Valencia, 1982.

García-Ballester, Luis, Lola Ferre, and Eduard Feliu. "Jewish Appreciation of Fourteenth-Century Scholastic Medicine." *Osiris,* 2nd ser., 6 (1990): 85–117.

García Ballester, Luis, and Michael R. McVaugh. "Nota sobre el control de la actividad médica y quirúrgica de los barberos (*barbers, barbitonsores*) en los *furs* de Valencia de 1329." In *Homenatge al doctor Sebastià Garcia Martínez,* I:73–88. Valencia, 1988.

García-Ballester, Luis, Michael R. McVaugh, and Agustín Rubio-Vela. *Medical Licensing and Learning in Fourteenth-Century Valencia. Transactions of the American Philosophical Society* 79, part 6 (1989).

Garosi, A. "Perizie e periti medico legali in alcuni capitoli di legislazione statuaria medioevali." *Rivista di Storia delle Scienze Mediche e Naturali* 29 (1938): 157–67.

Gaya Massot, Ramón. "Por qué se retardó la fundación de la Universidad de Barcelona." *AST* 25 (1952): 165–73.

———. "Provisión de cátedras en el estudio general de Lérida." *AST* 30 (1958): 233–96.

Getz, Faye Marie. "Archives and Sources: Medical Practitioners in Medieval England." *Social History of Medicine* 3 (1990): 245–83.

———. "Black Death and the Silver Lining: Meaning, Continuity, and Revolutionary Change in Histories of Medieval Plague." *Journal of the History of Biology* 24 (1991): 265–89.

Giménez Soler, Andrés. *Don Juan Manuel.* Zaragoza, 1932.

Girona i Llagostera, Daniel. "Itinerari de l'infant Pere (després Pere III) (1319–1336)." *EUC* 18 (1933): 336–56; 19 (1934): 81–262.

Given, James Buchanan. *Society and Homicide in Thirteenth-Century England.* Stanford, 1977.

Glick, Thomas R. "*Muhtasib* and *Mustasaf*: A Case Study of Institutional Diffusion." *Viator* 11 (1971): 59–81.

Goltz, Dietlinde. *Mittelalterliche Pharmazie und Medizin, dargestellt an Geschichte und Inhalt des Antidotarium Nicolai. Veröffentlichungen der internationalen Gesellschaft für Geschichte der Pharmazie,* n.s., 44 (1976).

González Antón, Luis. "Las cortes aragonesas en el reinado de Jaume II." *Anuario de Historia del Derecho Español* 47 (1977): 523–682.

González Hurtebise, Eduardo, ed. *Libros de tesorería de la casa real de Aragón.* Vol. I. Barcelona, 1911.

González y Sugrañes, Miquel. *Contribució a la historia dels antichs gremis dels arts y oficis de la ciutat de Barcelona.* Vol. I. Barcelona, 1915.

Gottfried, Robert S. *Doctors and Medicine in Medieval England, 1340–1530.* Princeton, 1986.

"English Medical Practitioners, 1340–1530." *Bulletin of the History of Medicine* 58 (1984): 164–82.

Gouron, André. *La réglementation des métiers en Languedoc au moyen âge.* Geneva/ Paris, 1958.

Grau i Monserrat, Manuel. "Medicina a Besalú (s. xiv) (metges, apotecaris i manescales)." *Annals Patronat d'Estudis Històrics d'Olot i Comarca 1982–3,* pp. 105–11. Olot, 1984.

"Metges jueus a Besalú (s. XIV)." *Actes,* I Assemblea d'Estudis sobre el comtat de Besalú, 1968, pp. 29–33. Olot, 1972.

Grayzel, Solomon. *The Church and the Jews in the XIIIth Century.* Philadelphia, 1933; rev. edn, New York, 1966.

Green, Monica. "Problems of Documenting Medieval Women's Medical Practice." Forthcoming.

"Women's Medical Practice and Health Care in Medieval Europe." *Signs* 14 (1989): 434–73.

Grewe, Rudolf, ed. *Libre de Sent Sovi.* Barcelona, 1979.

Guilleré, Christian. "Assistance et charité à Gérone au début du XIVème siècle." In *La pobreza y la asistencia a los pobres en la Cataluña medieval,* ed. Manuel Riu, I:191–204. Anuario de Estudios Medievales, anejo 9. Barcelona, 1980.

"Une famille de médecins au XIVe siècle: Les ça Riera." Unpublished paper.

Hamarneh, S. K. "Origin and Function of the Ḥisbah System in Islam and its Impact on the Health Professions." *Sudhoffs Archiv* 48 (1964): 157–73.

Hammond, E. A. "Incomes of Medieval Doctors." *Journal of the History of Medicine* 15 (1960): 154–69.

Henderson, John. "The Hospitals of Late-Medieval and Renaissance Florence: A Preliminary Survey." In *The Hospital in History,* ed. Lindsay Granshaw and Roy Porter, pp. 63–92. London/New York, 1989.

Hillgarth, J. N. *The Spanish Kingdoms 1250–1516.* 2 vols. Oxford, 1976.

Hillgarth, J. N., and Giulio Silano. *The Register Notule Communium 14 of the Diocese of Barcelona.* Toronto, 1983.

Hippocratic Writings. Edited by G. E. R. Lloyd. Harmondsworth, 1978.

Hoffman, Gerda. "Beiträge zur Lehre von der durch Zauber verursachten Krankheit und ihrer Behandlung in der Medizin des Mittelalters." *Janus* 37 (1933): 129–44, 179–92, 211–20.

Horden, Peregrine. "A Discipline of Relevance: The Historiography of the Later Medieval Hospital." *Social History of Medicine* 1 (1988): 359–74.

Huici Miranda, Ambrosio, and María Desamparados Cabanes Pecourt. *Documentos de Jaume I de Aragón.* Vol. IV. Textos Medievales, no. 55. Zaragoza, 1982.

Hunt, Tony. *Popular Medicine in Thirteenth-Century England.* Cambridge, 1990.

Iglesies Fort, José. "El fogaje de 1365–1370: Contribución al conocimiento de la población de Cataluña en la segunda mitad del siglo XIV." *Memorias de la Real Academia de Ciencias y Artes de Barcelona* 34, no. 11 (1962): 249–356.

Jackson, Stanley W. "Unusual Mental States in Medieval Europe. I: Medical Syndromes of Mental Disorder." *Journal of the History of Medicine*, 27 (1972): 262–97.

Jacquart, Danielle. "Medical Explanations of Sexual Behavior in the Middle Ages." *Homo Carnalis, Acta*, 14 (1987): 1–21.

Le milieu médical en France du XIIe au XVe siècle. Geneva, 1981.

"La réception du Canon d'Avicenne: Comparaison entre Montpellier et Paris au XIIIe et XIVe siècles." *Actes du 110e Congrès national des sociétés savantes – Montpellier, 1985*, 2:69–77. Paris, 1985.

Supplément to Ernest Wickersheimer, *Dictionnaire biographique des médecins en France au moyen âge.* Geneva, 1979.

Jacquart, Danielle, and Claude Thomasset. *Sexuality and Medicine in the Middle Ages.* Princeton, 1988.

James, Montague Rhodes. *A Descriptive Catalogue of the Manuscripts in the Library of Peterhouse.* Cambridge, 1899.

Jaume d'Agramunt. *"Regiment de preservació de pestilència" de Jacme d'Agramont (S. XIV).* Edited by Joan Veny i Clar. Tarragona, 1971.

Jeanselme, E. "Comment l'Europe, au Moyen Age, se protégea contre la lèpre." *Bulletin de la Société Française d'Histoire de la Médecine* 25 (1931): 1-155.

Jenks, Stuart. "Medizinische Fachkräfte in England zur Zeit Heinrichs VI (1428/29–1460/61)." *Sudhoffs Archiv* 69 (1985): 214–27.

Johannes de Sancto Amando. *Expositio supra Antidotarium Nicolai.* In *Ioannis Mesuae Medici Clarissimi Opera*, 2 vols. in one, II:ff. 192–232. Venice, 1581.

Jordan, William Chester. *The French Monarchy and the Jews.* Philadelphia, 1989.

Jordi, R. "Curioso documento inédito de año 1333 y muerte burocrática de la triaca." *Athena*, no. 72 (Oct. 1977): 4–12.

Jordi González, Ramón. "Viejos papeles del siglo XIV: 1312–1316–1339–1336." *Boletín Informativa de Circular Farmaceutica* 80 (1976): 1–7.

"Viejos papeles del siglo XIV: 1334–1344–1354." *Boletín informativa de Circular Farmaceutica* 79 (1975): 55–60.

Juan Manuel, Don. *Libro de la caza.* Edited by José María Castro y Calvo. Barcelona, 1947.

Libro de los estados. Edited by R. B. Tate and I. R. Macpherson. Oxford, 1974.

Libro infinido. Edited by Pascual de Gayangos. *Biblioteca de autores españoles*, 51:264–75. Madrid, 1860; rpt., Madrid, 1952.

Kantorowicz, Hermann. "Cino da Pistoia ed il primo trattato di medicina legale." *Archivo Storico Italiano* 37 (1906): 115–28. (Reprinted in Kantorowicz, *Rechthistorische Schriften*, ed. Helmut Coing and Gerhard Immel, pp. 287–97. Karlsruhe, 1970.)

Karl, Ludwig. "Théodoric de l'ordre des prêcheurs et sa chirurgie." *Bulletin de la Société Française d'Histoire de la Médecine* 23 (1929): 140–83.

"Theodoric der Katalane und seine Chirurgie." *Zeitschrift für romanische Philologie* 49 (1929): 236–72.

Kealey, Edward J. *Medieval Medicus: A Social History of Anglo-Norman Medicine.* Baltimore/London, 1981.

Kibre, Pearl. "The Faculty of Medicine at Paris, Charlatanism and Unlicensed Medical Practices in the Later Middle Ages." *Bulletin of the History of Medicine* 27 (1953): 1–20.

Kieckhefer, Richard. *Magic in the Middle Ages*. Cambridge, 1989.

Kristeller, Paul Oskar. *Studi sulla scuola medica salernitana*. Naples, 1986.

La Torre y del Cerro, Antonio de, ed. *Documentos para la Historia de la Universidad de Barcelona*. Vol. I: Preliminares (1289–1451). Barcelona, 1971.

Ledesma Rubio, María Luisa, and María Isabel Falcón Pérez. *Zaragoza en la baja edad media*. Zaragoza, 1977.

Lerner, Robert E. "The Pope and the Doctor." *Yale Review* 78 (1988–9): 62–79.

Lladonosa Pujol, Josep. *Lérida medieval*. 2 vols. Lerida, 1974.

Llull, Ramon. *Libre de contemplació en Deu*, vol. III. Published as *Obres de Ramon Lull*, vol. IV. Palma de Mallorca, 1910.

Libre de Evast e Blanquerna. Edited by Salvador Galmés. 2 vols. Barcelona, 1935–47.

López de Meneses, Amada. "Documentos culturales de Pedro el Ceremonioso." *Estudios de Edad Media de la Corona de Aragón* 5 (1952): 669–771.

McVaugh, Michael R. "Arnau de Vilanova's *Regimen Almarie* (*Regimen castra sequentium*) and Medieval Military Medicine." *Viator* 23 (1992): 201–13.

"Bernat de Berriacho (*fl.* 1301–43) and the *Ordinacio* of Bishop Ponç de Gualba." *Arxiu de Textos Catalans Antics* 9 (1990): 240–54.

"The Births of the Children of Jaime II." *Medievalia* (Barcelona) 6 (1986): 7–16.

"The *Experimenta* of Arnald of Villanova." *Journal of Medieval and Renaissance Studies* 1 (1971): 107–18.

"Further Documents for the Biography of Arnau de Vilanova." *Dynamis* 2 (1982): 363–72.

"Islamic Medicine in the Kingdom of Aragon in the Early Fourteenth Century." *Proceeding of the Third International Conference on Islamic Medicine*, pp. 63–7. Kuwait, 1984.

"The Nature and Limits of Medical Certitude at Early Fourteenth-Century Montpellier." *Osiris*, 2nd ser., 6 (1990): 62–84.

"Nota sobre las relaciones entre dos maestros de Montpellier: Arnau de Vilanova y Bernardo Gordon." *Asclepio* 25 (1973): 331–6.

"Quantified Medical Theory and Practice at Fourteenth-Century Montpellier." *Bulletin of the History of Medicine* 43 (1969): 397–413.

"Royal Surgeons and the Value of Medical Learning: The Crown of Aragon, 1300–1350." In *Practical Medicine from Salerno to the Black Death*. Cambridge, forthcoming.

"The Two Faces of a Medical Career: Jordanus de Turre of Montpellier." In *Mathematics and Its Applications to Science and Natural Philosophy in the Middle Ages*, ed. Edward Grant and John E. Murdoch, pp. 301–24. Cambridge, 1987.

McVaugh, Michael R., and Luis García Ballester. "The Medical Faculty at Early Fourteenth-Century Lerida." *History of Universities* 8 (1989): 1–25.

Makowski, Elizabeth. "The Conjugal Debt and Medieval Canon Law." *Journal of Medieval History* 3 (1977): 99–114.

Martí de Barcelona, P. "Regesta de documents arnaldians coneguts." *Estudis Franciscans* 47 (1935): 261–300.

Martínez Ferrando, J. Ernesto. *El Archivo de la Corona de Aragón.* Barcelona, 1944.
"La camera real en el reinado de Jaime II." *Anales y Boletín de los Museos de Arte de Barcelona* 11 (1953–4): 1–230.
"Los correos de la curia regia en la Corona de Aragón a principios del siglo XIV." *AST* 17 (1944): 97–113.
Jaime II de Aragón: Su vida familiar. 2 vols. Barcelona, 1948.
Jaume II o el seny català; Alfons el benigne. 2nd edn. Barcelona, 1963.
Martínez Loscos, Carmen. "Orígenes de la medicina en Aragón: Los médicos árabes y judíos." *Zurita* 6–7 (1954): 7–67.
Martorell, F. "Inventari dels bens de la cambra reyal en temps de Jaume II (1323)." *Anuari de l'Institut d'Estudis Catalans* 4 (1911–12): 553–67.
Menéndez y Pelayo, Marcellino. *Historia de los Heterodoxos Españoles,* vol. VII. Edited by Enrique Sánchez Reyes. *Edición nacional de las obras completas de Menéndez Pelayo,* ed. Angel González Palencia, vol. XLI. Santander, 1948.
Meyerhof, Max. "The History of Trachoma Treatment in Antiquity and during the Arabic Middle Ages." *Bulletin of the Ophthalmological Society of Egypt* 29 (1936): 26–73. (Reprinted in Max Meyerhof, *Studies in Medieval Arabic Medicine.* London, 1984.)
Miquel Parellada, José María, and José Sanchez Real. *Los hospitales de Tarragona.* Tarragona, 1959.
Miret i Sans, Joaquim. "Escolars catalans al estudi de Bolonia en la XIIIa centuria." *BRABLB* 8 (1915–16): 137–55.
El forassenyat primogènit de Jaume II. Barcelona, 1957.
"Itinerario del rey Alfonso III de Cataluña IV en Aragón." *BRABLB* 5 (1909–10): 3–15, 57–71, 114–23.
"Le massacre des Juifs de Montclus en 1320." *Revue des Etudes Juives* 53 (1907): 255–66.
Sempre han tingut béch les oques. 2 vols. Barcelona, 1905–6.
Miró i Borràs, Olaguer. *El receptari de Manresa i la mort de l'infant Jaume, comte d'Urgell.* Manresa, 1913.
"Salaris dels antics metjes de Manresa." *Butlletí del Centre Excursionista de la Comarca de Bages* 6 (1910): 1–6.
Moliné, Enric. "Un diagnòstic mèdic del 1372 a La Seu." *Església d'Urgell* 183 (July–Aug. 1989): 5–6.
Mollat, Michel. *The Poor in the Middle Ages.* Translated by Arthur Goldhammer. New Haven/London, 1986.
Monticolo, Giovanni. *I capitolari delle arti Veneziane.* Vol. I. Rome, 1896.
Moore, R. I. *The Formation of a Persecuting Society.* Oxford/ New York, 1987.
Morel-Fatio, Alfred. *Catalogue des manuscrits espagnols et des manuscrits portugais.* Paris, 1892.
Mundy, John H. "Charity and Social Work in Toulouse, 1100–1250." *Traditio* 22 (1966): 203–57.
Murray, Jacqueline. "On the Origins and Role of 'Wise Women' in Causes for Annulment on the Grounds of Male Impotence." *Journal of Medieval History* 16 (1990): 235–49.
Mutgé Vives, Josefa. *La ciudad de Barcelona durante el reinado de Alfonso el Benigno (1327–1336).* Madrid/Barcelona, 1987.

Murdoch, John Emery, and Edith Dudley Sylla. *The Cultural Context of Medieval Learning*. Dordrecht/Boston, 1975.

Naso, Irma. *Medici e strutture sanitarie nella società tardo-medievale: Il Piemonte dei secoli XIV e XV*. Milan, 1982.

Neugebauer, Richard. "Medieval and Early Modern Theories of Mental Illness." *Archives of General Psychiatry* 36 (1979): 477–83.

Neuman, Abraham A. *The Jews in Spain: Their Social, Political and Cultural Life during the Middle Ages*. 2 vols. Philadelphia, 1942.

Nicaise, E. *Chirurgie de Maître Henri de Mondeville*. Paris, 1893.

La grande chirurgie de Guy de Chauliac. Paris, 1890.

Nutton, Vivian. "Continuity or Rediscovery? The City Physician in Classical Antiquity and Mediaeval Italy." In *The Town and State Physician in Europe from the Middle Ages to the Enlightenment*, ed. Andrew W. Russell, pp. 9–46. Wolfenbüttler Forschungen, vol. 17. Wolfenbüttel, 1981.

O'Boyle, Cornelius. *Medieval Prognosis and Astrology*. Cambridge, 1991.

Olmos y Canalda, Elias. *Pergaminos de la Catedral de Valencia*. Valencia, 1961.

Ortalli, Edgardo. "La perizia medica a Bologna nei secoli XIII e XIV: Normativa e pratica di un istituto giudiziario." *Deputazione di Storia Patria per le Province di Romagna: Atti e Memorie*, n.s., 17–19 (Bologna, 1969): 223–59.

Ottosson, Per-Gunnar. *Scholastic Medicine and Philosophy*. Naples, 1984.

Pagel, Julius Leopold. "Die Chirurgie des Heinrich von Mondeville (Hermondaville)." *Archiv für klinische Chirurgie* 40 (1890): 253–311, 653–752, 869–904; 41 (1891): 122–73, 467–504, 705–46, 917–68; 42 (1891): 172–228, 426–90, 645–708, 825–924.

"Raymundus de Moleriis und seine Schrift de impedimentis conceptionis." *Janus* 8 (1903): 530–7.

Palmer, Richard. "The Church, Leprosy and Plague in Medieval and Early Modern Europe." In *The Church and Healing*, ed. W. J. Sheils, pp. 79–99. Oxford, 1982.

Paniagua Arellano, Juan Antonio. "L'Arabisme à Montpellier dans l'œuvre d'Arnau de Vilanova." *Le Scalpel* 117 (25 July 1964): 631–7.

El maestro Arnau de Vilanova médico. Valencia, 1969.

"La psicoterapia en las obras médicas de Arnau de Vilanova." *Archivo Iberoamericano de Historia de la Medicina y Antropologia Médica* 15 (1963): 1–15.

"Las traducciones de textos medicos hechas del arabe al latín por el maestro Arnau de Vilanova." *Actas del XXVII Congreso Internacional de Historia de la Medicina*, pp. 321–6. Barcelona, 1981.

ed. Arnau de Vilanova, *El maravilloso regimiento y orden de vivir*. Zaragoza, 1980.

Pansier, P. "La pratique de l'ophthalmologie dans le moyen-âge latin." *Janus* 9 (1904): 3–26.

Park, Katharine. *Doctors and Medicine in Early Renaissance Florence*. Princeton, 1985.

"Healing the Poor: Hospitals and Medical Assistance in Renaissance Florence." In *Medicine and Charity before the Welfare State*, ed. Jonathan Barry and Colin Jones, pp. 26–45. London/New York, 1991.

"Medicine and Society in Medieval Europe, 500–1500." In *Medicine in Society: Historical Essays*, ed. Andrew Wear, pp. 59–90. Cambridge, 1992.

Pelling, Margaret. "Medical Practice in Early Modern England: Trade or Profession?" In *The Professions in Early Modern England*, ed. Wilfrid Prest, pp. 90–128. London/ New York/Sydney, 1987.

"Occupational Diversity: Barber-Surgeons and the Trades of Norwich, 1550–1640." *Bulletin of the History of Medicine* 56 (1982): 484–511.

Pelling, Margaret, and Charles Webster. "Medical Practitioners." In *Health, Medicine and Mortality in the Sixteenth Century*, ed. Charles Webster, pp. 165–235. Cambridge, 1979.

Perarnau i Espelt, Josep. "Activitats i fórmules supersticioses de guarició a Catalunya en la primera meitat del segle XIV." *Arxiu de Textos Catalans Antics* 1 (1982): 47–78.

L' "Alia informatio beguinorum" d'Arnau de Vilanova. Barcelona, 1978.

"Una hypòtesi relativa a Bernat de Barriac." *Arxiu de Textos Catalans Antics* 10 (1991): 277–83.

"L'"Ordinacio studii Barchinone et rectoris ejusdem' del Bisbe Ponç de Gualba (8 novembre 1309)." *Revista Catalana de Teologia* 2 (1977): 151–88.

Pere III of Catalonia. *Chronicle*. Translated by Mary Hillgarth with introduction and notes by J. N. Hillgarth. 2 vols. Toronto, 1980.

"Ordenacions fetes per lo molt alt senyor en Pere terç rey Darago sobra lo regiment de tots los officials de la sua cort." Vol. V of *Colección de documentos inéditos del archivo general de la corona de Aragón*, ed. Próspero de Bofarull y Mascaró. Barcelona, 1850.

Pérez Santamaría, Aurora. "El hospital de San Lázaro o Casa dels Malalts o Masells." In *La pobreza y la asistencia a los pobres en la Cataluña medieval*, ed. Manuel Riu, I:77–115. Anuario de Estudios Medievales, anejo 9. Barcelona, 1980.

Pérez Vidal, José. *Medicina y dulcería en el "Libro de buen amor."* Madrid, 1981.

Peset, V. "Terminología psiquiátrica usada en los estados de la corona de Aragón en la baja edad media." *Archivo Iberoamericano de Historia de la Medicina* 7 (1955): 431–42, 561–88; 10 (1958): 305–47; 11 (1959): 65–84.

Pifarré Torres, Dolors. "Dos visitas de comienzos del siglo XIV a los hospitales barceloneses d'En Colom y d'En Marcús." In *La pobreza y la asistencia a los pobres en la Cataluña medieval*, ed. Manuel Riu, II:81–93. Anuario de Estudios Medievales, anejo 11. Barcelona, 1982.

Pingree, David. "The Diffusion of Arabic Magical Texts in Western Europe." In *La diffusione delle scienze islamiche nel medio evo europeo*, pp. 57–102. Rome, 1984.

Piquer, Josep Joan. "Metges i malalties en els miracles del procés de canonització de Sant Ramon de Penyafort." *Actes*, II Congrés d'Història de la Medicina Catalana, II:41–2. Barcelona, 1975.

Pita i Merce, Roderic. "Metges Jueus als regnes de la Corona d'Aragó." *Gimbernat* 2 (1984): 133-58.

Pladevall, Antoni. "La disminució de poblament a la Plana de Vich a mitjans del segle XIV." *VI Assemblea d'Estudis Comarcals*, pp. 23–35. Vich, 1962. (Also published in *Ausa* 4 [1961–3]: 361–73.)

Pleyan de Porta, José. *Apuntes de historia de Lérida*. Lerida, 1873.

Pons, Antoni. "Constitucions e ordinacions del regne de Mallorca." *Bolletí de la Societat Arqueológica Lulianà* 22 (1929): 350–4.

Pons i Guri, Josep Maria. "Constitucions conciliars Tarraconenses (1229 a 1330)." *AST*

47 (1974): 65–124; 48 (1975): 241–63. (Reprinted in Pons i Guri, *Recull d'estudis d'història jurídica catalana*, II:223–387. Barcelona, 1989.)

"Constitucions de Catalunya." In Pons i Guri, *Recull d'estudis d'història jurídica catalana*, III:55–76. Barcelona, 1989.

"Un fogatjament desconegut de l'any 1358." *BRABLB* 30 (1964): 323–498.

Porter, Roy, ed. *Patients and Practitioners*. Cambridge/New York, 1985.

Rafat Selga, Juan. "Aspectos de la medicina en Manresa (siglos XIII al XVII)." *Actes*, I Congrés Internacional d'Història de la Medicina Catalana, I:91–126. Barcelona, 1970.

Rahola i Sastre, Josep. "Els odontòlegs dels segles XIV i XV a Barcelona." *Actes*, I Congrés Internacional d'Història de la Medicina Catalana, I:293–300. Barcelona, 1970.

Rashdall, Hastings. *The Universities of Europe in the Middle Ages*. 3 vols. Edited by F. M. Powicke and A. B. Emden. Oxford, 1936.

Rawcliffe, Carole. "The Hospitals of Later Medieval London." *Medical History* 28 (1984): 1–21.

"The Profits of Practice: The Wealth and Status of Medical Men in Later Medieval England." *Social History of Medicine* 1 (1988): 63–78.

Régné, Jean. *History of the Jews in Aragon: Regesta and Documents 1213–1357*. Edited by Yom Tov Assis. Jerusalem, 1978.

Renan, Ernest. "Les écrivains juifs français du XIVe siècle." *Histoire Littéraire de la France* 31 (1893): 351–789.

Renaud, H. P. J. "Un chirurgien musulman du royaume de Grenade: Muhammad al-Safra." *Hesperis* 20 (1935): 1–20.

Requejo Díaz de Espada, Elena. "La vida conventual del cabildo de la Seo de Zaragoza en 1292 . . . ' *Zurita* 23–24 (1972–3): 123–89.

Rius, Josep. "Més documents sobre la cultura catalana medieval." *EUC* 13 (1928): 135–70.

Rius Serra, José. "Aportaciones sobre médicos judíos en Aragón en la primera mitad del siglo XIV." *Sefarad* 12 (1952): 337–50.

ed. *San Raimundo de Penyafort, Diplomatario*. Barcelona, 1954.

Roca, Joseph Ma. *Johan I d'Aragó*. Barcelona, 1929.

"Johan I y les supersticions." *BRABLB* 10 (1921): 125–69.

La medicina catalana en temps del rey Martí. Barcelona, 1919.

"Notes medicals històriques: Frau quirúrgich." *Anals de Ciencies Mediques* 18 (1924): 66–7.

"Notes medicals historiques: Medicaments reyals." *Anals de Ciencies Mediques* 17 (1923): 51–2.

Ordinacions del hospital general de la Santa Creu de Barcelona. Barcelona, 1920.

Roca Traver, Francisco A. *El justicia de Valencia*. Valencia, 1970.

Ordenaciones municipales de Castellón de la Plana durante la baja edad media. Valencia, 1952.

Rodrigo Pertegás, José. *Hospitales de Valencia en el siglo XV*. Madrid, 1927.

Roger Bacon. *De erroribus medicorum*. In *Rogeri Baconi De retardatione accidentium senectutis*, ed. A. G. Little and R. Withington, pp. 150–79. Oxford, 1928; rpt., Farnborough, 1966.

Romano, David. "Les juifs de la couronne d'Aragón avant 1391." *Revue des Etudes Juives* 141 (1982): 169–82.

Rosen, Edward. "The Invention of Eyeglasses." *Journal of the History of Medicine and Allied Sciences* 11 (1956): 13–46, 183–218.

R[ubió] y B[alaguer], J. "Metges y cirurgians juheus." *EUC* 3 (1909): 489–97.

Rubió y Lluch, Antoni. "Contribució a la biografía de l'infant Ferràn de Mallorca." *EUC* 7 (1913): 291–379.

"La cultura catalana en el regnat de Pere III." *EUC* 8 (1914): 213–47.

Documents per l'historia de la cultura catalana mig-eval. 2 vols. Barcelona, 1908–21.

"Joan I Humanista i el primer període de l'humanisme català." *EUC* 10 (1917–18): 12–18.

"Notes sobre la ciencia oriental a Catalunya en el XIVèn sigle." *EUC* 3 (1909): 389–98, 485–8.

Rubio Vela, Agustín. "Un hospital medieval según su fundador: El testamento de Bernat dez Clapers (Valencia, 1311)." *Dynamis* 3 (1983): 373–87.

Peste negra, crisis y comportamientos sociales en la España del signo XIV: La ciudad de Valencia (1348–1400). Granada, 1979.

Pobreza, enfermedad y asistencia hospitalaria en la Valencia del siglo XIV. Valencia, 1984.

Ruggiero, Guido. "The Cooperation of Physicians and the State in the Control of Violence in Renaissance Venice." *Journal of the History of Medicine and Allied Sciences* 33 (1978): 156–66.

Ruíz Moreno, Aníbal. "El juicio de insanía de Don Ginés Rabaza, diputado por Valencia, al Conclave de Caspe." *Archivos Iberoamericanos de Historia de la Medicina* 6 (1952): 3–39.

La medicina en la legislación medioeval española. Buenos Aires, 1946.

Russell, Josiah Cox. *Medieval Regions and Their Cities.* Bloomington, 1972.

Sablonier, Roger. "The Aragonese Royal Family around 1300." In *Interest and Emotion: Essays on the Study of Family and Kinship,* ed. Hans Medick and David Warren Sabean, pp. 210–39. Cambridge, 1984.

Sainz de Baranda, Pedro. *España Sagrada.* Vol. XLVII. Madrid, 1850.

Salvador de los Borges. *Arnau de Vilanova moralista.* Barcelona, 1957.

Santi, Francesco. *Arnau de Vilanova: L'obra espiritual.* Valencia, 1987.

Sarasa Sánchez, Esteban. *Las cortes de Aragón en la edad media.* Zaragoza, [1979].

Sarret i Arbos, Joaquim. *Historia de la industria, del comerç i dels gremis de Manresa.* Monumenta Historica Civitatis Minorisae, no. 3. Manresa, 1923.

Scarlata, Marina, and Laura Sciascia. *Documenti sulla luogotenenza di Federico d'Aragona 1294–1295.* Acta Siculo-Aragonensia, no. 2. Palermo, 1978.

Schipperges, Heinrich. "Zur Sonderstellung der jüdischen Ärzte im spätmittelalterlichen Spanien." *Sudhoffs Archiv* 57 (1973): 208–11.

Schwarz, Karl. *Aragonische Hofordnungen im 13. und 14. Jahrhundert. Abhandlungen zur mittleren und neueren Geschichte,* vol. LIV. Berlin, 1914.

Secall i Guell, Gabriel. "Metges i cirurgians hebreus de Santa Coloma de Queralt (s. XIV–XV)." *Gimbernat* 4 (1985): 339–48.

Segura, Joan. "Aplech de documents curiosos é inedits fahents per la historia de las costums de Catalunya." *Jochs Florals de Barcelona* 27 (1885): 119–287.

Sevillano Colom, Francisco. "Apuntes para el estudio de la cancillería de Pedro IV el Ceremonioso." *Anuario de Historia del Derecho Español* 20 (1950): 137–241.

"De la institución del mustaçaf de Barcelona, de Mallorca y Valencia." *Anuario de Historia del Derecho Español* 23 (1953): 625–38.

Valencia urbana medieval a través del oficio del mustaçaf. Valencia, 1957.

Shatzmiller, Joseph. "Doctors' Fees and Their Medical Responsibility." In *Sources of Social History: Private Acts of the Late Middle Ages*, ed. Paolo Brezzi and Egmont Lee, pp. 201–8. Toronto, 1984.

Médecine et justice en Provence médiévale. Aix-en-Provence, 1989.

Sider, David, and Michael McVaugh. "Galen *On Tremor, Palpitation, Spasm, and Rigor.*" *Transactions and Studies of the College of Physicians of Philadelphia* 1 (1979): 183–210.

Las siete partidas del rey don Alfonso el Sabio. Madrid, 1807.

Sigerist, Henry E. "Bedside Manners in the Middle Ages: The Treatise *De Cautelis Medicorum* Attributed to Arnald of Villanova." In *Henry E. Sigerist on the History of Medicine*, ed. Felix Martí-Ibáñez, pp. 131–40. New York, 1960. (Originally published in *Quarterly Bulletin*, Northwestern University Medical School, 20 [1946]: 135–43.)

tr. Arnald of Villanova, *The Earliest Printed Book on Wine.* New York, 1943.

Simili, Alessandro. "The Beginnings of Forensic Medicine in Bologna." In *International Symposium on Society, Medicine and Law; Jerusalem, March 1972*, ed. H. Karplus, pp. 91–100. Amsterdam/London/New York, 1973.

Simon de Guilleuma, Josep Maria. "De l'ús de les ulleres en els països de la Confederació Catalano-Aragonesa en el segle XIV." *III Congreso de Historia de la Corona d'Aragón*, 1:485–501. Valencia, 1923.

Siraisi, Nancy G. *Medieval and Early Renaissance Medicine.* Chicago, 1990.

"The Physician's Task: Medical Reputation in Humanist Collective Biographies." in *The Rational Arts of Living*, ed. A. C. Crombie and Nancy Siraisi, pp. 105–33. Northampton, Mass., 1987.

Smith, Cyril E. *The University of Toulouse in the Middle Ages.* Milwaukee, 1958.

Smith, Robert S. "Fourteenth-Century Population Records of Catalonia." *Speculum* 19 (1944): 494–501.

Sobrequés Callicó, Jaime. "La peste negra en la península ibérica." *Anuario de Estudios Medievales* 7 (1970–1): 67–102.

Soldevila, Ferran, ed. *Les quatre grans cròniques.* 2nd edn. Barcelona, 1983.

Sorní Esteva, Javier, and José Maria Suñé Arbussá. "Algunas noticias de Guillem Jordà, boticario de Jaume II, a comienzos del siglo XIV." *Boletín de la Sociedad Española de Historia de la Farmacia* 36 (1985): 213–16.

"Barcelona. Baja edad media. ¿Especieros o boticarios?" *Boletín de la Sociedad Española de Historia de la Farmacia* 34 (1983): 139–50.

"Un boticario barcelonés del siglo XIII–XIV." In *Homenaje al profesor Guillermo Folch Jou*, pp. 11–13. Madrid, 1982.

"La farmacia en Barcelona desde Alfons el Benigne a Pere el Ceremoniós (1327–1387)." *Boletín de la Sociedad Española de Historia de la Farmacia* 36 (1985): 67–79.

"La farmacia en Barcelona desde Jaume I a Jaume II (1213–1327)." *Boletín de la Sociedad Española de Historia de la Farmacia* 34 (1983): 59–68.

Steele, R. "Dies Aegyptiaci." *Proceedings of the Royal Society of Medicine*, Sec. Hist. Med., 12 (1919): 108–21.

Steinschneider, Moritz. *Die hebraeischen Übersetzungen des Mittelalters und die Juden als Dolmetscher*. Berlin, 1893; rpt., Graz, 1956.

Talbot, C. H. *Medicine in Medieval England*. London, 1967.

Temkin, Owsei. *The Falling Sickness*. 2nd edn., revised. Baltimore/ London, 1971.

Teodorico. *Chirurgia*. In Guy de Chauliac, *Ars Chirurgica* (Venice, 1546), ff. 134v– 184.

Thorndike, Lynn. "Advice from a Physician to His Sons." In Thorndike, *University Records and Life in the Middle Ages*, pp. 154–60. New York, 1944; rpt., New York, 1971.

A History of Magic and Experimental Science. 8 vols. New York/London, 1923–58.

ed. *The Herbal of Rufinus*. Chicago, 1946.

Thorndike, Lynn, and Pearl Kibre. *A Catalogue of Incipits of Mediaeval Scientific Writings in Latin*. Revised and augmented edn. Cambridge, Mass., 1973.

Tintó i Sala, Margarida. *Els gremis a la Barcelona medieval*. Barcelona, 1978.

de la Toree y del Cerro, Antonio. *Documentos para la historia de la Universidad de Barcelona*. Vol. I. Barcelona, 1971.

Tractenberg, Joshua. *The Devil and the Jews*. New Haven, 1943.

Udina Martorell, Federico. *Guia histórica y descriptiva del Archivo de la Corona de Aragón*. Madrid, 1986.

Ussery, Huling. *Chaucer's Physician*. Tulane Studies in English, no. 19. New Orleans, 1971.

Utrilla Utrilla, Juan F. "El monedaje de Huesca de 1284." *Aragón en la Edad Media* 1 (1977): 1–50.

Van den Berg, W. S. *Eene middelnederlandsche Vertalung van het Antidotarium Nicolaï*. Leiden, 1917.

Vilaseca Anguera, Salvador. *Metges, cirurgians i apotecaris reusencs dels segles XIII–XVI*. Reus, 1961.

Villanueva, Joaquín Lorenzo. *Viage literario a las iglesias de España*. Vol. V. Madrid, 1806.

Vincke, Johannes. "Sobre la caça amb falcons pels reis de Catalunya-Aragó els segles XIII i XIV." *Estudis d'Història Medieval* 5 (1972): 55–70.

"El trasllat de l'arquebisbe Joan d'Aragó de la seu de Toledo a la de Tarragona." *AST* 6 (1930): 127–30.

Vinyoles, Teresa-Maria. *Les barcelonines a les darreries de l'edat mitjana (1370–1410)*. Barcelona, 1976.

Voigts, Linda E., and Michael R. McVaugh. *A Latin Technical Phlebotomy and Its Middle English Translation. Transactions of the American Philosophical Society* 74, part 2, 1984.

Wack, Mary F. *Lovesickness in the Middle Ages*. Philadelphia, 1990.

Welborn, Mary Catherine. "The Long Tradition: A Study in Fourteenth-Century Medical Deontology." In *Medieval and Historiographical Essays in Honor of James Westfall Thompson*, ed. James Lea Cate and Eugene N. Anderson, pp. 344–57. Chicago, 1938.

Wickersheimer, Ernest. *Dictionnaire biographique des médecins en France au moyen âge*. Geneva, 1936.

"Organisation et législation sanitaires au royaume franc de Jérusalem (1099–1291)." *Archives Internationales d'Histoire des Sciences* 16 (1951): 689–705.

Wolff, Philippe. *Commerce et marchands de Toulouse (vers 1350–vers 1450)*. Paris, 1954.

"Recherches sur les médecins de Toulouse au XIVe et XVe siècles." In Wolff, *Regards sur le Midi médiéval*, pp. 125–42. Toulouse, 1978.

Zeissberg, Heinrich R. v. "Das Register Nr. 318 des Archives der aragonesischen Krone in Barcelona." *Sitzungsberichte der philosophisch-historischen Classe der kaiserliche Akademie der Wissenschaften* 140, part 1 (1899).

Zurita, Jerónimo. *Anales de la Corona de Aragón*, ed. Angel Canellas López. Zaragoza, 1972.

Index

In general, this index lists persons by their first names. Since these names have not always been converted from the way they appear in the documentation to a standard spelling, individuals ought to be looked for under the various forms of their names: Jacme/Jacobus/Jaume; Michael/Miquel; Çulema/Salomo/Solamon, etc. Names of patients have ordinarily not been included.

266